LPN to RN Transitions
6th Edition
Transitions
Achieving Success in Your New Role

LPN to RN Transitions

6th Edition

Achieving Success in Your New Role

Linda Lee Phelps, DNP, RN
Assistant Professor
Nursing Education Department
Palomar College
San Marcos, California

Wolters Kluwer

Philadelphia • Baltimore • New York • London
Buenos Aires • Hong Kong • Sydney • Tokyo

Not authorised for sale in United States, Canada, Australia, New Zealand, Puerto Rico, and U.S. Virgin Islands.

Vice President and Segment Leader, Health Learning & Practice: Julie K. Stegman
Director, Nursing Education and Practice Content: Jamie Blum
Senior Acquisitions Editor: Susan Hartman
Senior Development Editor: Meredith L. Brittain
Editorial Coordinator: Varshaanaa SM
Marketing Manager: Wendy Mears
Editorial Assistant: Sara Thul
Manager, Graphic Arts and Design: Stephen Druding
Art Director, Illustration: Jennifer Clements
Senior Production Project Manager: Bridgett Dougherty
Manufacturing Coordinator: Margie Orzech
Prepress Vendor: Straive

6th edition

Copyright © 2025 Wolters Kluwer.

Copyright © 2019 Wolters Kluwer. Copyright © 2013, 2009 by Lippincott Williams & Wilkins, a Wolters Kluwer business. Copyright © 2003 by Lippincott Williams & Wilkins. Copyright © 1996 by Lippincott-Raven Publishers.

All rights reserved. This book is protected by copyright. No part of this book may be reproduced or transmitted in any form or by any means, including as photocopies or scanned-in or other electronic copies, or utilized by any information storage and retrieval system without written permission from the copyright owner, except for brief quotations embodied in critical articles and reviews. Materials appearing in this book prepared by individuals as part of their official duties as U.S. government employees are not covered by the above-mentioned copyright. To request permission, please contact Wolters Kluwer at Two Commerce Square, 2001 Market Street, Philadelphia, PA 19103, via email at permissions@lww.com, or via our website at shop.lww.com (products and services).

Nursing diagnoses in this title are ICNP® nursing diagnoses. ICNP® is owned and copyrighted by the International Council of Nurses (ICN). Reproduced with permission of the copyright holder.

9 8 7 6 5 4 3 2 1

Printed in Mexico

Library of Congress Cataloging-in-Publication Data
Names: Phelps, Linda Lee, author. | Harrington, Nicki. LPN to RN transitions.
Title: LPN to RN transitions : achieving success in your new role / Linda Lee Phelps.
Description: 6th edition. | Philadelphia : Wolters Kluwer, [2025]. | Preceded by LPN to RN transitions / Nicki Harrington, Cynthia Lee Terry. 5th edition. [2019] | Includes bibliographical references and index. | Summary: "Make the most of your personal and financial investment and learn how to effectively balance career, school, and personal pursuits on your journey to success as an RN. A proven guide to personal and professional achievement, LPN to RN Transitions, 6th Edition, eases the return to academic life and helps licensed practical and vocational nurses effectively balance career, school and personal pursuits on the journey to success in registered nursing programs"—Provided by publisher.
Identifiers: LCCN 2024023721 (print) | LCCN 2024023722 (ebook) | ISBN 9781975241919 (print) | ISBN 9781975241940 (epub)
Subjects: MESH: Nursing | Career Mobility | Nurse's Role | Nurses—psychology | Case Reports | Examination Questions | BISAC: MEDICAL / Nursing / LPN & LVN
Classification: LCC RT82 (print) | LCC RT82 (ebook) | NLM WY 18.2 | DDC 610.7306/9—dc23/eng/20240701
LC record available at https://lccn.loc.gov/2024023721
LC ebook record available at https://lccn.loc.gov/2024023722

This work is provided "as is," and the publisher disclaims any and all warranties, express or implied, including any warranties as to accuracy, comprehensiveness, or currency of the content of this work.

This work is no substitute for individual patient assessment based upon healthcare professionals' examination of each patient and consideration of, among other things, age, weight, gender, current or prior medical conditions, medication history, laboratory data and other factors unique to the patient. The publisher does not provide medical advice or guidance and this work is merely a reference tool. Healthcare professionals, and not the publisher, are solely responsible for the use of this work including all medical judgments and for any resulting diagnosis and treatments.

Given continuous, rapid advances in medical science and health information, independent professional verification of medical diagnoses, indications, appropriate pharmaceutical selections and dosages, and treatment options should be made and healthcare professionals should consult a variety of sources. When prescribing medication, healthcare professionals are advised to consult the product information sheet (the manufacturer's package insert) accompanying each drug to verify, among other things, conditions of use, warnings and side effects and identify any changes in dosage schedule or contraindications, particularly if the medication to be administered is new, infrequently used or has a narrow therapeutic range. To the maximum extent permitted under applicable law, no responsibility is assumed by the publisher for any injury and/or damage to persons or property, as a matter of products liability, negligence law or otherwise, or from any reference to or use by any person of this work.

LWW.com

To the compassionate souls embracing the noble journey of nursing, may your hearts be as resilient as your hands are gentle. May you find strength in every challenge, solace in every care, and fulfillment in the healing touch you bring to those in need.

I hope you will find inspiration within these pages to fuel your unwavering commitment to healing, kindness, and the profound impact you will make on countless lives. This book is dedicated to the caregivers, the healers, and the future leaders of the healthcare world. Your journey begins here; may it be filled with compassion, courage, and boundless love.

—Linda Lee Phelps

Preface

Choosing to reenter the rigors of academic life is a monumental decision for any LPN/LVN returning to school. Doing so is both a personal and a financial investment and can be characterized by extreme highs and lows. This new path challenges the aspiring associate degree nurse (ADN) to operate in a sometimes chaotic new world that calls for nonlinear thinking, balancing many simultaneous challenges, and a global perspective. It also requires the nurse to be an independent practitioner while functioning collaboratively within an expanded and more specialized healthcare team. *LPN to RN Transitions: Achieving Success in Your New Role*, 6th Edition, serves as a guide to prepare students for a successful journey.

The previous five editions of this book were authored by Nicki Harrington and Cynthia Lee Terry. Their dedication and expertise helped countless LPN students successfully transition to an RN program. The 6th edition welcomes a new author, Linda Lee Phelps. This updated edition incorporates contemporary research, evidence-based practices, and real-world scenarios to reflect the dynamic nature of healthcare. Each chapter guides students through the complexities of role transition, addressing the challenges and opportunities unique to this professional evolution. The inclusion of cutting-edge information, current healthcare policies, and advancements in nursing education ensures that learners are well prepared for the realities of modern nursing practice. This text is designed to be used by students in a variety of adult learning settings, including independent study, classroom collaborative workgroups, online discussions, and interactions in virtual learning spaces. Whether you are a student embarking on this transformative journey or an educator guiding others through it, this textbook was developed to be a comprehensive and indispensable resource, providing the knowledge and support needed for a successful transition from LPN to RN.

Today's nurse must be resourceful, inquisitive, politically active, and must consistently seek additional knowledge, competencies, and career growth to meet the needs of a rapidly changing world. Through the lens of changing societal trends, students are asked to think critically about their personal and professional viewpoints and values. This text encourages the application of evidence-based research, critical thinking, and clinical judgment as the student confronts challenges as a critical member of the healthcare team. The content of this book promotes learning for diverse student populations with a variety of learning styles and experiential backgrounds. In addition, it provides students with useful tools and practical strategies for balancing their job, school, and personal lives while achieving their educational and professional goals.

FEATURES

This textbook has been thoughtfully revised and updated to provide aspiring nurses with the latest information, insights, and best practices in the field. Features that students and educators value include case studies of student experiences at the beginning of each chapter, which assist the reader in realizing that the journey to associate degree nursing is not an isolated one—it is shared by other students of all ages and life backgrounds. Students may recognize their own experiences in one or more of these case studies and realize that others face similar challenges.

Strategies used throughout the text to help the student with role transition to the ADN program include interactive student exercises and the development of a personal education plan based on the student's own experience along with their program's philosophy, curricular framework, and student learning objectives. The "Thinking Critically" feature provides students with opportunities to reflect on presented material, to examine application of theoretical content to the clinical practice setting, and to share perspectives with peers and in a group setting. Other helpful features are learning outcomes, sample NCLEX-RN style questions, and "On the Web" boxes that refer readers to useful resources.

Each chapter employs evidence-based practice techniques to enhance clinical judgment and to foster success in the transition to the professional role. Updated resources, websites, case studies, and real-world examples provide students with the opportunity to further explore individual topics and to enhance their learning by incorporating the latest advancements, research findings, and educational methodologies. These revisions ensure that the content is relevant, engaging, comprehensive, and aligned with the changing landscape of the nursing profession. This book serves as a dynamic platform for students to deepen their knowledge, to foster critical thinking skills, and to stay abreast of the evolving developments within nursing, ultimately preparing them for success in their academic and professional journeys.

TEXT ORGANIZATION

Unit I, The Transition Process, empowers learners with the knowledge and skills necessary to navigate the transformative phase in their nursing careers from LPN/LVN to RN. Updated college success strategies address a more diverse, multicultural student population. Support and resource information is included for underrepresented communities, individuals of color, men, LGBTQIA+ individuals, and students for whom English may not be their first language.

Chapters 1 through 6 explore the significance of continuous learning in the evolving field of nursing. As aspiring RNs embark on this journey, understanding the intricacies of role development becomes paramount to their success in assuming the responsibilities and expectations of an RN. The text explains how students can assess their preferred learning styles and also covers emotional intelligence, study skills, and organizational skills. Recognizing that each individual's journey is unique, each chapter equips students with the knowledge and skills essential for success in their educational pursuits and provides guidance on tailoring a plan that aligns with personal and professional goals.

The concepts of "role overload" and "role transition" are expanded to provide additional support for contemporary students experiencing financial difficulties, extended work commitments, and personal challenges exacerbated by the ongoing effects of the COVID-19 pandemic and the prevailing economic conditions. Support resources are included for students reentering academia who may face challenges navigating web pages and virtual learning spaces. Resources and coping strategies are explored for veterans pursuing nursing programs who may face additional challenges as they adjust to both the student role and civilian life.

Chapter 7 has been extensively updated to provide students with the latest information and insights essential for success in taking exams in the revised Next-Generation NCLEX (NGN) format. The NGN marked a transformative shift in the nursing licensure examination as well as a crucial evolution in nursing education and practice. The NGN was introduced with the primary objective of enhancing clinical judgment skills among nursing professionals and better aligning the examination with the realities of contemporary clinical practice, ultimately advancing the level of public safety in healthcare. The updated chapter not only describes the modifications to the examination but also describes the new perspectives, case studies, and scenarios that mirror the challenges and nuances of real-world clinical practice.

Unit II, Core Competencies for Professional Nursing Practice, explores the core competencies and knowledge essential for the modern that allow them to handle the complexities of professional practice. The nursing student learns to navigate the regulatory frameworks and standards that guide nursing practice, and they gain valuable insights into ethical considerations that form the foundation of nursing practice. Students are encouraged to examine the cognitive processes that are integral to nursing decision-making. They hone advanced critical thinking skills and clinical judgment skills that nurses must possess to respond effectively to complex situations in the dynamic and fast-paced healthcare environment.

UNIT III, Role Concepts Essential for RN Practice, is divided into three parts:

- Part A, "Provider of Care," explores the essential role concepts for RN practice, emphasizing assessment, communication, and teaching as integral components of the nurse's role. Chapter 10 examines the foundational aspects of the nursing process, focusing on the critical role of assessment in delivering comprehensive and patient-centered care. Students explore the process in which nurses translate assessment findings into meaningful actions that address the holistic needs of their patients. In Chapter 11, from active listening to conveying empathy, students learn various communication strategies essential for establishing trust and fostering collaboration in diverse healthcare settings. Chapter 12 discusses the nurse in the pivotal role of educator. From assessing learning needs to developing effective teaching plans, students explore a comprehensive framework for nurses to impart knowledge and to empower individuals to take an active role in their health. With a focus on individualized teaching strategies, students discover how to adapt their educational approach to diverse patient populations, fostering a collaborative and informed healthcare experience.
- Part B, Manager of Care, provides an in-depth exploration of the managerial aspects of nursing, focusing on individualized client care, efficient time management, conflict resolution, and managing resources. These chapters empower the nursing student with the knowledge and skills necessary to excel in their role as a manager of care, navigating the complexities of healthcare delivery with competence and professionalism. In Chapter 13, students discover the intricacies of managing unique client care, taking into account factors such as cultural background, age, and specific health conditions, and emphasizing the nurse's role as a dynamic and adaptable caregiver. From personalized care assessments to the coordination of interdisciplinary efforts, students explore practical insights into optimizing the quality of care delivery. Chapter 14 discusses efficient time management, conflict resolution, and managing resources, which are all paramount in allowing nurses to prioritize tasks while ensuring quality patient care. Students gain valuable insights about how to identify, address, and resolve conflicts, fostering a collaborative and supportive work environment.

- Part C, Member of the Discipline of Nursing, encompasses the professional, legal, and ethical dimensions that shape the nursing discipline. These chapters equip nursing students with the knowledge and ethical decision-making skills necessary to uphold the highest standards of professionalism, legal accountability, and ethical conduct within the dynamic and evolving healthcare landscape. Students explore the core tenets that define the profession, including standards of practice, continuing education, and professional development. These chapters emphasize the importance of upholding ethical standards, maintaining competence, and engaging in collaborative efforts to advance the nursing discipline. Students gain insights into the diverse responsibilities that characterize their professional commitment, from understanding the scope of practice to contributing to the evolution of healthcare policies. To gain an understanding of legal accountability in nursing practice, students navigate legal frameworks, licensure requirements, and the implications of negligence and malpractice in nursing. In addition, these chapters examine ethical considerations that are intrinsic to the fabric of nursing practice such as end-of-life care decisions, resource allocation, and cultural competence.

INCLUSIVE LANGUAGE

A note about the language used in this book. Wolters Kluwer recognizes that people have a diverse range of identities, and we are committed to using inclusive and non-biased language in our content. In line with the principles of nursing, we strive not to define people by their diagnoses, but to recognize their personhood first and foremost, using as much as possible the language diverse groups use to define themselves, and including only information that is relevant to nursing care.

We strive to better address the unique perspectives, complex challenges, and lived experiences of diverse populations traditionally underrepresented in health literature. When describing or referencing populations discussed in research studies, we will adhere to the identities presented in those studies to maintain fidelity to the evidence presented by the study investigators. We follow best practices of language set forth by the *Publication Manual of the American Psychological Association,* 7th Edition, but acknowledge that language evolves rapidly, and we will update the language used in future editions of this book as necessary.

A COMPREHENSIVE PACKAGE FOR TEACHING AND LEARNING

To further facilitate teaching and learning, a carefully designed ancillary package has been developed to assist faculty and students.

RESOURCES FOR INSTRUCTORS

Tools to assist you with teaching your course are available upon adoption of this text at http://thePoint.lww.com/Phelps6e.

- An **e-book** gives you access to the book's full text and images online.
- A **Test Generator** lets you put together exclusive new tests from a bank containing hundreds of questions to help you in assessing your students' understanding of the material. Test questions link to chapter learning objectives.
- **PowerPoint Presentations** provide an easy way for you to integrate the textbook with your students' classroom experience, either via slide shows or handouts.

Multiple-choice and true/false questions are integrated into the presentations to promote class participation and allow you to use i-clicker technology.
- An **Image Bank** allows you use the illustrations and tables from this textbook in your PowerPoint slides or as you see fit in your course.
- Sample **Syllabi** provide guidance for structuring your course.

RESOURCES FOR STUDENTS

A set of free resources is available to help students review material and become even more familiar with vital concepts. Students can access these resources at http://thePoint.lww.com/Phelps6e using the codes printed in the front of their textbooks.

- **NCLEX-Style Review Questions** for each chapter help students review important concepts and practice for the NCLEX.
- **Journal Articles** offer access to current research available in Wolters Kluwer journals.

Acknowledgments

I extend my heartfelt gratitude to the incredible individuals who made the creation of this book possible. To family, friends, and mentors who provided unwavering encouragement and support throughout this journey: Your belief in me has been a constant source of strength. To my students: Your curiosity and enthusiasm inspired the content; I learn from all of you every day. To my colleagues: Your collaboration and valuable insights greatly enriched the material.

I would like to extend my gratitude to the previous authors of this book, whose dedication and expertise laid the foundation for this edition. To Nicki Harrington and Cynthia Lee Terry: Your insightful content inspired me in this journey.

Special thanks to the dedicated editors and reviewers at Wolters Kluwer, especially Meredith Brittain, whose expertise and diligence shaped the manuscript into its final form: Your attention to detail and commitment to maintaining the highest standards have undoubtedly enhanced the quality of this book; I am deeply grateful for your patience, encouragement, and constructive feedback, which not only improved the manuscript but also enhanced my writing process.

—LINDA LEE PHELPS

Contents

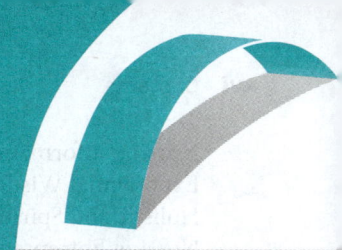

Preface vii
Acknowledgments xiii

Unit I The Transition Process — 1

1 Lifelong Learning: Returning to School — 3
Lifelong Learning in Nursing 5
The Reentry Process: Overcoming Barriers and Fears 5
Resuming the Student Role: "Returning to School Syndrome" 11
Diverse Learning Styles 13
Student Role: Strategies for Success 19
Conclusion 32

2 Role Development and Transition — 38
Definitions 39
Types of Roles 41
Role Development 42
Personal and Adult Development 45
Professional Role Development 49
Role Transition 55
Conclusion 60

3 Adapting to Change — 63
Change Defined 64
Process of Change 65
Individual and Organizational Change 65
Factors That Motivate Change 66
Types of Change 67
Stages of Planned Change 69
Effects of Change 71
Adjusting to Change 79
Positive Outcomes of Change 81
Conclusion 82

4 Transitions Throughout Nursing's History — 85
Development of Nursing 86
Professional Nursing Organizations 93
Evolution of Nursing as a Profession 99
The Discipline of Nursing 102
Evolution of Nursing Science 105
Transitions in Nursing Education 105
Factors That Have Influenced Trends and Transitions in Nursing 109

xv

Nursing Informatics and HIPAA — 121
Experiential Wisdom and Evidence-Based Practice — 122
Holistic and Spiritual Care — 123
Nursing Entrepreneurism — 124
Service Learning, Advocacy, and Policy Making — 125
Collaborative Practice and Nursing's Future — 125
Conclusion — 126

5 Learning at the ADN Level — 130

Adult Learning Theory — 131
Practical/Vocational and Associate Degree Nursing Education: A Comparison — 134
Learning Strategies for Success — 141
Transition Needs Unique to the LPN/LVN-to-ADN Student — 146
Differentiating ADN Student and LPN/LVN Practice Roles — 147
Conclusion — 149

6 Individualizing a Plan for Role Transition — 152

Assessing Preparedness for the Student Role — 154
Assessing Learning Style — 161
The Reflective Process: Assessing Adult Learner Uniqueness — 161
Assessing Prior Learning: Standardized and Nonstandardized Tests — 162
Instructor–Student Partnership — 164
Initiating Your Student Portfolio — 165
Conclusion — 165

7 Test Success and the Challenge of NCLEX-RN Questions — 172

Development of the NCLEX-RN — 173
Main Categories of the NCLEX-RN Test Plan — 175
Test Language: Key Components to a Test — 176
Bloom's Taxonomy and Level of Difficulty — 177
Clinical Judgment — 182
Test Item Formats — 184
Preparation for an NCLEX-RN Style Exam — 184
After the Exam: Decompressing, Reviewing, and Getting Help — 192
Conclusion — 193

Unit II Core Competencies for Professional Nursing Practice — 195

8 Practicing Within Regulatory Frameworks — 197

Regulations, Policies, and Standards — 198
Nurse Practice Acts — 201
Directed, Autonomous, and Collaborative Nursing Practice — 201
Mechanisms for Identifying Differences in Knowledge and Roles — 203
National Council Licensure Examinations — 205
Practical/Vocational Nursing Roles and Competencies — 206
Associate Degree Nursing Roles and Competencies — 207

Contents **xvii**

Licensed Practical/Vocational Versus Registered Nurse Knowledge, Skills, and Abilities	208
Conclusion	209

9 Critical Thinking, Clinical Reasoning, and Clinical Judgment in Nursing — 211

The Need for Critical Thinking	212
Critical Thinking Defined	213
Critical Thinking Versus Feeling	216
Critical Thinking and Creative Thinking	218
Metacognition, Reflective Thinking, and Self-Regulation	218
Critical Thinking in Nursing	220
Critical Thinking, Problem-Solving, and the Nursing Process	221
Clinical Reasoning, Intuition, and Clinical Judgment	222
Clinical Judgment and the Nursing Process	224
Critical Thinking and Holistic Nursing	225
Critical Thinking and Accountability	227
Critical Thinking and Nursing Education	228
Conclusion	231

Unit III Role Concepts Essential for RN Practice — 235

PART A PROVIDER OF CARE — 237

10 The Nursing Process: Assessment and Caring Interventions — 237

From Licensed Practical Nurse to Professional Nursing Practice	238
An Historical Overview of the Nursing Process and Nursing Language	239
The Nursing Process: Overview and Steps	240
Conclusion	259

11 The Nurse as Communicator — 261

Basic Communication Revisited	264
Communication in the Healthcare Setting	276
Conclusion	283

12 The Nurse as Teacher — 287

The Challenge of Client Education	288
Teaching, Learning, and Functional Literacy Defined	289
Principles of Teaching and Learning	289
Teaching Interventions	298
Steps in the Teaching–Learning Process	301
Documentation of Client Teaching	307
Clinical Application of the Teaching–Learning Process	308
Conclusion	310

PART B MANAGER OF CARE — 312

13 Managing the Care of Unique Clients — 312

Understanding Uniqueness	313
Uniqueness and Culture	314

Sensitively Assessing a Client's Uniqueness ... 316
Aspects of Client Uniqueness ... 318
Incorporating Uniqueness Into the Nursing Care Process ... 324
Conclusion ... 327

14 Decision-Making and Managing Time, Conflict, and Resources ... 329
Managing Time ... 331
Managing Conflict ... 343
Making Decisions ... 349
Managing Resources ... 351
Conclusion ... 352

PART C   MEMBER OF THE DISCIPLINE OF NURSING ... 355

15 Professional Responsibilities ... 355
Advocacy ... 357
Accountability ... 359
Professional Growth ... 362
Advancing Nursing as a Profession ... 369
Professional Stewardship ... 372
Conclusion ... 374

16 Legal Accountability ... 378
Sources of Law ... 380
Classifications of Law ... 382
Accountability ... 386
Liability, Negligence, and Malpractice ... 389
Risk Management ... 391
Legally Sensitive Areas That Affect Nursing Practice ... 393
Confidentiality and the Right to Privacy ... 395
Defamation of Character ... 396
Conclusion ... 398

17 Ethical Issues ... 401
Ethics and History ... 402
Ethical Dilemmas and Moral Distress ... 403
Ethics and the Law ... 404
Ethics and Religion ... 404
Nursing Ethics ... 405
Ethical Decision-Making in Nursing ... 414
Conclusion ... 416

Appendix   Answers to "The NCLEX-RN Might Ask" Questions ... 419

Index 425

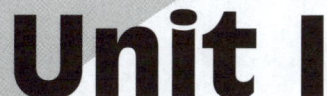

Unit I

The Transition Process

Lifelong Learning: Returning to School

CHAPTER 1

LEARNING OUTCOMES

By the end of this chapter, the student will be able to:
1. Describe the importance of lifelong learning in nursing.
2. Describe the process of reentry into the role of student.
3. Outline the stages of the return to the student role.
4. Design a plan for working effectively with your instructor.
5. Describe diverse learning styles.
6. Assess personal learning style.
7. Compare personal learning style with those described by theorists.
8. Develop beginning strategies for being successful in college.
9. Summarize learning resources that enhance the student's ability to be successful.
10. Examine methods to manage time effectively.
11. Give examples of effective study skills and strategies.
12. Design a win/win agreement with significant others for successful time management.
13. Design an individualized plan for a successful return to school.

KEY TERMS

abstract conceptualization
active experimentation
active learner
assertiveness
clinical reasoning
concrete experimentation
creative thinking
critical thinking
curriculum threads
disintegration
diverse learning styles
educationally mobile
evidence-based practice
honeymoon stage
interprofessional collaborative team
learning style
lifelong learning
netiquette
program philosophy
reflective observation
reintegration
resolution
returning to school syndrome (RTSS)
student learning outcomes (SLOs)
win/win agreements

Case STUDY

Sandy Martin has been a licensed practical nurse (LPN) for 10 years. Although she has always wanted to go back to school for her registered nurse (RN), marriage and a full-time job at a skilled nursing facility have kept her more than busy since graduation. In addition to raising two children, she has a mortgage, aging parents, and all the responsibilities that come with life. She never seems to have time for herself. Finally, with her two children

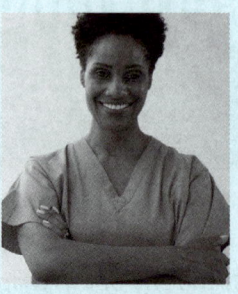

now in middle and high school and the nursing shortage at its highest in years, Sandy has decided to reduce her full-time work schedule and go back to school part time to seek an Associate Degree in Nursing (ADN). However, as Sandy waits to talk to the nursing advisor about class requirements and prerequisites, she begins to worry. Can she really meet her current obligations and earn her degree? It is going to take her at least 3 to 5 years to finish her degree, which is a bit discouraging. Also, will she have retained enough information after all these years? From the time she was studying to be an LPN, she remembers the struggles she had with anatomy, physiology, and pharmacology, as well as her fear of clinical rotations and assignments. She also worries about whether she will "fit in" with the younger students. She hopes the nursing advisor will be able to help alleviate her concerns and help her through this journey.

Remember when you first made the decision to be a nurse? For many people, the desire to be a nurse revolved around wanting to help people who could not help themselves and putting caring into action. However, with your experience in the world of nursing as a licensed practical nurse/licensed vocational nurse (LPN/LVN), your vision and opinions of nursing may have changed somewhat. Perhaps your view of nursing differs from the views of other nurses. Your reasons for returning to school reflect changes in your life. Your reasons may include the desire to have more job opportunities, increase your job satisfaction, and expand the scope of your responsibilities, or you may be seeking self-improvement.

The fact that you are returning to school reflects the positive impact of the many changes that have occurred in your life and in society. At one time, attaining a license in practical/vocational nursing was seen as a terminal process; an LPN/LVN would not seek higher education. If an LPN/LVN wanted to continue their nursing education, it often meant starting over. Conversely, changes in the educational system have enhanced your ability to further your education, building on your prior knowledge, skills, and experience. The attrition rate of RNs is high, with many leaving in the first year of practice because of high-stress environments, lack of acceptance by peers in the clinical setting, and undesirable quality of working life (Mayes & Cochran, 2023; Norful et al., 2023; NSI, 2023). However, your foundation as an LPN/LVN has given you a preview to what registered nursing practice will be, and your choice to pursue professional registered nursing licensure and an associate or baccalaureate degree in nursing has been made with this basis of knowledge of the workplace. Such experiential knowledge is already a foundation for your success in the ADN or Baccalaureate of Science in Nursing (BSN) program you are entering in pursuit of a higher, professional degree. It must be noted that this too will not be a "terminal" process; professional development is an ongoing part of a professional RN's role. You may find you want to eventually pursue a graduate degree or specialize in a clinical specialty that requires advanced training. The unlimited possibilities for career diversity and advancement helps keep nurses vibrant and excited about the profession.

LIFELONG LEARNING IN NURSING

The National League for Nursing identifies **lifelong learning** as integral to the profession. As an RN, you will progress along a continuum of developing greater and greater clinical expertise. Your nursing judgment will expand as you engage in **evidence-based practice** as a professional nurse and work collaboratively with other healthcare professionals to refine and strengthen patient care.

Today's nurse must be committed to lifelong learning and the use of new evidence and best practices to continuously provide high-quality care to patients. As you embark on your registered nursing educational path, lifelong learning and changes in practice based on new evidence will be essential not only to your ability to exercise best practices but also to the ongoing revitalization of your professional identity.

Advances in the healthcare industry, technological advances, societal trends, nursing research, and changes in practice due to evidence-based research processes all require the professional nurse to engage in lifelong learning to update their knowledge and practices. As you return to school, you will likely find a new learning environment where faculty use teaching strategies that help you develop your competencies as a lifelong learner. You may find the learning environment different than when you were a student in an LPN/LVN program. Today's learning environment includes the use of case studies, group activities, clinical simulations, technology-supported activities such as online threaded discussions regarding patient care, and other computer-managed educational systems. Additionally, the use of student portfolios assists today's nursing students in reflecting on their practice, connecting theory to that practice, employing **critical thinking** and **clinical reasoning** skills, developing judgment, and raising questions for ongoing evidence-based practice advancements. This new learning environment may cause you anxiety, but this text and the strategies you employ working with your nursing advisor will ease your concerns in returning to school. Such skills and competencies include those identified by Longworth (2003) and shown in Box 1.1. These needed skills and competencies are still true today.

THE REENTRY PROCESS: OVERCOMING BARRIERS AND FEARS

Although you may be as hesitant as Sandy Martin about the prospect, your return to school is important. It is also a challenge and an adventure. Whether you have been out of school for only a brief time or for many years, you will probably have fears; however, these should diminish after a few months. Returning to academic life is not easy. The thought of new risks or the return to old roles may be frightening.

Another factor that may cause anxiety may be your desire to be highly successful in the educational process while also wanting to be successful in other roles, such as an employee, a caregiver, or a spouse. Each person has individual issues as they return to school, but you may find you have many things in common with others. It is important to examine what it means to return to school and to determine what strategies will best help you cope, succeed, and achieve satisfaction in the process.

When you return to the role of student nurse, you may have barriers and fears to overcome. The Thinking Critically activity in this section allows you to examine your own issues, and Chapter 6 provides you with an opportunity to develop a personal

> **BOX 1.1**
>
> **Basic Skills and Competencies for Lifelong Learning**
> - Information handling
> - Presenting–communicating formally
> - Discussing–communicating informally
> - Learning to learn
> - Listening and memorizing
> - Entrepreneurial skills
> - Making-practical skills
> - Critical judgment and reasoning
> - Decision-making
> - Problem solving
> - Self-esteem, self-management, and self-awareness
> - Empathy and tolerance for others
> - Creativity, a sense of humor
> - Meditation skills
> - Flexibility, adaptability, and versatility
> - Thinking, vision, and planning
>
> Adapted from Longworth, N. (2003). *Lifelong learning in action: Transforming education in the 21st century* (p. 140). Routledge/Falmer.

education plan (PEP), individualizing it for your success. Establishing short- and long-term goals will both motivate and inspire you in your return to school.

AGE
One perceived barrier in returning to school may be your age. You may believe that it has been too many years since you were in school. You may also fear that the other students will be much younger and that you might have little in common with them; you will find that this is almost definitely not the case. You may think that your academic ability is less than what is needed and worry because you have not had to study intensively for a long time. Attaining a college degree may seem like an out-of-reach dream. As an older student, you may fear that the math and science knowledge you once had has diminished over time or that younger students will think you are inferior or out of place.

Although you have been an LPN/LVN for some time now, you may feel that your extensive experience is not being valued; you may be seen as a new student nurse and feel like you are "starting over." Established nurses sometimes bully and ostracize new nurses, which Anthony (2020) describes as the phenomenon of lateral and horizontal violence. This phenomenon can contribute to a lack of self-confidence and a sense of discouragement and anxiety for an older student entering a new clinical setting.

ETHNICITY, GENDER, AND SEXUAL ORIENTATION CONSIDERATIONS
You may be fearful that your ethnicity, gender, or sexual orientation may set you apart from others and that you will have little in common with your classmates. However, as you return to school, you may find that faculty and staff have become more diverse and

that this diversity is more greatly valued than it was at the time of your LPN/LVN training; the diversity among both students and faculty has expanded to mirror the diversity of the general population, including males, those from underrepresented groups, and LGBTQIA+ (lesbian, gay, bisexual, transgender, questioning or queer, intersex, asexual, and allies) representatives. Remember that everyone brings unique strengths and perspectives to nursing and education. Navigating the diverse landscape of education can be a rewarding but sometimes challenging experience. Here are some suggestions for students to effectively handle differences in culture, ethnicity, and socioeconomic status as they enter academia:

- Learn about the cultures and backgrounds of other students to better understand cultural norms, values, and communication styles.
- Participate in events that celebrate different cultures such as festivals, conferences, seminars, and workshops.
- Participate in initiatives or student organizations that promote diversity, equity, and inclusion.
- Engage in open and respectful communication to bridge cultural and ethnic gaps.
- Be willing to listen and learn from others' perspectives.
- Seek mentors and faculty from diverse backgrounds; they can provide valuable insights and support as you progress through your academic journey.

By actively engaging with diversity, you not only enrich your own learning experience but contribute to the creation of a more inclusive and welcoming academic environment for everyone (Bradbury-Hael & McGarvey, 2024; Luhanga et al., 2023).

The percentage of nurses who are men has slowly increased from less than 1% in 1966 to around 11.2% in 2022 (Smiley et al., 2023). Today, male nursing pursue both clinical specialties and higher degrees for nursing faculty positions. Male students in nursing have experienced such challenges as a lack of information and support from guidance counselors, lack of role models on campus and in the workplace, the stigma that nursing is not viewed as a respectable profession for men, and the lack of teaching strategies among nursing faculty for male students (Guy & van der Krogt, 2021; Kane et al., 2021). National organizations such as the American Association for Men in Nursing (AAMN) provide a voice for male nurses. AAMN attracts and supports expert practitioners based on characteristics and principles, not racial or gender demographics (AAMN, n.d.). Through local chapters, AAMN showcases narratives of men in nursing and provides personalized resources (AAMN, n.d.).

The nursing workforce has also become more ethnically diverse; according to a 2022 survey conducted by the National Council of State Boards of Nursing (NCSBN) and the Forum of State Nursing Workforce Centers, nurses from underrepresented ethnic groups represent 19.9% of the U.S. registered nurse (RN) workforce (Smiley et al., 2023). Academic settings have also benefited from such diversity because students have more opportunities to learn from each other's experiences and worldviews and to relate to a more diverse client population. Students from underrepresented groups, including those who identify as LGBTQIA+, may have experienced classroom bias from both faculty and peer students, as well as a sense of isolation in classroom and clinical settings. As both collegiate settings and the nursing workforce become increasingly diverse, these barriers are lessening. Additionally, there are more resources for the diverse nursing workforce; examples include *Minority Nurse* magazine and website (http://minoritynurse.com), and websites with resources to support nursing practice for

LGBTQIA+ individuals and communities, such as The American Academy of Family Physicians (https://www.aafp.org/family-physician/patient-care/care-resources/lbgtq.html). Various journal articles, associations, and websites can be found through any online search engine for a wide array of diverse issues that may be of interest to you. Your faculty advisor, counselor, and college librarians are also good resources to assist you in finding literature on your specific areas of concern. These individuals have participated in professional development activities to expand their understanding of, and support for, students of diverse backgrounds.

FEAR OF NURSING FACULTY, TECHNOLOGY, AND TODAY'S CLASSROOM

As a returning student, you may be anxious about interacting with nursing faculty. This fear may be related to previous experiences with nursing instructors or stories you may have heard from other students. Note that nursing faculty have become increasingly diverse and have participated in professional development themselves to diversify their teaching strategies to meet a wider range of students' learning styles and needs and to foster critical thinking. Some instructors may intimidate you or expect you to know more than you do. Some may treat you as a novice, whereas others will treat you as the adult learner that you are, who brings to the learning environment many life experiences and practical nursing knowledge. You will undoubtedly find that you relate well with some of the faculty and have difficulty relating to others. Nursing faculty members are similar to you—unique and imperfect but dedicated to their profession as nurses and nurse educators.

Ellis (2022b) describes the need to enroll instructors in your success. In each class, it is important to get to know your instructor. Introduce yourself and set up a visit during the instructor's office hours. Get to know the instructor's style and how they wish to be contacted should the need arise. Always be respectful, show interest in class, form your own opinions of the instructor (instead of listening to those of other students), draw your own conclusions, accept criticism, and submit professional work. When communicating electronically (e-mail, text, etc.) with your instructor, be professional and respectful. Always proofread your correspondence to ensure accuracy and respectful language, and use proper **netiquette** (e-mail/text etiquette). If you are unsure what that involves, contact your advisor or college library staff for a resource to review the details of effective, professional electronic correspondence.

You may be intimidated by today's technology and classroom environment. Perhaps your LPN/LVN program theory content was delivered in an all-lecture format. Today's registered nursing students are active participants in teaching–learning environments that use computer technology, internet research, collaborative work groups, online classrooms, discussion boards, case studies, learning contracts, portfolio development, role-playing, debates, and other interactive processes to foster critical and **creative thinking** and to develop lifelong learning skills. The instructor's role is to impart professional experiential knowledge and facilitate learning, to ensure relevance and inclusiveness of the diversity of learners, and to assist students with attitudes and techniques to strengthen their motivation to learn. A variety of learning styles will be addressed, and you may find yourself at ease with some learning activities more than others. However, it is helpful to gain experience with a variety of teaching and learning methods to diversify your learning style. (For more on learning styles, see the "Diverse Learning Styles" section later in this chapter.)

If you are expecting to merely listen to lectures and passively take notes, it may take you several months to become comfortable in this more active student role. Important skills for today's classroom environment include strengthening your computer literacy (including becoming familiar with current technology and conducting research online using library databases and web-based search engines), learning how to write professional papers, and working in teams with classmates on group projects. Often, the LPN/LVN returning to school to become an RN enters the program thinking they will only need to learn more complex treatments and procedures, yet you will be asked to think in a whole new way. As an **active learner**, you will be expected to draw on knowledge and research from a wide array of subject areas and case studies to synthesize, think critically, problem solve, and exercise judgment in nursing diagnoses and determining client care needs. This preparation for transition from a practical to a professional role will be covered in more depth later in this book.

FINANCIAL AND/OR FAMILY CONSTRAINTS

Another stressor to your return to school may be financial constraints. Tuition, fees, books, student uniforms, and commuting costs are large burdens. The necessity to remain employed and/or to find and finance childcare may add to these pressures; many returning students are also single caregivers and/or the sole breadwinner or family caretaker. The COVID-19 pandemic and its extremely slow recovery may have exacerbated your financial constraints as a retuning student. Reduced employment opportunities, possible job loss, increased financial strain due to healthcare expenses, and financial uncertainty may have influenced the decision to delay or alter educational plans. The economic crisis that followed caused some families to "double up" in housing, and extended family members and/or multigenerational households have become more prevalent. Financial obligations have expanded, credit standards have tightened, and accessing loans has become more difficult. This may cause you additional strain as you return to school and may cause you to have to work more hours, impeding your ability to devote study time needed to be successful as a returning student. Fortunately, many financial assistance programs are in place for students, and many scholarships are available for nursing students in particular.

In addition to financial constraints, returning students at times experience family constraints. Children, spouses, partners, or other family members may need your time and support. Although accommodating of your desire to return to school, they may also want life to remain unchanged. Another related factor is that life does not stop while you are in school. Illnesses, life events, and crises may occur. Although you have likely planned for many things, the unexpected and unplanned may occur over the next months and/or years as you pursue your degree. College campuses have many resources for students, including scholarships and programs targeted to assist first-generation college students, students of color, and students who are socioeconomically disadvantaged. Federal, state, and local support programs with which you may not yet be familiar are commonly found in colleges; these include TRIO (a government outreach program to low-income households for which you need to meet one of the three qualifications to be eligible), Student Support Services, Puente, and MESA (Mathematics, Engineering, Science Achievement). Special support services are also available for veterans and for students needing physical or learning disability accommodation. Talk to your nursing advisor or college counselor if you are in need financial or other support services.

Unfortunately, many students wait to seek such resources until they have missed classes or clinical, or have received failing grades. Seeking help early can make the difference between success and failure in your coursework.

FEAR OF FAILURE

The final barrier to returning to school that will be discussed in this chapter is the fear of failure itself. You have invested a lot of time and effort to be where you are today. Taking exams and being observed in the clinical area can be frightening. You may have developed shortcuts to clinical skills or bad habits that will need to be corrected. The fear of not being successful as a student nurse can be overwhelming; it may stem from previous school experiences or from lack of self-confidence. You may also find yourself hesitant or uneasy in new clinical settings. Adult learners are typically hard on themselves because they not only want to be successful, but they often also want to be perfect. It takes frequent reminders that the learning and transition processes need not be perfect, only positive. In addition, many factors are involved as a student progresses through a nursing program, including learning at a professional practice level that requires nursing diagnosis, critical thinking, and judgment not required at the LPN/LVN level. There may be times where you feel that you have forgotten everything you learned in LPN/LVN training or that you are "starting over." These are common experiences of returning students. It is important that you share these issues or concerns with your nursing advisor, who can give you reassurance and suggest strategies to address your particular situation. It is important to remember that faculty want to see you succeed as much as you want to succeed. They will do all they can to support you, but to be able to assist you, they must be aware you are struggling.

It is beneficial to identify your fears and concerns as you return to school. Later in this chapter, some strategies for success and minimizing fears are presented. Remember that the barriers and fears you may be experiencing are real; you may find that they are shared by others and that together you can find answers and solutions. For instance, as you get to know your classmates, you will find that your age, experience, and unique qualities are valuable to other class members. It may be advantageous to have had certain experiences, such as participating in certain cultural/ethnic traditions or raising children. Your concerns about studying may be the same as those of your fellow students, and you may find that you will be able to assist each other. You may also find

THINKING CRITICALLY

After reading the previous section, you may have found yourself nodding your head in recognition or wondering why your particular fears and concerns were not voiced. At this point, identify the barriers and fears that you face as you return to school. Include all of them, regardless of whether they have been mentioned. If you have identified some coping strategies or possible solutions, include those as well. As a next step, talk with a fellow student or another nurse at work who returned to school to determine whether you share common concerns. You may also find it useful, as did the student in the vignette, to share these concerns with your nursing advisor. This is a beginning step in preparing for success when returning to school.

that your study skills did not disappear. In fact, you may be more organized and better able to complete the assigned work than you anticipated. Other students may provide insight into particular courses or instructors. Many students experience financial concerns; you may find that you can share commuting costs, childcare, or other resources. It may also be reassuring to know that you are not alone. As you develop your individual educational plan and discuss these issues with your advisor, success strategies will emerge.

RESUMING THE STUDENT ROLE: "RETURNING TO SCHOOL SYNDROME"

Donea L. Shane (1983) identified the process of reentry as the "**returning to school syndrome**" **(RTSS)**. Although Shane's research was conducted more than 30 years ago, it is still applicable to today's returning student. In studying educationally mobile nursing students as they returned to school, she was able to identify stages that comprise an entire syndrome. **Educationally mobile** nurses are those who are returning to school or at least contemplating such a return. Shane's work was derived from stories and data collected during a 6-year period from those studying to become RNs. Those students were able to "share their insecurities, sorrows, failures, and anxieties as well as their triumphs, humor, and joy" (p. vii). The results of her work remain valuable today.

Shane (1983) defined RTSS as up-and-down emotional swings that are experienced by nursing students who are returning to school. These swings occur because returning students are familiar with their nursing roles within the work setting yet are taking on a different role by becoming nursing students again. The RTSS model depicts a series of sequential stages. She notes, "However, an individual nurse may not proceed through these phases in a linear fashion. The usual progression is an irregular one, with relapses, detours, and expressways through certain stages" (p. 73). Shane identified three major stages within the RTSS syndrome (Table 1.1).

TABLE 1.1 Returning to School Syndrome

Stage	Description
Honeymoon	Individual is happy and delighted about being back in school; does not see any problems with the process.
Conflict	Characterized by high anxiety: individual feels conflict about educational process and role changes.
a. Disintegration	a. Individual represses feelings of anger and hostility; may become depressed and sullen.
b. Reintegration	b. Person becomes outwardly hostile and angry, particularly with nursing faculty; individual is frustrated with the educational program.
Resolution	There are various forms in the process of resolving conflicts.
a. Chronic conflict	a. The student nurse maintains angry feelings and fails to see anything worthwhile or valuable in the educational process.
b. False acceptance	b. Individual pretends to accept the changes in role but actually does not understand or see any difference.
c. Oscillation	c. The educationally mobile nurse vacillates between stages; generally involves regression if a stressful event occurs; once the stressor is resolved, the person moves to a more positive resolution.
d. Biculturalism	d. A positive resolution in which the individual accepts the differences and role values and is challenged to grow within the professional role.

STAGE 1: HONEYMOON

Typically, the shortest and most benign stage is called the **honeymoon stage**. It is a somewhat blissful time in which the reality of a situation has not quite been absorbed. Individuals are generally happy about being in school and see the experience as congenial. The end of the honeymoon usually occurs when the educationally mobile nurse is enrolled in her or his first clinical nursing course. At this point, the student may become intimidated and begin to fear that her or his experience is no longer of value. In particular, the dreaded clinical evaluation looms ahead, causing the individual increasing anxiety.

STAGE 2: CONFLICT

Shane (1983) suggested that the longest and most intense phase is conflict. It is a difficult time that can be emotionally exhausting and overwhelming. In general, the educationally mobile nurse experiences conflicts with beliefs, family roles, work roles, prior knowledge versus new knowledge, and nursing faculty. Such nurses may believe that there is no difference in the educational programs, that they already know what they need to know to be RNs, or that they are already better than the graduates of this program, and thus, nothing will change by continuing the educational process. Work role conflicts arise from realism versus idealism. Working nurses know and understand the real-work world, and so they dispute the idealistic presentations or experience guilt at not being able to practice idealistically. Other conflicts also arise, such as stressful relationships with clinical faculty, dealing with various teaching styles, and adjusting to new ways of learning in the nursing program.

The conflict stage is subdivided into two parts (Shane, 1983):

- **Disintegration** is characterized by a state of anxiety in which the individual turns their anxious feelings inward. This can result in several negative feelings that are potentially harmful: depression; sadness; withdrawal from friends, family, and others; and attitudes of obstinacy and gloom. It is remarkable that significant people who have contact with this person are able to overlook these behaviors or do not notice them.
- **Reintegration** is marked by outwardly intense feelings of frustration and hostility that are directed toward those around the individual, especially the faculty. This anger is the result of the individual's frustrations with the nursing program or with the whole educational process. Although these outbursts are difficult to handle, they are healthier than the repression of feelings that is seen in disintegration.

STAGE 3: RESOLUTION

The third and final stage, **resolution**, is a variable phase because each individual experiences it for different lengths of time, and its outcomes can differ. Shane (1983) presented a few of the forms that resolution can take:

- **Chronic conflict.** This resolution is the least effective because these nurses become stuck in a quagmire of anger. They may continue with their nursing education, but they fail to recognize the value of that education or the inherent worth of the role change. They spend valuable energy and time being angry and belligerent, with little energy put into creating a positive outcome.
- **False acceptance.** This resolution is also not considered positive. Educationally mobile nurses play games of deceit and pretense. They may claim to accept the

differences in the former work role and the present educational role and the value of the new role but do not actually recognize any difference. They also cannot perceive the positive aspects of education and transition. In some regard, they become their own victims by not realizing any difference or usefulness in the process.
- **Oscillation.** Individuals who fall into this category vacillate between the various resolutions. To some degree, their oscillation occurs because they have experienced each resolution in various forms. Fortunately, oscillation is reversible. An oscillation (most frequently a regression to a more negative state) usually occurs because of some unusual stressor, such as failure on an exam, an illness at home, or an unfortunate interchange with a faculty member.
- **Biculturalism.** This resolution is the most positive. These educationally mobile nurses have positive feelings about their previous educational experiences. They also value their current education and their growth within the nursing profession. It is important to them to be challenged and to develop their professional roles.

The RTSS presents an interesting way to view the reentry process. You may recognize the various emotional states. However, Shane (1983) also found that some educationally mobile nurses deny that any of the RTSS concepts apply to them. These nurses resent being analyzed and categorized. Behavior and role changes are not uniformly valued in the educational process. It is even more difficult to identify your own emotions and feelings. The value of understanding this syndrome is that it provides you with some insights into the conflicts and concerns that can arise when you are dealing with role change and changes in your own beliefs and it can affirm that these are normal responses.

THINKING CRITICALLY

After reading about the RTSS, consider how these phases apply to you in your own LPN/LVN-to-RN role transition. For example, recall your practical/vocational nursing education experience. Was it positive or negative? In thinking about the role change from LPN/LVN to RN, what do you value about this process? Have you experienced any of the emotions described in the explanation of RTSS? As you consider these questions, write down what you are experiencing and why. You may find it helpful to keep a journal as you progress through this role transition or make a note on your calendar to review this material again after taking your first clinical course.

DIVERSE LEARNING STYLES

The process of learning often seems formidable, particularly if the learner has not been engaged in formal learning activities for several years or if previous experiences were not especially positive. Adults have long been occupied with the tasks of returning to educational settings in pursuit of further educational degrees. Many adults fear that they will not be capable of learning new information or that they will not be able to focus on their educational program due to other commitments or interests that demand their attention. However, for most adults, it is a pleasant surprise to find that not only are they still able to learn but that they are also more focused and dedicated than in previous educational endeavors. They also may experience again their love for learning and a renewed interest in the nursing profession and the value of their nursing practice.

Much research has been conducted over the past few decades to determine the ways in which people learn; these are called "**learning styles**." One categorization of learning styles is to examine one's preference for learning through visual, auditory, or kinesthetic delivery mechanisms. For example, some individuals learn better when information is provided visually. Use of graphs, charts, visual aids, DVDs, internet, or video streaming modes of delivery is more effective for these individuals. Some of us learn faster, or retain more, when information is accessed in an auditory manner. Acquiring information through a lecture, DVD, or other method where listening is involved are auditory learning processes. A third learning style is the preference for "doing" things to learn new information and concepts. Assembling three-dimensional objects, building conceptual models, role-playing, and "learning by doing" all align with this learning style.

As the research on teaching and learning has progressed, it has become evident that there are many **diverse learning styles**; they are much more complex, varied, and interdependent than just these three. Additionally, we are influenced by our social and cultural context, age, and other factors so that our learning styles do not always remain the same. You may find as you return to school that you no longer learn in the same way(s) you did in LPN/LVN training. You are older and have had more life and nursing experiences from which you can draw when acquiring new information, applying research to practice, or engaging in evidence-based practice.

Ellis (2022a) describes that learning styles are based on both how we perceive new information and how we process new information, leading to four styles of learning. An overview of these concepts is presented in the "Four Styles of Learning" section later in this chapter. Ellis (2022b) provides a simple Learning Styles Inventory whereby learners can begin to gain insight into their preferences for learning. He examines one's learning profile based on four key learning preferences: feeling (concrete experience), watching (**reflective observation**), thinking (**abstract conceptualization**), and doing (**active experimentation**). He also acknowledges the interrelatedness of these preferences into four "modes"—that is, the kinds of behaviors that feel most comfortable and familiar to an individual who is learning something—as follows: Mode 1 (a blend of feeling and watching), Mode 2 (a blend of watching and thinking), Mode 3 (a blend of thinking and doing), and Mode 4 (a blend of doing and feeling). The more you can reflect on your patterns of learning over time, and understand how you learn best, the more successful you will be in your educational pursuits at any level. You may wish to take Ellis's Learning Style Inventory to learn more about your own learning style(s), preference(s), and mode. You can then develop and/or apply study techniques that will maximize your success as you return to school.

ADULT LEARNING STYLES

In addition to understanding your inherent learning style since youth, it is important to also note that you will likely experience learning differently as an older/adult returning student. Learning styles of adults differ from those of children. Adults have a different and clearer sense of themselves, what their purpose is in a particular educational endeavor, and what is worthwhile and what is not. Adults are able to draw on their experiences to gain a deeper and more meaningful understanding and, therefore, have a greater capacity to apply theoretical concepts to practical situations. Adults pursue educational opportunities because there is a desire or need to attain new learning for job acquisition, career advancement, or personal gratification or self-actualization (Sarver et al., 2020). Covey (2004, 2013) describes that to develop effective habits, such as those needed for studying and learning, one must possess the knowledge, skills, and desire for that learning. He notes that finding meaning and your own voice (i.e., why you are going back to school, your true aspirations) will yield greater success. Additionally, learning achievement will be stronger if motivation is intrinsic, coming from within yourself rather than from external forces.

Learning from experience changes what we do and how we view things. You may find differences between what you have learned from experience as an LPN/LVN and what you read in preparation for class assignments. This is to be expected because, just as patients bring with them a unique array of personal attributes, you as an adult learner bring with you various life experiences. Your learning in the RN program will involve an active process in which you will engage in activities that further your knowledge, practice, and abstract skills.

PERCEIVING AND PROCESSING TASKS

Styles of learning are the methods that the learner prefers to use for perceiving and processing new information (Ellis, 2022a, 2022b). It is advantageous to be aware of one's learning styles to recognize that there are differences, to use strengths, and to adapt when the learning styles of others are predominant. Ellis identifies styles of learning as involving two tasks: perceiving and processing. He summarizes two methods of perceiving and two methods of processing information (see Box 1.2). As Ellis emphasizes, these categories are not absolute, and successful learners benefit from participating in all four styles of learning. (Refer to Box 1.3 for a review of terms used in this section.)

FOUR STYLES OF LEARNING

When considering the different styles of perceiving and processing, four distinct styles of learning emerge (Ellis, 2022a, 2022b). The following material has been adapted from Ellis's (2022a) *Becoming a Master Student: Making the Career Connection*. Each learning style is intended to serve as a guide for you to begin thinking about your own learning preferences. There is no hierarchal design in the four learning styles; each has validity and usefulness. It is helpful to review each style and identify the characteristics that best describe your own learning preferences. This is intended to assist you in increasing your self-awareness. You will discover that you probably draw from all four categories and that it often depends on the particular situation, the context, or your experiences.

Style 1 Learners

Perception of new information is best accomplished with concrete experiences. These learners prefer to find examples of how particular information applies to their world. They use reflective observation to process new learning. Characteristics may include the following:

- Viewing concrete situations from different points of view
- Approaching events as observers
- Reflecting on situations rather than taking action
- Enjoying experiences that necessitate creation of ideas
- Using imagination
- Working for harmony and developing support
- Placing importance on concerns, caring, and trust in others

BOX 1.2 Methods of Perceiving and Processing

Methods of Perceiving

Some people perceive by:
- Using concrete experimentation
- Dealing with situations with an intuitive ability to problem solve
- Sensing and feeling
- Taking the initiative in unstructured settings

Other people perceive by:
- Using abstract conceptualization
- Thinking about things completely and analytically
- Using a scientific approach to problem solving
- Functioning well within structured settings
- Along with styles of perception, Ellis also delineated two styles of processing

Methods of Processing

Some people process new information by:
- Using active experimentation
- Applying new information in practical situations
- Seeing results despite potential risks

Other people process by:
- Using reflective observation
- Considering various points of view
- Presenting different ideas about a specific situation

Adapted from Ellis, D. (2022a). *Becoming a master student: Making the career connection* (17th ed.). Cengage Learning; Ellis, D. (2022b). *The essential guide to becoming a master student: Making the career connection* (6th ed.). Cengage Learning.

BOX 1.3 Review of Terminology Related to Perceiving and Processing Tasks

Active experimentation: a method to process information that involves a hands-on approach to be able to apply new information; implies that an individual wants to work with an idea or concept to determine if it makes sense

Abstract conceptualization: a mode of perceiving new knowledge that entails an ability to analyze, think through, and organize theoretical material in a logical way

Concrete experimentation: a means to perceive new information in a more passive way; involves approaching situations in a more observational manner, preferring to look at a situation from several viewpoints and ponder various ideas

Experiential learning: a process of learning that evolves and is evolving as an individual matures and has a wider range of experiences: involves adaptation and growth, and increased self-awareness

Learning style: a preferred method to perceive and process new information

Reflective observation: a method of processing information that involves careful observation and pondering about those observations and judgments that occur after the individual has contemplated several alternatives

Goals: being involved in important issues and bringing harmony

Favorite questions: Why? Why do I need to know this? Why should I attend this class? How do these concepts relate to my life?

Skills: valuing—brainstorming, listening, speaking, interacting, feeling, data gathering, and imaging

Preferred skill: problem identification

Style 2 Learners

These learners perceive best through abstract conceptualization. Explanations through lecture style are favored, particularly if a theoretical base is included. They process new information generally by reflective observation. Characteristics may include the following:

- Understanding a broad range of information
- Compiling information in a concise and logical form
- Being interested more in abstract ideas and less in people
- Favoring theory that is logical as opposed to practical
- Preferring traditional learning settings that include lectures and reading assignments and do not include open-ended tasks
- Being industrious and goal oriented with attention to detail

Goal: understanding things on an intellectual level

Favorite questions: What? What is important to learn from this particular class?

Skills: thinking—observing and analyzing, classifying, theorizing, organizing, conceptualizing, and testing theories

Preferred skill: solution identification

Style 3 Learners

Perceiving knowledge is best done through abstract conceptualization. Traditional modes of lecture and listening to theory are most preferred. New learning is best processed through active experimentation. Characteristics may include the following:

- Being skilled at applying ideas and theories for practical use
- Answering questions and demonstrating problem-solving and decision-making skills
- Enjoying technical tasks, as opposed to contemplating social issues
- Discovering how things work, including experimentation and tinkering
- Preferring plans and schedules

Goal: putting new information into use in their work and daily living tasks

Favorite questions: How does this thing operate? How can I use this information to make a positive difference in my life?

Skills: deciding—manipulating, tinkering, improving, applying, experimenting, and goal setting

Preferred skill: selecting a workable solution from all possibilities

Style 4 Learners

These learners perceive information by using concrete experience. They also use active experimentation to process new information. They prefer to explore ideas to determine if they can make sense of them or apply them in a practical way. Characteristics may include the following:

- Learning best from hands-on methods
- Carrying out plans

- Being involved in new and different experiences
- Relying on gut feelings, as opposed to logical analysis
- Taking risks
- Feeling comfortable in new situations
- Encouraging others to be independent thinkers
- Drawing conclusions without necessarily having logical reasons

Goals: bringing action to ideas and encouraging creativity

Favorite questions: What if? If I am learning important and accurate information, how does it apply to my own life? What else does it mean?

Skills: activity—modifying, adapting, risking, collaborating, committing, influencing, and leading

Preferred skill: implementing a selected solution

Being aware of your learning preferences will help you have a greater understanding of your learning needs and strengths. By appreciating your own individuality and recognizing that there are many learning styles, you should be open to situations that are not conducive to your style of learning. You will be exposed to different modes of education and instruction. You also will care for a range of clients who will have educational needs and styles of learning that are different from yours. Having the knowledge that there are various learning styles provides you not only with flexibility but also with an ability to meet your own needs and the needs of others. The following example illustrates this truth.

EXAMPLE 1.1 A student nurse is assigned to care for a client who has recently been diagnosed with hypertension. The client has begun a regimen of antihypertensives and a low-sodium diet. The student nurse observes the dietitian reviewing diet pamphlets and a list of low-sodium foods with the client. The dietitian instructs the client to read the materials and jot down any questions. After the dietitian leaves, the client tells the student nurse that they are confused. The student nurse, who believes the instructional methods were appropriate, asks the client what would help them learn the information. The client tells, "I don't learn well when I just have to read about it." The student nurse recognizes that a more visual method of instruction might be beneficial to this client and arranges for them to view a video and to learn to recognize low-sodium foods by reading their labels.

THINKING CRITICALLY

After reading the preceding material and determining which characteristics apply to you, list your preferred learning styles. Identify which of the four styles is the most predominant for you. Give several examples of why that style is your most preferred. You may use examples that demonstrate when you have enjoyed or deplored a particular learning situation. Share this information with a partner, and discuss observations about yourself and each other that back your selection of a learning style. It also may be helpful for you to share this with your faculty advisor.

STUDENT ROLE: STRATEGIES FOR SUCCESS

The key to being a successful student rests with you. Although methods and techniques to assist you in your endeavors are available, only you can make them work. This will require that you assume responsibility for your academic efforts and use assertive behavior to meet your goals. **Assertiveness** is a positive skill because it provides you with the courage and stamina to meet your needs. Assertiveness does not mean confrontation or aggression; rather, it implies that you are able to communicate in a positive and constructive manner. Assertive behavior assists you in exploring possibilities, asking for more information and clarification, considering various viewpoints, and making informed decisions. It will be important that you are assertive in building a relationship with faculty and in seeking their feedback on what you are doing well and where you need to improve. This will assist you in setting clear goals for yourself for success. Several strategies to support your success are discussed in the sections that follow.

COLLEGE SUCCESS COURSES AND RESOURCES

Colleges today provide you with many opportunities to sharpen your academic skills. For instance, you may find it helpful to take a course that provides you with study skills, test-taking skills, or an improved ability to write professional term papers. If you have been away from an academic setting for a while, or were overwhelmed by previous academic experiences, it may be extremely beneficial to enroll in a course designed for college success. In addition, computer literacy and library research courses may be helpful. Many colleges require or strongly suggest that you take these courses. Again, you may be pleasantly surprised that some of the obstacles that you believed had prevented you from being successful were not as much of a problem as you anticipated, given the right tools and college success strategies. You may also discover that relearning and/or refining your academic and study skills is not especially difficult and perhaps even more rewarding than it was in prior experiences due to your current motivation and desire for success.

On your return to school, take advantage of any courses that are available to assist you in being more successful in your nursing program. Research shows that students who take college success courses as they enter or reenter college do better in their course work. Such courses often include content on time management, note-taking, study skills, writing skills, using technology effectively, and accessing college support services. If you are not able to take a course in these areas, online programs and a wide array of college success texts on these subjects can be found in your college library and through online search engines. Smaller, inexpensive resources are available that have been authored by independent publishers. *The Study Skills Handbook: How to Ace Tests, Get Straight A's, and Succeed in School* (Hollins, 2021); *How to Succeed in Nursing School: Before, During, and After* (Thomas, 2011); and *Ten Strategies and Survival Tips for Managing Nursing School* (Mingo, 2023) give practical tips on such topics as time management, organizing your study notes, test-taking strategies, and approaching clinical rotations.

WORKING WITH A FACULTY ADVISOR

Once enrolled in a program of nursing, you will be assigned to a faculty advisor, most likely a member of the nursing faculty. You should introduce yourself to your advisor as early as possible so that both of you get to know each other. Exchanging telephone numbers and e-mail addresses will help you keep in closer contact and can be invaluable in the event of illness or a personal emergency. Your faculty advisor is available to you throughout the length of the program. Many students have primary contact with their advisors when it is time to register for the next term's classes. This contact may consist of getting a signature on the registration or add–drop form. However, there are many other reasons to have contact with a faculty advisor. Students often consult with their advisors when they are experiencing academic or personal difficulties. Faculty advisors are knowledgeable about finding appropriate resources for students to improve their academic performance or cope with personal concerns. For example, if a student finds that they are having trouble taking multiple-choice exams, the advisor may refer the student to college resources that can teach the student ways to be successful with that type of exam or to someone who can review past exams with the student and develop methods for taking future exams. Some faculty advisors are also skilled in these methods and assist the student directly.

Some students also seek assistance from faculty advisors if they believe that they are not skilled at taking notes in class or grasping the most important material from text and/or online assignments. Again, discussing these issues with an advisor may help the student focus on topics that are outlined in the study guides or that are main themes in a text or web source. The advisor may also refer the student to other college resources for improving study and note-taking skills.

Other reasons for students to see advisors are related to personal problems at home or in the college environment. Advisors are generally skilled at listening to problems and, although they are not trained counselors, will be able to discuss coping strategies and refer the student to an appropriate resource. If the problem involves another faculty member, the advisor may choose not to hear that issue completely but may suggest that the student speak directly with the faculty person, counselor, or program administrator.

An advisor can be most helpful if you meet them as soon as possible, instead of waiting until you have an insurmountable or overwhelming situation. It is highly advantageous to schedule an individual appointment at the start of the term to develop a rapport with your advisor. Advisors can be many things, but they are not mind readers, miracle workers, or saviors. If you begin to experience academic problems, you are expected to proactively seek help early in the process so that the difficulty can be remedied before failure. Advisors can help only as much as you are willing to seek help. Advisors are not always immediately available because of other academic commitments. In most instances, it is advisable to make an appointment to meet with your advisor, rather than trying to deal with an issue before or after class. This provides for a more relaxed, focused interaction with your advisor and their undivided attention. If you have an urgent issue, other faculty members may need to be involved if the advisor is not available. If you find that you have difficulty relating to your advisor, you may be able to change advisors by speaking with the program administrator.

RESOURCE MATERIALS

As you begin your nursing program, many different resources are available to you that will enhance your success. The following is a brief summary of some of the most important resources as you return to school.

Student Handbooks

A college student handbook is designed specifically for students at that designated college or university. Additionally, most nursing programs have a Nursing Student Handbook. It is important to read and familiarize yourself with these handbooks, as they contain important information about the academic calendar, important dates, student policies, attendance policies, grading procedures, and resources available on campus. Becoming familiar with the handbooks will help you avoid conflict and issues during the program that can occur if you do not know college or program policies and procedures. When a question arises, always refer to your handbook rather than asking a fellow student, who may give you inaccurate, incomplete, or outdated information.

Program Philosophy and Curriculum

Faculty for each nursing program have developed a **program philosophy** that presents the concepts, themes, and **curriculum threads** for the nursing program. Generally, nursing education philosophies are composed of beliefs about nursing, the education of nurses, and the various recognized levels of nursing education. They may include philosophical approaches to the education of adults and the responsibilities of adult students. In many instances, the program philosophy carries out the principles stated in the college or university philosophy. It is also helpful to explore this in terms of your own evolving philosophy about nursing. The curriculum is designed based on the program's philosophy, the standards governing nursing licensure, the NCLEX-RN test plan, and accreditation standards of both the institution and the nursing program. Each program will adopt certain concepts as "curriculum threads" that will be woven into each course in the program.

Student Learning Outcomes

The nursing program will also have identified **student learning outcomes (SLOs)** for students as they progress through the course work. SLOs are identified for each course, program, and degree in the institution. SLOs are required by accrediting bodies for the institution and the program and will be found in the college catalog, student handbook, and course syllabi. Learning outcomes portray the knowledge, skills, and abilities expected of all program participants as they complete coursework, graduate, and proceed to higher educational degrees or enter the workforce. Individual courses and their learning activities are designed to facilitate the student achieving these learning outcomes as they progress through the curriculum of the program.

Course Syllabus

A course syllabus is an outline and summary of material that will be covered in a particular course, including the expected SLOs, and often includes structure of the course, learning activities, guidelines for assignments, grading criteria, and important due dates. Reading assignments, web-based resources, and other useful information is often included. It is important to read the course syllabus carefully and ask clarifying questions if needed. The syllabus becomes a roadmap for the course and outlines how your progress and performance in the course will be assessed and evaluated.

Faculty and Course Web Pages

Today's student must be adept in the use of electronic environments. Many schools require students to have access to either a computer, a tablet, or an internet access device. If this is an area of discomfort for you, it is highly recommended that you take a course or workshop at the college to strengthen not only your use of such environments but also your confidence in troubleshooting any technological difficulties you may experience. Many faculty maintain a home page online with e-mail addresses, other contact information, announcements, reminders, and other important information for students. Whether online or traditional face-to-face, most nursing programs present courses using a learning management system (LMS) such as Canvas, Blackboard, or Desire2Learn that contains the course syllabus, course calendar, school policies, assignment information, discussion boards, and other helpful tools vital to student success in the course. Many faculty require assignments to be submitted electronically and expect students to access and review the LMS daily for important information about the course and any changes in course assignments, meetings, class cancellations, etc. If you are unfamiliar with these learning technologies, talk to your faculty advisor for assistance in locating an orientation session, class, or other forum for becoming familiar with using these online resources. It is also important to turn in all assignments in advance of the due date/time to avert being late due to any technical difficulties that sometimes arise.

Personal Professional Library

Collecting nursing texts, resources, and web-based materials can be confusing, overwhelming, and expensive. Students returning to school are often tempted to purchase all the books they can, with the hope that each book might be helpful. There are many excellent resource books, but you do not need all of them. The course syllabus generally lists required and recommended texts. The faculty members usually select recommended texts to assist you in acquiring more knowledge about a particular topic. In general, students are generally required to attain a comprehensive medical dictionary, a drug resource manual, a laboratory manual, and possibly a text that assists with the nursing process and the development of care plans. Although many textbooks also have online student resources, computer-based resources are also available from websites specifically for student nurses. Other resources that students may want to purchase are current anatomy, physiology, and pathophysiology texts, and those about a particular subject in which they have a strong interest. The nursing textbooks and other resources you acquire will be valuable after completing the program when you prepare for the NCLEX-RN. Other resources that may be helpful are pharmacology and nutrition texts, state board review books, CDs, DVDs, and computerized programs. Before purchasing anything, you may find it helpful to discuss your choices with faculty and recent graduates of the nursing program. Your college's library will have additional resources, and many more are available via interlibrary loan and online.

Periodical Subscriptions and Web Resources

Many nursing journals are available both by subscription and online. It is often difficult to choose which journals are appropriate for you. Again, talking with faculty and other students may assist you. Many nursing journals are available at campus libraries, in hospital libraries, and online, which is a less expensive and easier way to become familiar with nursing journals as resources of information. As a student nurse, you will have many opportunities to read journal articles as part of course requirements. This will help you decide whether you want to subscribe to a particular journal. If you use an online resource, make sure it is reputable. Not all information on the web is accurate; therefore, if you are unsure of the accuracy of a website, consult your instructor or the college learning resource center.

RESOURCES FOR UPDATING YOUR RESEARCH SKILLS

Web resources have greatly expanded over the past decade. In completing your general education and nursing course requirements and writing professional papers, you will find general resources—such as a dictionary, thesaurus, and standards for writing professional papers—readily available online. Search engines and directories are abundant, including those available in other languages if English is not your first language. You will need to become skilled at using these resources, and many students enhance their abilities in this area via a college success or library use course, or by working with the college library staff. Although it may take some time for you to become comfortable in this environment, you will find your time saving is extensive once you are adept at online research. Examples of web resources are available with this text.

If you have not been in an academic setting recently, you will discover that performing research for assignments and term papers has also become a more technical process because most libraries now have computerized records and online databases. There also are several sources from which to obtain particular articles, journals, and books, depending on what you are researching. You must become familiar with using the college's library and its computer system to research a topic properly. As part of your initial orientation to academic life, make sure that a library orientation is provided or independently orient yourself to the college's library. Although you may feel "technologically challenged" initially, you will find that technology actually expedites and expands your research capability and often allows you to do your research at home and at times most convenient to you. When you begin to use the library, do not be afraid to ask the library staff for assistance, as that is their purpose of being there, and like others at the institution, they want students to be successful. You will soon be able to access many resources, which will enable you to research a topic thoroughly. These skills will be critical to your lifelong learning as an RN, as well as to your pursuit of advanced degrees and/or clinical certification.

VALUING PRIOR LEARNING

As stated previously, adults often return to school with the fear that they will not do well, that they will appear foolish, or that the rest of the students will be more advanced. For the LPN/LVN, it is also difficult to be removed from an environment that values clinical skills and to be placed in an environment that values skills necessary for academic success. However, the value of your experiences as an LPN/LVN and your life experiences in general are immeasurable. You will probably find that your view of the world and of nursing has been greatly influenced by your many experiences.

Educators of adult students have long recognized the value of prior learning. You will find that your experiences enable you to perceive course work in a different way and to place a higher value on your efforts. The life experience you bring to your classes is valuable and will equip you to ask meaningful questions and to make solid connections between theory and practice (Ellis, 2022a).

Valuing who you are and your life, work, and educational experiences provides you with a foundation for continued growth and development in your career as a nurse and as a person. You remain capable of acquiring new knowledge and of adapting to the educational process. Everything that you have learned before returning to school will serve you well. Instead of despairing about what you may not know or understand, rejoice in the knowledge that you can achieve your goals with hard work and a reliance on the skills and knowledge that put you where you are today.

Langridge et al. (2023) stress the importance of students in professional careers developing personal portfolios. A portfolio is an organized compilation of materials and records that showcases and provides evidence of an individual's skills, achievements, experiences, and qualifications. Because documents in your portfolio are self-selected, they reflect your individuality, autonomy, and unique attributes. A professional portfolio is a snapshot of accomplishments and should be tailored to a specific use—for example, for a student to showcase academic accomplishments or for a professional nurse to acquire a job following licensure (Langridge et al., 2023; Marino, 2023; Siddiqui et al., 2023). A portfolio can be used with your nursing advisor to introduce yourself and to identify strengths and areas where you may need further mentoring or development. Items that may be useful to assemble for your portfolio when meeting with your nursing advisor include sample nursing care plans, clinical skills checklists, papers you have written, case study projects, and other documents or projects you have completed as an LPN/LVN and/or returning student that demonstrate your critical thinking ability and work as a healthcare professional.

The PEP you design in Chapter 6 of this text is an excellent document to include in your portfolio when working with your nursing advisor. Maintaining and adding to your portfolio throughout the nursing program will continue to bring value to your portfolio as you customize it for job applications upon graduation. After graduation, as a professional nurse, maintaining a portfolio will showcase your unique skills, knowledge, and abilities as a member of the profession and as a member of **interprofessional collaborative teams**.

TIME MANAGEMENT

One of the biggest challenges that returning students face is the lack of time to perform all roles adequately. There never seems to be enough time to manage everything and to do it well, but developing a plan will assist you in managing your time more effectively. Research has shown that there is a direct correlation between class attendance and student success. Good time management will ensure you have strong attendance and thereby support your success in nursing school. (For more information on time management, see Chapter 14.)

Balancing Personal, Career, and Student Roles

It is particularly helpful to plan a weekly schedule to see the entire picture. Some blocks of time are inflexible, such as work and class schedules. You must also remember to make time for other activities, such as sleeping, eating, exercising, family time, and studying. Once you have the weekly plan in place, it is helpful to formulate a daily "to-do" list to keep yourself organized and to be realistic about your time commitments. Successful students neither procrastinate nor work from morning to night without a break for personal "down time." Breaking tasks down into smaller achievable units and managing time wisely are both critical to success.

It is not necessary that you do everything as you did before you started school. Involve your significant others in your scheduling plan. Delegate some tasks or hire others to help. Give up some tasks until there is time to do them, and learn to be flexible so that you can take care of unexpected needs that arise. Let your family and friends know your schedule so that they have a better understanding of your needs. Enlist family and significant others in chores traditionally done by you. The decision for you to return to school must be an "all-family" decision, as it is disruptive not only to you but also to your family. Acknowledge the extra burden on everyone and work out a schedule where everyone feels consulted and part of the plan. Share the academic calendar, your scheduled exams, etc., so that they are aware of when extra support will be needed. This may also need to be the year you decline roles you may have held in the past as the organizer of events or activities in your personal life (professional organizations, clubs, boards, charitable organizations, etc.).

Do not give up all your exercise and recreation activities; you may need to modify what you do or when you do it, but continue to find time for yourself. Exercise is not only healthy but also reduces your stress level. Some students find it helpful to walk or jog between classes, plan a physical activity with a friend, or take a physical education class. You also will find it beneficial to designate some periods of quiet time for reflection and/or meditation. Students often feel guilty about taking time for a walk or quiet time, but it can actually rejuvenate you and make your work and study time more productive. Reading for pleasure, watching television or a movie, listening to music, meditating, or even just taking a walk may help you regroup and recharge.

Returning students need to be prepared to spend 2 to 3 hours of studying and preparing for every hour spent in class or clinical. If you are carrying a full-time student load, you will need to plan 20 to 30 hours per week for reading, studying, and completing assignments. This does not need to be done in huge blocks of time; most people generally study best in 1- to 2-hour blocks of time spent at the library or another quiet place without distractions. The benefits will be realized at exam time or when a project is due because you will not have to have marathon study times to prepare or complete the work. Retention of information is also improved when you avoid "cramming" at the last minute. For some students, carrying a full academic load is not feasible, and so they choose to attend school on a part-time basis. This will reduce both the workload and stress of multiple role responsibilities.

It is also helpful to communicate early with your employer regarding your needs and potential scheduling difficulties. Although most employers will support your decision to return to school, they also have to manage an entire staff, multiple work schedules, and many other details. Most students find that it is advantageous to reduce the number of work hours to the lowest number that is absolutely necessary to maintain financial commitments. With a full course load, it is recommended that you work only 1 to 2 days/shifts per week. Students who complete their general education and science course work before entering the nursing program, however, may find that they can work half time while attending college. Box 1.4 summarizes 10 hints for time management (Efron, 2023; Pitre & Pugh, 2023).

Reassessing Commitments

When you are rationing your time, besides creating a "to-do" list (see Box 1.4), consider also creating a "not-to-do" list. This list should include tasks that are not a priority and those that can be done by others while you are in school. For instance, if you serve on a committee at your child's school, consider resigning and giving someone else the opportunity to serve. If you volunteer for a local nursing home, you may decide to take a leave of absence. When you finish school, there will always be opportunities to be a member of a board or committee or a chance to do volunteer work. One student who returned to school referred to his time in school as "the years to say no."

THINKING CRITICALLY

Track your time commitments for 1 week. Think in terms of 15-minute blocks of time so that you can account for short activities. Account for all 24 hours of a day, and include adequate personal time and study time to avoid cramming assignments and exams. Carry the plan with you, and at the end of the week, examine what you did, and modify your plan for the following week so that you are organizing and using your time more efficiently.

> **BOX 1.4**
>
> ### Ten Hints for Time Management
>
> 1. Be realistic about how much time projects may take. Don't overcommit, underestimate the amount of work that has to be done, or overbook yourself to the point where you become overstressed.
> 2. Include "safe time" in your schedule. Allow yourself some "wiggle room" in case of computer malfunctions, automobile issues, or other unforeseen circumstances that can push you behind schedule, result in missed deadlines, or leave you unprepared for an exam.
> 3. Use a calendar to plan your activities. Make a weekly schedule that includes time allocated for all of your responsibilities (student, spouse, caregiver, employee, volunteer, and, most importantly, yourself).
> 4. When reading, studying, writing papers, or working on projects, find a calm, clutter-free area and let people know that's where you're going to be working.
> 5. Remember that life is about more than just academics. Make time for your classes and other necessities, but don't forget to prioritize time for your family, friends, and health.
> 6. Establish weekly priorities, then work throughout the week so that you don't have too many tasks on any one day. Put off chores that aren't absolutely necessary for your achievement.
> 7. Break large projects into smaller tasks to maintain a positive outlook, make progress, and gain a sense of accomplishment.
> 8. Learn to say "no," propose an alternative, or delegate tasks.
> 9. Group similar tasks together to reduce the mental effort required to switch between different types of activities.
> 10. Regularly review your time management strategies by identifying what works well and what needs adjustment. Be willing to adapt your approach to better suit your needs.

Adapted from Efron, N. (2023). Ten tips for efficient academic time management. *Clinical & Experimental Optometry, 106*(7), 691–693. https://doi.org/10.1080/08164622.2022.2139592; Pitre, C. J., & Pugh, C. M. (2023). Reclaiming the calendar: Time management for the clinician educator. *Journal of Graduate Medical Education, 15*(1), 117–118. https://doi.org/10.4300/JGME-D-22-00939.1.

Using the Win/Win Agreement

Stephen Covey (1989, 2004) formulated a method to reach agreements in which there is mutual benefit or satisfaction from the agreement for all involved. **Win/win agreements** create an environment in which each party thinks in terms of cooperation, as opposed to competition. Win/win is conceived on the idea that "there is plenty for everybody, that one person's success is not achieved at the expense or exclusion of the success of others" (p. 207). Such agreements are useful in working out arrangements with significant others while you are in nursing school.

Covey identified five dimensions that are interdependent and relational:

1. **Character:** This is the foundation of win/win and consists of three traits:
   - Integrity: the value you place on yourself; a commitment to yourself and others
   - Maturity: the maintenance between the ability to express your opinions and attitudes and the respect for the opinions and attitudes of others
   - Abundance mentality: the notion that there is enough or plenty for everyone; requires the individual to have strong integrity and maturity

2. **Relationships:** Win/win involves a level of trust in the process and in the person(s) that are involved with the formulation of an agreement. It also involves an ability to listen and to communicate with respect for the person(s) and the various points of view.
3. **Agreements:** Win/win requires that each party have a clear understanding of the limits and scope of the process. The agreements include an understanding of the desired results, any guidelines that are needed, an awareness of all available resources, accountability by all those involved in the agreement, and an evaluation of the process with possible consequences.
4. **Systems:** For win/win agreements to work, there must be support for the process. Each individual involved must feel equal responsibility for achieving goals and results and, therefore, solutions.
5. **Processes:** Win/win solutions are best achieved if each person looks at the problem from the other's perspective; this gives the other person a chance to be heard. It is then essential to name the concerns and issues that are involved. Each person next presents possible results that would be acceptable solutions to the problem. As a last step, various options could be determined for achieving the specific results.

Win/win agreements do not need to be elaborate or lengthy. The process can actually be simple, particularly if each person is committed to the process. An example of a win/win agreement within a family is illustrated in the following example.

EXAMPLE 1.2 When Sandy, an LPN, returned to school, she recognized that her time would be more restricted because she would be in class for 6 hours a week and clinical practice for 15 hours a week. Her study and preparation time would require 20 to 30 hours a week. She also needed to work two 8-hour shifts per week to pay certain bills and maintain benefits and seniority. Her husband works full time (Monday to Friday, 9 AM to 5 PM). Their son and daughter are 10 and 16 years old, respectively. Historically, Sandy has taken care of many of the household chores, particularly housecleaning, preparing meals, and the majority of errands. The other family members helped but not on a regular basis and often only with much persuasion. With classes and studying, Sandy realized that she could no longer be responsible for all of these tasks. Sandy's family developed the following win/win agreement:

Sandy will do the housecleaning in the living room, dining room, and kitchen. The son and daughter will be responsible for the bedrooms, and the husband will be responsible for the bathrooms. They agree that these jobs will be done without reminders and in a timely manner. The daughter will have Sandy's car 2 days a week and, for that privilege, will be responsible for doing most of the weekly errands and transporting her mother to and from school. The son and husband will do the weekly grocery shopping. Everyone will share in meal preparation and cleanup, with assigned days for those tasks. The children will receive compensation for their work, and the parents will put aside an equal amount so that they can have an occasional evening out. On Sunday evenings, they will have a brief family meeting to plan for the coming week and evaluate how things are going based on the agreement.

The wins for Sandy are more time to devote to classes and studying and fewer responsibilities at home. The wins for the family members are that Sandy will have some time to spend with them, and everyone benefits from sharing responsibilities without having to be reminded or badgered. There are financial and social benefits for all. The consequences of failure are also made clear: If a person does not uphold their responsibilities, they will not receive the agreed-on compensation. They have built in some flexibility by planning ahead each week to account for special activities and needs. At the end of this chapter, you have an opportunity to develop a win/win agreement to assist you in developing methods to manage your time more effectively.

DEVELOPING STUDY SKILLS

Forming and refining study skills can be a challenge for returning students. The difficulty is often related to previous experiences in which adequate study skills were not formed or because there are many other distractions for adult learners than for students directly out of high school. Another difficulty may be that past study skills involved rote memory, whereas you now will be asked to analyze, synthesize, and think critically about the material presented and to write papers and design care comprehensive care plans for your clients. In *The Essential Guide to Becoming a Master Student*, Ellis (2022b) provides an excellent summary of strategies for success as you enter the academic arena. Ellis (2022b) covers a variety of topics on study skills, using today's technology effectively, time management, and maximizing learning through your most successful learning styles. The texts *How to Survive & Thrive in College* (Bennet, 2022) *and Insider's Guide to College Success: The Underground Playbook for Making Great Grades, Having More Fun, and Studying Less* (Stemmle, 2021) provide valuable contemporary strategies for success in college. Reading texts such as these, and completing student exercises, will be money well spent to support your success in returning to school in today's collegiate environment.

Time and Place for Study

A first step in developing good study habits is to create study time. The specific time will depend on your other demands, but it will be most helpful if you can select a time of day in which you learn best or when you can be assured of minimal or no interruptions. Plan to study in short blocks of time (1 to 2 hours) with 5- to 10-minute breaks. Many students also plan study time between classes or other activities.

A place to study is also essential. Instead of trying to read while reclining on the sofa with the television on, try to find a quiet area in your home or go to the library. Your family and friends need to be aware that your study time and place are off-limits so that you can study without interruption. Turn off your cell phone and plan to return calls on breaks or after the study time.

Another useful study skill is to plan your time so that you know what you want to accomplish each day. Short-term goals are often less intimidating than long-term goals. Once your overall weekly plan is established, break up large or lengthy assignments into "small bites" that can be accomplished in 1- to 2-hour time blocks. You will be surprised at how much progress you will make using this strategy.

Procrastination

Another common challenge for adults returning to school is procrastination. As an LPN/LVN, your time outside of work hours has been filled with family time and/or other interests. You may find you procrastinate when faced with heavy reading assignments, writing papers and nursing care plans, and other assignments. Delaying

BOX 1.5 Suggestions for Overcoming Procrastination

- Define clear, achievable goals for your tasks. Knowing what you need to accomplish provides direction and motivation.
- Divide larger tasks into smaller, more manageable steps. This makes the workload seem less overwhelming and helps you focus on one aspect at a time.
- Develop a realistic and structured schedule. Allocate specific time slots for tasks, including breaks, and stick to the schedule as closely as possible.
- Identify and prioritize tasks based on their importance and deadlines. Focus on high-priority items first to ensure you address critical responsibilities.
- Use time management techniques such as working in short, focused intervals with breaks.
- Minimize potential distractions by creating a dedicated workspace, turning off notifications, and staying away from social media during work periods.
- Envision the positive outcomes and benefits of completing a task.
- Establish deadlines for yourself that are achievable. Self-imposed deadlines create a sense of urgency.
- Share your goals and deadlines with someone who can hold you accountable, such as a friend, family member, or study buddy.
- Reward yourself for completing tasks. Once you've accomplished a specific goal, treat yourself to a break, a small snack, or an enjoyable activity.
- Remind yourself that everything doesn't have to be "perfect." Focus on completing tasks rather than striving for perfection.
- Begin your work with a small, manageable task to create momentum and to make it easier to transition to more challenging assignments.
- Identify the potential negative consequences of procrastination, such as the impact on your grades or your well-being.

Adapted from Hinton, S. T., & Cherry, B. (2023). Managing time: The path to high self-performance. In B. Cherry & S. R. Jacob (Eds.). *Contemporary nursing: Issues, trends, & management* (9th ed., pp. 460–475). Elsevier; How to Stop Procrastinating. (n.d.). MindTools. https://www.mindtools.com/a5plzk8/how-to-stop-procrastinating; Mingo, S. (2023). Ten strategies and survival tips for managing nursing school. *Nursing Made Incredibly Easy!, 21*(6), 7–11. https://doi.org/10.1097/nme.0000000000000005

tasks often results in rushed and below-average work that negatively affects overall academic success. Identifying the cause of your procrastination and working to overcome it will improve your time management skills, reduce stress, and enhance your academic performance. Strategies to help you overcome procrastination are listed in Box 1.5.

Reading, Note-Taking, and Writing Skills

Many study habits you will need to develop are those that will assist you in improving or strengthening your reading, note-taking, and writing skills. For example, in reading textbooks, there are a few methods that will help make your reading time more productive. Many educators recommend that you take a few minutes to scan a reading assignment before reading it. This enables you to get a feel for the subject and to identify the main themes of the material. You can also decide how much time is needed to complete the assignment. Some material requires in-depth concentration, whereas other texts and reading assignments can be skimmed. In addition, a focus on reading with the course objectives and learning outcomes in mind will help pinpoint information that requires application and mastery.

Other strategies involve taking notes while you read. This can be in the form of an outline, or it can be more elaborate if the material is complex. Some students find it helpful to highlight or underline so that when they review the material, they can focus on these sections. It may also be useful to make notes in the margins or to write questions. For visual learners, flash cards, mind-mapping, and drawing models of conceptual relationships among content themes may be helpful. Instructors usually start their lectures by asking for student questions; this would be a perfect time to ask for clarification of your reading materials. Of course, this requires having read and jotted down questions in advance of class. Make use of the chapter objectives, terminology list, summaries, and review questions. These help clarify and reiterate certain concepts. Some students find it helpful to read aloud to maintain their focus. Finally, review your readings frequently so that the material will not look new just before an exam.

Note-taking in class is another necessary skill to master. One of the most useful note-taking skills is to complete the reading assignments before attending class. Thus, the material will not sound foreign, and you might be able to reduce or simplify the notes you take. It also helps you focus on the class content, ask questions, and synthesize information attained from multiple resources rather than worrying that you are missing something. Another important aspect of note-taking is to sit where you will not be distracted and where you can focus on what you need to do. Maintaining your concentration is also related to having sufficient supplies, having everything in good working order, and running on a "full battery." If an instructor is agreeable, you may want to record their classes as an adjunct to note-taking; you can use the recording to clarify certain points or as a way to review if you have a long commute. Some faculty videostream their lectures and/or post them to their websites so that students may review them again later for this same purpose. If you have strong keyboarding skills, taking a portable laptop to class may expedite your note-taking ability.

Other tips for note-taking are related to format and responding to clues. Note-taking can be done in many forms; you have probably seen various methods. Generally, whether you outline or write in narrative form, it is best to be as brief as possible. It does not matter whether you use complete sentences or words as long as you write in a way that you can decipher later. Using abbreviations is helpful, but be consistent with the abbreviations that you use. A helpful abbreviation strategy for remembering nursing concepts is acronyms. Underline or star important points; instructors often emphasize or state what is particularly important and may repeat a key issue. It is useful to copy information from slides, computer presentations, or whiteboards, although the information does not need to be verbatim. Develop your own system of shortcuts, abbreviations, and coding. Many computer software programs now provide note-taking, highlighting, and other editing features that will assist you in organizing your notes. Lastly, it is also important to review your notes within 1 to 2 days, rather than waiting until time for an exam.

Writing skills will also be required as you return to school. Hacker and Sommers (2021) and Foster (2022) provide information for success in writing and reviews common errors made in punctuation, verb tense, pronouns, modifiers, and diction. Matthews (2023) provides a step-by-step approach to writing essays and academic papers, from developing a foundation for the essay—what it is about and how to develop your thesis—to developing an outline, writing paragraphs, and finalizing your essay.

Preparation for Tests

Developing study skills also includes preparing for tests and exams. This can be stressful for many students, and so it is beneficial to use methods that will aid the process. Reading assignments and notes should be reviewed on a regular basis to keep familiar with the course content. This does not substitute for a comprehensive review before a test, but it does enhance the process. It can help to review your previous exams to learn from your mistakes and to get a feel for how the instructor asks questions. If you have difficulty with the type of exams your instructor uses, consult with the tutoring center on campus, where useful tools are available to assist you in perfecting your test-taking skills.

Most nursing schools have adopted testing styles similar to the Next Generation NCLEX (NGN), which the National Council of State Boards of Nursing (2023) developed to better measure clinical judgment and decision-making abilities. The NGN features real-world patient scenarios that are constructed to measure your critical thinking and clinical judgment. To prepare you for this exam, your instructor may assign case studies or include case-study questions on exams and quizzes.

Developing study skills is an important component of student success. Again, the process depends on you. Being a proactive student means that you accept responsibility for achieving your goals. If you are having difficulty studying or taking exams, or if you experience test anxiety, you must seek help from appropriate sources. Asking for help is not a weakness; rather, it is strength. Your advisor, counselor, and many text- and computer-based programs can all be resources to support your success. For those who specifically are having difficulty with math or who have math anxiety, the campus tutoring center can provide assistance to decrease stress and review math concepts that are particularly applicable to healthcare (measurements, drug calculations, etc.).

Cultivating Study Groups and Mentors

Study groups and mentors can be extremely valuable resources. Although you may feel that you don't have time for a study group, the discussion of various reading assignments, making connections between and among concepts, and applying past experiential knowledge to new concepts can improve retention and also build confidence. Additionally, peer students may explain complex topics in different ways and share their use of different study strategies (from different learning styles) that may benefit you and vice versa. Another rewarding strategy is to form a study group, sharing in common struggles and successes. The group needs to have a spirit of cooperation, as opposed to competition, to be beneficial. The group's meeting cannot be a social gathering because the purpose must be to study. The best approach is to join a group with students who have similar goals and study habits and who seem to have the same focus in classes. If the group is larger than five or six people, it will probably be too unwieldy. A "study buddy" can be helpful in motivating you during times of procrastination and can also suggest coping and accommodation strategies for challenges you face.

The format of study group meetings should include reviewing material, comparing class notes, testing each other with review questions, or asking questions based on the readings or notes. A study group can be used for developing projects or reviewing members' written work. Nursing students find it useful to develop nursing care plans to help each other understand the process and to strengthen the comprehensiveness of such plans.

It may also be helpful for you to develop a mentor as you enter the program. A mentor is generally defined as a wise and trusted counselor. It is a person for whom you have respect and admiration and from whom you feel you will receive guidance and support. As you begin the nursing program, you may find that a faculty member, a nurse where you work, or even a more advanced student is someone with whom you are able to consult or use as a role model. This relationship may provide you with the courage to explore other options or discuss new ideas. More information on developing mentors is presented in Chapter 6.

Characteristics of Highly Successful Students

Being successful as an adult learner is not just about grades—it's also about personal growth. Finding a balance that works for you is key to a fulfilling college experience. Returning to college often demands adaptability and strong organizational skills. Many adult learners face the challenge of reacquainting themselves with academic expectations, technological advancements, and evolving learning methods. Skills such as information literacy, critical thinking, and effective communication become important tools for navigating coursework successfully. Returning students must cultivate resilience and a growth mindset, embracing the learning curve and persevering through challenges.

Characteristics of successful students are described in Box 1.6. Developing these characteristics can positively impact not only academic performance but also personal and professional growth. Although these traits contribute to academic success, remember that each student is unique, and success can be defined in various ways.

Fagan and Coffey (2023) and Mingo (2023) describe the current academic environment as one that moves at a faster pace, with more diverse teaching strategies requiring today's student to think critically, to engage in group activities, and to use technology effectively. Students who are curious, open-minded, and self-disciplined often develop learning and study strategies that foster their success (Box 1.7).

In examining nursing students in specific, Thomas (2011) surveyed nursing faculty from colleges and universities across the nation to ascertain what characteristics they believe lead to success for student nurses. Thomas stressed how important it is for nursing students to let their faculty members know as early as possible if they are struggling with something. A summary of faculty responses to questions about student success is included in her text *How to succeed in nursing school: Before, during, and after*. These responses provide insights into the experiential knowledge of nursing faculty working every day to help students be successful.

CONCLUSION

Returning to school as an adult is not easy. The strategies presented in this chapter provide you with a means to facilitate the educational process and to make the journey more successful and enjoyable; they also put you in the driver's seat. Preparing for your return to school will be time well spent; it will build self-confidence and strengthens the likelihood of your academic success.

Do not be intimidated by the process; your prior learning and work experiences have provided you with a sturdy foundation. As an adult learner and a returning student, you have a wealth of knowledge and experience that will support your efforts. Now, you must continue to maximize your skills and abilities. Remember Sandy Martin? She involved her job and family to help meet her needs. She sought guidance from her nursing advisor and took a proactive approach to her learning experience. Together, they have built a strong foundation on which she can build her continued success.

BOX 1.6 Characteristics of Highly Successful Students

Self-motivation and self-discipline	Successful students often have a genuine passion for learning and, beyond external rewards, are internally motivated to succeed. They demonstrate self-discipline, resist the temptation to procrastinate, and stay focused on their academic goals.
Goal setting	Successful students set clear, achievable goals for themselves, providing direction and motivation. They maintain a healthy balance between academic commitments and personal well-being, recognizing the importance of physical and mental health.
Time management	Successful students effectively manage their time, prioritize tasks, and adhere to deadlines. They excel in managing their time efficiently, balancing academic and personal responsibilities.
Adaptability and resilience	Successful students can adapt to challenges, adjust to different learning environments, and overcome obstacles. They bounce back from setbacks, learn from failures, and maintain a positive attitude despite challenges.
Continuous active learning	Successful students actively engage in the learning process, participate in class discussions, ask questions, and seek additional resources. They have a curiosity for continuous learning beyond the classroom and seek opportunities for personal and professional growth.
Effective study habits	Successful students demonstrate a commitment to their studies and consistently put in the effort required to succeed. They employ effective study techniques, create study schedules, use diverse learning resources, and practice active recall.
Organization	Successful students are well-organized, keeping track of assignments, deadlines, and other responsibilities.
Seeking help when needed	Successful students are not afraid to seek help when faced with challenges, whether that assistance is from professors, tutors, or counseling services. They build positive relationships with professors, classmates, and professionals, and they recognize the value of networking for future opportunities.

Adapted from Hollins, P. (2021). *The study skills handbook: How to ace tests, get straight A's, and succeed in school.* petehollins.com; Jantzen, D. (2022). Getting grounded: Educational foundations for nurses lifelong learning. *Journal of Professional Nursing, 39,* 34–40. https://doi.org/10.1016/j.profnurs.2021.12.009; Mulolli, D., & Gothberg, J. (2023). How doctoral students with low GRE scores succeed: A grounded theory study. *The Qualitative Report, 28*(1), 14–32. https://doi.org/10.46743/2160-3715/2023.5672; Sarver, W., Seabold, K., & Kline, M. (2020). Building a foundation of evidence to support nurses returning to school: The role of empowerment. *Nursing Education Perspective, 41*(5), 285–290. https://doi.org/10.1097/01.NEP.0000000000000704

BOX 1.7 Strategies of Successful Students

Strategy	Example
Set realistic long-term and short-term goals	• Be specific • Start small • Set reasonable time limits
Manage time	• Study in time blocks • Don't cram for exams • Create schedules
Prevent procrastination	• Stay organized • Set realistic goals • Meet challenges first
Practice self-care	• Exercise regularly • Get enough sleep • Eat a healthy diet
Use nursing program resources	• Schedule office hours with faculty • Seek assignment clarification • Utilize textbook resources
Utilize campus support systems	• Consult with student advisors • Request librarian assistance • Attend social events
Think positively	• "I can do this" • "I will be successful" • Trust you intuition
Stay motivated	• Visualize success • Reward yourself • Track your progress
Manage anxiety	• Be prepared • Read assignment instructions carefully • Practice breathing exercises
Participate in study groups	• Prepare lecture notes to share • Utilize campus study rooms • Maintain a distraction-free environment
Develop critical thinking	• Draw concept maps • Take practice exams • Review rationales for interventions

Adapted from Fagan, J. M., & Coffey, J. S. (2023). Despite challenges part II: Bridging the gap to success. *Journal of College Student Retention: Research, Theory & Practice*, 152102512311702. https://doi.org/10.1177/15210251231170297; Jantzen, D. (2022). Getting grounded: Educational foundations for nurses lifelong learning. *Journal of Professional Nursing, 39*, 34–40. https://doi.org/10.1016/j.profnurs.2021.12.009; Mingo, S. (2023). Ten strategies and survival tips for managing nursing school. *Nursing Made Incredibly Easy! 21*(6), 7–11. https://doi.org/10.1097/nme.0000000000000005

STUDENT *Exercises*

Exercise 1.1

Consider the relationship you have with family and significant others from whom you will need support in your return to school. Develop a win/win agreement that encompasses the following:

1. Who needs to be involved with determining the win/win agreement?
2. What are the desired results of the agreement?

3. What perspectives would you anticipate that each individual has of how they contribute to reaching the results desired?
4. What perspective do you have?
5. What guidelines can you identify to guide the agreement?
6. What resources might be necessary to carry out the agreement?
7. What is the win for each individual?
8. What are the consequences if the agreement is not followed?

Capture what you have identified in writing and review it together. Make adjustments as needed. An effective agreement will be extremely helpful in managing your time and commitments as you return to school.

Exercise 1.2

Reflect on the attributes needed for success as you enter the professional nursing program. It is now time for you to design and assemble your first professional portfolio to be used as you meet with your nursing advisor. Consider the following:

1. What are the documents you will include that provide tangible evidence of your accomplishments and the knowledge, dispositions, and skills that you possess?
2. What documents or projects have you completed as an LPN/LVN and/or returning student that can be included to demonstrate your critical thinking ability and work as a healthcare professional?
3. How will you assemble your portfolio in such a way to introduce yourself as the unique student nurse that you are, highlighting your strengths and areas where you may need further mentoring or development as a growing professional?

REFERENCES

Anthony, M. R. (2020). Nurse leaders as problem-solvers: Addressing lateral and horizontal violence. *Nursing Management, 51*(8), 12–19. https://doi.org/10.1097/01.NUMA.0000688928.78513.86

Bennet, P. (2022). *How to survive & thrive in college*. Canyon Press.

Bradbury-Hael, N., & McGarvey, B. (2024). *The freshman survival guide: Soulful advice for studying, socializing, and everything in between* (revised ed.). Center Street.

Covey, S. (1989). *The seven habits of highly effective people*. Simon & Schuster.

Covey, S. R. (2004). *The 8th habit: From effectiveness to greatness*. Free Press.

Covey, S. R. (2013). *The seven habits of highly effective people* (25th Anniversary ed.). Simon & Schuster.

Efron, N. (2023). Ten tips for efficient academic time management. *Clinical & Experimental Optometry, 106*(7), 691–693. https://doi.org/10.1080/08164622.2022.2139592

Ellis, D. (2022a). *Becoming a master student: Making the career connection* (17th ed.). Cengage Learning.

Ellis, D. (2022b). *The essential guide to becoming a master student: Making the career connection* (6th ed.). Cengage Learning.

Fagan, J. M., & Coffey, J. S. (2023). Despite challenges part II: Bridging the gap to success. *Journal of College Student Retention: Research, Theory & Practice*, 152102512311702. https://doi.org/10.1177/15210251231170297

Foster, N. (2022). *How to write in plain English. A writing guide that saves time, is easy to read and helps readers understand your message*. Grammatika.

Guy, M., & van der Krogt, S. (2021). Supporting male nursing students—What works best? *Kai Tiaki Nursing New Zealand, 27*(2), 22–24.

Hacker, D., & Sommers, N. A. (2021). *A writer's reference* (10th ed.). Bedford/St. Martin's.

Hinton, S. T., & Cherry, B. (2023). Managing time: The path to high self-performance. In B. Cherry & S. R. Jacob (Eds.), *Contemporary nursing: Issues, trends, & management* (9th ed., pp. 460–475). Elsevier.

Hollins, P. (2021). *The study skills handbook: How to ace tests, get straight a's, and succeed in school.* petehollins.com

How to Stop Procrastinating. (n.d.). MindTools. https://www.mindtools.com/a5plzk8/how-to-stop-procrastinating

Jantzen, D. (2022). Getting grounded: Educational foundations for nurses lifelong learning. *Journal of Professional Nursing, 39*, 34–40. https://doi.org/10.1016/j.profnurs.2021.12.009

Johnson, B. (2020). Observational experiential learning: Theoretical support for observer roles in health care simulation. *Journal of Nursing Education, 59*(1), 7–14. https://doi.org/10.3928/01484834-20191223-03

Kane, D., Rajacich, D., & Andary, C. (2021). Exploring the contextual factors surrounding the recruitment and retention of men in a Baccalaureate nursing program. *Nursing Forum, 56*(1), 24–29. https://doi.org/10.1111/nuf.12504

Langridge, N., Welch, H., Jones, D., Small, C., Lynch, G., & Ganatra, B. (2023). Portfolios in practice: Developing advancing practice within a musculoskeletal competency-based model. *Musculoskeletal Science & Practice, 63*, 102689. https://doi.org/10.1016/j.msksp.2022.102689

Longworth, N. (2003). *Lifelong learning in action: Transforming education in the 21st century*. Routledge/Falmer.

Luhanga, F., Maposa, S., Puplampu, V., Abudu, E., & Chigbogu, I. (2023). "You have to strive very hard to prove yourself": Experiences of Black nursing students in a Western Canadian province. *International Journal of Nursing Education Scholarship, 20*(1), 1–15. https://doi.org/10.1515/ijnes-2022-0094

Lyu, X., Akkadechanunt, T., Soivong, P., Juntasopeepun, P., & Chontawan, R. (2022). A qualitative systematic review on the lived experience of men in nursing. *Nursing Open, 9*(5), 2263–2276.

Marino, M. (2023). Building on the competency pivot: Helping students build job portfolios for employment. *Business and Professional Communication Quarterly*, 232949062311655. https://doi.org/10.1177/23294906231165565

Matthews, J. (2023). *How to write a 5-paragraph essay step-by-step: Step-by-step study skills*. Independently Published.

Mayes, C. G., & Cochran, K. (2023). Factors influencing perioperative nurse turnover: A classic grounded theory study. *AORN Journal, 117*(3), 161–174. https://doi.org/10.1002/aorn.13880

Mingo, S. (2023). Ten strategies and survival tips for managing nursing school. *Nursing Made Incredibly Easy! 21*(6), 7–11. https://doi.org/10.1097/nme.0000000000000005

Mulolli, D., & Gothberg, J. (2023). How doctoral students with low GRE scores succeed: A grounded theory study. *The Qualitative Report, 28*(1), 14–32. https://doi.org/10.46743/2160-3715/2023.5672

National Council of State Boards of Nursing, Inc. (2023). *Next generation NCLEX: An enhanced NCLEX.* https://www.nclex.com/next-generation-nclex.page

Norful, A. A., Cato, K., Chang, B. P., Amberson, T., & Castner, J. (2023). Emergency nursing workforce, burnout, and job turnover in the United States: A national sample survey analysis. *Journal of Emergency Nursing, 49*(4), 574–585. https://doi.org/10.1016/j.jen.2022.12.014

NSI Nursing Solutions Incorporated. (2023). *2023 NSI national health care retention & RN staffing report.* https://www.nsinursingsolutions.com/Documents/Library/NSI_National_Health_Care_Retention_Report.pdf

Pitre, C. J., & Pugh, C. M. (2023). Reclaiming the calendar: Time management for the clinician educator. *Journal of Graduate Medical Education, 15*(1), 117–118. https://doi.org/10.4300/JGME-D-22-00939.1

Sarver, W., Seabold, K., & Kline, M. (2020). Building a foundation of evidence to support nurses returning to school: The role of empowerment. *Nursing Education Perspective, 41*(5), 285–290. https://doi.org/10.1097/01.NEP.0000000000000704

Shane, D. L. (1983). *Returning to school: A guide for nurses*. Prentice-Hall.

Siddiqui, Z. S., Fisher, M. B., Slade, C., Downer, T., Kirby, M. M., McAllister, L., Isbel, S. T., & Wilson, C. B. (2023). Twelve tips for introducing E-portfolios in health professions education. *Medical Teacher, 45*(2), 139. https://doi.org/10.1080/0142159X.2022.2053085

Smiley, R. A., Allgeyer, R. L., Shobo, Y., Lyons, K. C., Letourneau, R., Zhong, E., Kaminski-Ozturk, N., & Alexander, M. (2023). The 2022 national nursing workforce survey. *Journal of Nursing Regulation, 14*(1), S1–S90. https://doi.org/10.1016/S2155-8256(23)00047-9

Stemmle, D. (2021). *Insider's guide to college success: The underground playbook for making great grades, having more fun, and studying less*. College Success Academy Press.

The American Association for Men in Nursing. (n.d.). *Our values.* https://www.aamn.org/our-values

Thomas, C. P. (2011). *How to succeed in nursing school: Before, during, and after*. CreateSpace Independent Publishing Platform.

On the WEB

American Association of Colleges of Nursing. *The essentials: Core competencies for professional nursing education.* https://www.aacnnursing.org/AACN-Essentials

The American Association for Men in Nursing. http://www.aamn.org

Drugs.com. Provides information on pharmacology, drug interactions, pill identification, and more. http://www.drugs.com

Minority Nurse: A website for underrepresented groups in nursing, including men. http://www.minoritynurse.com

National Library of Medicine—National Center for Biotechnology Information. http://www.ncbi.nlm.nih.gov

The Online Writing Center: Formats references into APA, MLA, and Chicago/Turabian formats. http://www.bibme.org

Purdue University's Online Writing Lab: A resource for writing; includes a section on APA format and style. http://owl.english.purdue.edu

CHAPTER 2

Role Development and Transition

LEARNING OUTCOMES

By the end of this chapter, the student will be able to:
1. Differentiate between ascribed and acquired roles.
2. Differentiate between change and transition.
3. Describe the process of role choice in personal development.
4. Compare and contrast the stages of selected theorists describing personal and adult development.
5. Identify family developmental stages and the effects of individual issues on family development.
6. Apply the stages of professional role development to your current status in nursing.
7. Apply stage development theories to your personal roles.
8. Describe the phases of role socialization.
9. Apply the phases of role transition to your current situation.
10. Differentiate between intrapersonal and interpersonal aspects of role conflict.
11. Discuss methods for conflict management.
12. Analyze your personal status in role transition to professional nursing.
13. Design a personal plan with strategies to minimize role conflict and to support transition to the professional nursing role.

KEY TERMS

acquired roles	family development	role conflict
ascribed roles	moral development	role development
balance	professional role	role strain
cognitive development	socialization	role stress
commitment	role	role transition
experiential knowledge	role change	transition

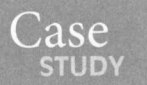

Juan Martinez, LVN, is a 25-year-old who lives alone and works in an outpatient clinic for the Veterans Administration. He is also an accomplished guitarist and plays music frequently with friends. Although he has been practicing vocational nursing only 4 years, Juan has become bored with his role and does not feel it offers him the challenges it did when he first started. Some of his discontent stems from wanting to further develop his assessment skills, do more procedures, acquire management skills, and increase his income. Although no one in his family has ever attended college, he believes he could be successful in a college degree program. After visiting with a college counselor, Juan enrolls in his local community college to pursue registered nursing and attain his ADN. As he progresses through the program, he finds he is in fact successful and finds his course work challenging and fulfilling. Once again, he is excited about nursing and his emerging new role as an RN. He is enjoying being a student, learning, and applying new theories to client care.

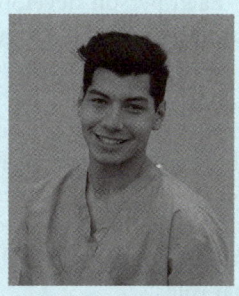

The notion of role development and transition is typically not part of the decision-making process of returning to school. These terms imply a very formal mode of thinking, when the actual reasons for returning to school may be much more pragmatic. In making the decision to pursue a degree in professional nursing, you acknowledge that a major life change is going to take place, but you likely are unaware of the full impact the transition process from this change will have on your values, world view, and who you area as a person. The realities of role development and role transition will be covered in this chapter.

DEFINITIONS

This section defines important terms related to roles. At the end of this section, Box 2.1 offers a quick recap of these definitions.

ROLE

Role is often defined as a person's particular function as it relates to others' functions. Certain behaviors must be learned so roles and functions become part of a whole. For example, one of your roles may be that of the oldest sibling. This role is defined by the fact that there are younger siblings. Behaviors for this role are learned; there are expectations of helping with the care of the younger children or having more responsibilities because you are the oldest. When a person is placed into a new situation, one often feels awkward and unfamiliar because of the uncertainty regarding the role and its obligate behaviors. You may recall how you felt as a new LPN/LVN in your first job or how you are now feeling on your return to school. For each role, expected behaviors are learned for survival and success.

ROLE DEVELOPMENT

Role development refers to the growth that occurs as a person learns the functions, expectations, and behaviors for a particular role. In your practical/vocational nursing education, you were taught specific tasks and behaviors to function within that role. You developed the skills that were necessary to perform a specific job, and as a result, you grew and expanded your knowledge and abilities. Once employed as an LPN/LVN, you continued to expand your knowledge and skills, adding **experiential knowledge**.

Each person develops roles that relate to the roles of others. For example, you will develop as a student nurse in relation to nursing instructors, staff nurses, and other student nurses. You develop in a spousal role as you relate to your spouse.

Each individual also plays multiple roles. For example, you may be a caregiver, spouse, daughter or son, sibling, employee, member of a faith-based community, etc. There are expectations for each of these roles. These behaviors are learned as part of the role development process. In your return to school, you will learn the role expectations and behaviors needed to be an RN. This process will be influenced by your other roles and experiences, as well as by those already licensed in the profession who also carry that role.

Role development is not always a voluntary process. In the "Role Development" section later in this chapter, the concepts related to role development are discussed in more detail.

ROLE CHANGE

Role change consists of adding a new role, dropping an old role, or modifying the behaviors associated with an existing role. Throughout a person's life, there are many role changes. Experiences, expected behaviors, personal values, and the context of your situation (significant others, family, friends, etc.) influence development in each role change.

ROLE TRANSITION

Role transition refers to the process one experiences during change in moving from one place in one's life to another and the subsequent impact on values, world view, and who you are as a person. Role transition is this experiential process resulting from a role change, and is often a major change. It involves letting go of some functions while adding others. You may have experienced the necessity of being a caregiver for a parent or grandparent. In this transition, you recognize that you have lost some of the functions of being a child and added those of caregiving. In essence, the role change has caused role transition to occur.

The LPN/LVN role has involved certain role expectations and behaviors. In the process of acquiring the new knowledge, technical skills, critical thinking skills, and clinical reasoning ability needed at the professional nursing level, you will experience changes in the way you think, act, and are. The process of role transition is individual and not only will affect you but also may have a profound effect on others in your life. In the transition process, it is common for a person to experience role strain or stress. These concepts are examined in the "Role Transition" section later in this chapter.

> **THINKING CRITICALLY**
>
> Consider your current role change to that of student nurse. Analyze the behavior changes and expectations that you anticipate for this role. What is similar to your previous student experiences? What is different?

> **BOX 2.1**
>
> **Definitions of Role Terms**
>
> **Role:** A particular function that is defined by its relationship with other functions; expected behaviors for a role are learned.
>
> **Role development:** Growth within a particular role as a person learns the functions, expectations, and behaviors for that role.
>
> **Role change:** Addition or subtraction of a role or the modification of behaviors associated with a particular role.
>
> **Role transition:** Passage or shift from one role to another; involves changing the way one thinks and acts.

TYPES OF ROLES

Throughout our lives, we experience many roles. Sometimes we have a choice in the roles, and sometimes we do not. The sections that follow describe the various roles people experience.

ASCRIBED ROLES

Ascribed roles are roles that are not chosen. They are given to us based on our genetics or the environment/social milieu in which we live.

Genetic Roles

Many ascribed roles are genetic such as those related to sex assigned at birth, age, and skin color. Previously in this chapter, the example of being the oldest sibling was used to demonstrate the necessity to learn behaviors for each role. It is also an example of an ascribed role.

Social Milieu

Ascribed roles can also relate to the social milieu. This includes ethnic, religious, familial, or cultural roles, which have certain functions and expectations. For example, if you are born into a family with a particular religious affiliation, you are expected to learn the particular aspects of the religion, which may include the way you dress or eat, where you go to school, or who you marry. The ascribed roles related to social milieu carry with them expectations of certain behaviors and values. Ascribed and acquired roles are differentiated in Box 2.2.

ACQUIRED ROLES

Acquired roles are roles a person receives or takes on during a lifetime. These range from roles of choice, such as being a caregiver, to those over which there is little control, such as being a person with a physical disability. In your work as an LPN/LVN, you may have cared for clients who must adjust to a new role of being ill or disabled. It is not a role of choice, but it is an acquired role that involves similar issues of learning behaviors, expectations, and functions. Acquired roles can be personal, societal, or professional.

Personal Roles

Personal roles are those you assume as an individual. They can include relationship status, caregiving, or choice of friends. There are learned behaviors and expectations for each of these roles. The manner in which we behave depends on the relationship. Your role functions and expectations vary on any given day from being a caregiver to a spouse to a close friend.

BOX 2.2 Differentiation Between Ascribed and Acquired Roles

Ascribed Roles

Genetic	Social Milieu
Sex assigned at birth	Ethnicity
Age	Religion
Birth order	Family role
Skin color	

Acquired Roles

Personal	Societal	Professional
Relationship status	Religious organizations	Job role
Caregiving	Community organizations	Member of professional organization
Choice of friends	Political organizations	Professional appointment
Illness		

Societal Roles

Societal roles are those you assume as a member of a group. These may involve affiliations with religious, community, or political organizations. For example, you may have certain positions within a social organization: secretary of a church committee, school board member, or member of a political candidate's campaign organization. You are obligated to learn the expectations for each of these roles.

Professional Roles

Professional roles are those you assume related to your career or vocation. They may include job role, membership in a professional organization, or possibly a professional appointment to a committee or board. One of your reasons for returning to school is to acquire new knowledge and skills that will enhance your ability to take on new job roles and to join other professional organizations and boards. These roles require that certain expectations defined by a group and accepted by the individual are met.

THINKING CRITICALLY

Consider the many roles in your life. Differentiate between your ascribed and acquired roles. In what ways do the ascribed roles influence the acquired roles? Assess whether any of your acquired roles will be changing or modified as you return to school. Will any of your ascribed roles pose additional challenges for you? If so, how might you cope with these challenges?

ROLE DEVELOPMENT

Role development is discussed briefly in the beginning of this chapter. At this point, it is essential to examine this process more closely. The following text reviews concepts of role choice and personal, family, and professional development. These concepts will assist you in understanding your own role development and transition as you move from the role of an LPN/LVN to that of a professional nurse.

ROLE CHOICE

Your decision to become an RN was not one that you made on a whim. It has been a careful process of weighing the advantages and disadvantages, as well as determining the priorities in your life. Although you may have had some help with this decision, it can be a lonely and agonizing time. You have had to acknowledge that the decision will cause some disruption in your life and may have had to overcome some personal issues related to finances or child care, and/or perhaps your family did not support your decision to return to school. In the last chapter, the win–win agreement you developed with those that surround you will support your role choice and transition process. The educational road for some will be more difficult than for others. Your colleagues have different experiences and expectations. You may have noticed that your peer students may be very different from you. They may have more or less LPN/LVN experience, or who seem more or less knowledgeable than you. They may also have different ascribed and acquired roles than you. These factors may influence you in some way, but it is hoped that they will not deter you and that you will experience your own growth in valuing their differences.

THINKING CRITICALLY

Review your list of ascribed roles. Consider what these roles mean to you and how they may be an advantage to you achieving your goal. For example, if you feared your age would be a barrier to your success, in what ways might it be beneficial to you? How might you use these ascribed roles to your advantage as you enter the nursing program?

Acquired roles may involve choices. Your decision to continue your education has involved an active process on your part. Generally, you have not been able to sit back and let someone else make the choice for you. It is impossible to predict the implications that returning to school will have on you and your life. You have undoubtedly experienced a variety of emotional states in your decision-making process. Now that you are actually pursuing further education by returning to school, it is necessary for you to examine two aspects of this choice: commitment and balance.

Commitment

Commitment is the process of pledging to assume a role, perform a job, or accomplish a goal. Your decision to return to school initiated this process. However, you also have commitments to other ongoing roles that demand your attention. You have often heard that one must be able to set priorities. As you examine the commitment you have to your various roles (e.g., worker, caregiver, spouse), you will need to maintain a commitment to the highest priorities of each role and maintain balance in your life. You may also find you need to "unsubscribe" to certain acquired roles, such as your activity with a charitable organization or other chosen role, or at least reduce your time commitment to that particular role to prioritize the new role to which you have subscribed.

Balance

As you make a commitment to your new role as a returning student and adjust priorities among other roles, achieving overall **balance** in your life will again become a challenge. Stephen R. Covey (2004, 2013) identified the seven habits of highly effective people. His seventh habit, called "Sharpen the Saw," focuses on renewal and keeping ourselves in balance. Covey (2013) describes this habit as, "It's preserving and enhancing the greatest asset you have—you. It's renewing the four dimensions of your nature—physical, spiritual, mental, and social/emotional" (p. 300). Box 2.3 shows Covey's four dimensions of the seventh habit.

The need for balance in life transcends time and culture. As Sylvia Lee noted, "The Native American Medicine Wheel, in which life is only in balance when its physical, mental, emotional, and spiritual components are in balance, offers an old-world model for a new-world environment. Many other ancient models echo this theme—Taoist principles among them" (Longworth, 2003, p. vii).

THINKING CRITICALLY

You have already made some changes when you decided to return to school. What are those changes? How are these changes affecting your life's balance? What strategies can you use to restore balance to your life?

BARRIERS

You may experience some barriers in your educational journey. Some of these barriers are internal, and some are external. The following are examples of internal barriers to role development:

- Fear of failure
- Lack of confidence
- Confusion regarding new expectations
- Feelings of being overwhelmed

Fears common to college students include fear of failing, not understanding, being drawn into issues they would rather avoid, having their ignorance exposed or their prejudices challenged, or looking foolish in front of peers. For returning adult students, such as yourself, these fears may be exacerbated due to your age, length of time away from academia, and fear of technology, today's classroom environment, or new clinical settings, as discussed in the previous chapter. Such fears may serve as internal barriers

BOX 2.3 Steven R. Covey's Four Dimensions of Habit 7: Sharpen the Saw

Physical	Exercise, nutrition, stress management
Spiritual	Value clarification and commitment, study and meditation
Mental	Reading, visualizing, planning, writing
Social/emotional	Service, empathy, synergy, intrinsic security

Adapted from Covey, S. R. (2013). *The seven habits of highly effective people* (25th Anniversary ed.). Simon & Schuster.

to you being an active participant in class discussions, seeking new clinical experiences, using technology effectively, and experiencing success in the ADN program.

Other barriers to role development are external. They may include issues surrounding family needs, child care, financial concerns, job demands, and personal needs. These barriers have a tremendous impact on one's ability to succeed and are often more prevalent among returning adult students. Barriers and fears of the re-entry process, along with strategies to support your success, were discussed in Chapter 1. Subsequent chapters provide you with additional strategies for overcoming barriers by adapting to change and developing an individualized plan for role transition.

THINKING CRITICALLY
Identify internal and external barriers as you embrace role transition. Design a plan of action to deal with these barriers.

PERSONAL AND ADULT DEVELOPMENT

Researchers such as Erikson, Piaget, and others have proposed theories that provide an explanation for adult development. You may recall these theorists from your LPN/LVN education. Reflecting on these theories will assist you in more objectively examining your own development and personal journey, because you may be in a different stage of development than when you were an LPN/LVN student. Reviewing developmental theories will also provide you with a perspective to evaluate the stage of development of your clients and to recognize the effects of illness on their development.

ERIKSON
Erik Erikson (1963) is one of the earliest theorists to delineate development in terms of phases or stages. He views these stages in terms of psychosocial development throughout the lifespan. Personal development occurs with passage through each stage. Erikson theorized that a person develops by proceeding through developmental tasks or crises at each stage. Success or failure in resolving a crisis will influence a person's ability to deal with the next stage and may affect how they are able to handle crises as an adult (Erikson, 1963; Potter et al., 2023).

PIAGET
Jean Piaget is another early theorist who examined cognitive development, which is the process of understanding and knowing. He identified four stages related to intellectual development: sensorimotor (manipulation), preoperational (egocentric thought), concrete operations, and formal operations (abstract thought). Piaget theorized that **cognitive development** occurs in a continuum from infancy on; it is an additive process in which new experiences are understood as a result of previous knowledge (Piaget & Inhelder, 1972; Potter et al., 2023).

Formal operational thought is the highest level. To achieve this level, one must progress through the stages of manipulation and concrete thinking to consider all variables and solve problems. In his theory, this occurs in adolescence. Other theorists disagree, believing that abstract thinking or formal operations develop later in life with the appropriate experiences. These concepts are important to you for two reasons. First, your thought processes are more concrete as a result of your previous educational experiences. Second, these concepts are also important when considering the learning needs of your clients. Your approach for teaching a specific procedure will differ, depending on the age of the client and the ability of that individual (or the caregiver) to use formal or concrete operations. You may also find that some of your clients will revert to previous modes of thinking when they are faced with stress. This theory provides you with a framework to assess the learning needs of your clients and to then devise a realistic plan for teaching new information (Piaget & Inhelder, 1972; Potter et al., 2023).

KOHLBERG

The development of moral reasoning was researched extensively by Lawrence Kohlberg (1981). He determined that an integral part of socialization of a child from any culture is to teach the child the difference between right and wrong. This, in essence, gives the child a sense of values and constitutes his **moral development**. Kohlberg's concept of moral development is similar to the concepts of Erikson and Piaget. As a child identifies with caregivers, they are either positively or negatively reinforced for particular behaviors. If the reinforcement is consistent, a child's personal sense of values will be greatly influenced by the value system of the caregivers (Potter et al., 2023).

The first stage of preconventional moral thought signifies the beginning of value development in early childhood. The child is dependent on adults for survival and learns to view moral behavior as the avoidance of disapproval or punishment from adults. Conventional moral thought develops in the preteen years. At this time, the child is able to define the rules and expectations of society and better understands the consequences if the rules are broken. The last stage is called postconventional or principled moral thought. As the teenager moves into adulthood, they develop an abstract moral sense that enables them to determine what is just or unjust (Kohlberg, 1981). Of course, these stages of moral development are in the context of the ascribed roles of that individual and will vary from client to client. This will be important information for you as the professional nurse who must use clinical reasoning and judgment in designing care for the client.

Nurses develop a professional value system in much the same way (Taylor et al., 2023). Depending on your own stage of personal development and experiences, you may have some difficulty assimilating these factors. You are also faced with teachers, clients, and colleagues whose value systems may differ from yours. As you grow and develop in your professional role, you will be more sensitive to various beliefs. Later in this text, ethical decision-making is addressed. It will be helpful to apply Kohlberg's theory of moral development as you study ethical decision-making.

GILLIGAN

Early research in cognitive and moral development was conducted by males, with male subjects. However, in the early 1980s, important research was begun by females, with female subjects, that yielded interesting results counter to previous research. For example, as a student of Kohlberg and later as a colleague, Carol Gilligan (1982) objected to the generalization of his theory to women because his theory was based on work done with males and then applied to females. The similarities in their theories are that they both identify three stages of moral development. However, Kohlberg's theory is based more on rules and justice and the development of abstract thinking, whereas Gilligan asserts that women's development is seen more in terms of relationships, caring, and connectivity.

In Kohlberg's research with girls and women, he concluded that women were not able to reach the higher levels of moral development and that women were in some way deficient in their moral reasoning abilities. Gilligan based her research on the stories or "voices" of girls and women, finding that their sense of moral reasoning is based on relationships, responsibility, and caring. This countered Kohlberg's earlier work.

Gilligan's three stages of moral development are as follows:

1. **Orientation to individual survival:** The individual views the moral decision as one that is necessary for their own survival in terms of herself only. There is a sense of obligation to one's own needs.
2. **Goodness as self-sacrifice:** The individual makes a moral decision based on meeting the needs and expectations of others and not hurting others. The obligation is to others and not self in this process.
3. **Morality of nonviolence:** The individual determines that the moral choice must be responsible to self and others and must involve caring and not hurting. The individual remains obligated to nonviolence.

As the individual progresses through these stages, there is an emphasis on the relationships within a particular situation and the importance of caring, attachments, and connectedness.

THINKING CRITICALLY

Select one of the theories outlined in the preceding material. What theory and stage best describe your present status? Why? With what tasks are you most concerned? Do any issues remain unresolved or problematic? How is this stage impacted by your role transition to the student role and then to the professional nursing role?

The NCLEX-RN *Might Ask* 2.1

A nursing program utilizes nurse preceptors in some of its clinical experiences. The nurses who are chosen to be preceptors are considered proficient in their clinical area. To which of Benner's stages of novice to expert should a nurse preceptor belong?

a. Advanced beginner
b. Competent
c. Proficient
d. Expert

• See Appendix A for correct answer and rationale.

FAMILY DEVELOPMENT

In addition to personal development, individuals also grow and develop within the context of human relationships, which often involve a family unit. The study of **family development** provides us with contextual information that informs clinical reasoning when caring for an individual within a particular family unit. Evelyn Duvall and Murray Bowen were notable theorists who studied family development.

Duvall

Family development is perceived by some theorists in the context of a life cycle, with developmental stages and tasks similar to personal development. Duvall and Miller (1985) theorized that if a person understands who the family members are (including age, gender, and position in the family); what their status is in terms of ethnicity and social standing; and what stage they are in the family life cycle, much can be predicted about what is happening with the family at a particular time. Duvall described eight stages of family development within the framework of a family life cycle (Table 2.1).

With each stage, she delineated specific tasks requiring adaptation and acquisition of new responsibilities and challenges. For example, a family with young children has the task of adapting to members of the next generation. The parents must acquire parenting skills, adapt their own relationship to make room for children, and adjust relationships with other family members, such as aunts, uncles, and grandparents.

It is obvious that not all individuals and families fit into such predictable stages. Also, there are many variations of family units. Brief examples include the following:

- Couples without children
- Families who have children early in a marriage and then much later
- Same-sex and LGBTQIA+ (lesbian, gay, bisexual, transgender, questioning or queer, intersex, asexual, and allies) couples and families
- Children raised by grandparents or other caregivers
- Single-parent families
- Families with a member who is chronically ill or who has a disability

However, Duvall's theory provides a means to begin examining family relationships and roles and the impact of individual needs on family needs. For example, if there

TABLE 2.1 Stages of Family Development—Duvall

Stage	Developmental Tasks
Marriage of young couple; no children	Growth in marital relationship; adjustment to in-laws; decision regarding having children
Birth of children	Growth in caregiving roles; adjustment in marital relationship; resolution of conflicting roles: spouse, caregiver, daughter/son, sibling, employee
Family with preschool children	Adaptation to children who are very involved with their environment; adjustment in marital relationship; involvement of children in socialization activities, such as church and nursery school, and other activities
Family with school-age children	Encouragement of achievements of children in school and other activities; adjustment in marital relationship; coordination of child and adult activities
Family with adolescents	Promotion of teenagers' responsible independence; maintenance of communication with all family members; adjustment in marital relationship
Family with offspring who have left home	Adaptation to empty nest; adjustment in marital relationship; growth of relationships with married offspring and grandchildren
Family in early retirement	Adaptation to retirement and increased leisure activities; strengthening of marital ties; adjustment to being older
Family in old age	Maintenance of marital relationship; adjustment to widowhood and loss of friends; adaptation to aging

Adapted from Duvall, E. M., & Miller, B. C. (1985). *Marriage and family development* (6th ed.). Harper Collins.

is a sick family member during the school-age stage, it may prevent the family from participating in community and educational activities. It is not always possible to mesh individual and family needs. If a family does not quite conform to the expectations of the community, pressure may be placed on them. A young child with HIV may be isolated, along with the family. A biracial or same-sex couple may be shunned. These factors will interfere with the developmental tasks of the family. In addition, a caregiver with substance use disorder may place a heavy burden on other family members financially, socially, and developmentally.

Bowen
Murray Bowen (1985) proposed that the family is an interrelated and interdependent system that is influenced by each of its members and by external factors, such as the community, the environment, and life events. The interrelationships that exist between and among family members are so great that when one individual is changed, the whole family system will be affected. For instance, if a child becomes chronically ill, the caregivers will be focused on that child and may care for the siblings differently than they did before the child's illness. The siblings may begin to have behavior problems in school or vague physical ailments as a result of the first child's illness and the changed caregiving. All family members are affected by the condition of one member. Bowen's approach to family therapy consists of treating the individual not as an entity separate from the family, but rather as part of a family unit, all of whom should be involved in the counseling. In this way, family members are able to face issues and deal with them together, instead of making one member responsible (Bowen, 1985).

In your work as an LPN/LVN, you have already included family members when caring for an individual. As you move into the RN role, there will be an increased emphasis on the family unit. As healthcare delivery continues to evolve, the family plays a critical role. You must assess not only a person but also assess the family because the health status of individual members is affected by the function of the family. The family assessment will provide you with a clearer picture of the person's primary social context, family stressors, risk factors within the family, and the family's adaptation and coping mechanisms.

THINKING CRITICALLY
Review Duvall's stages of family development. Is there a stage that describes your current status? What is the same? What is different? What impact will your return to school have on your family's development? What impact will the situations of other family members have on your development as you return to school?

PROFESSIONAL ROLE DEVELOPMENT
Role development is defined in the beginning of this chapter. The addition of the word "professional" requires a brief explanation. To be a member of a profession, one must have special preparation and education to acquire knowledge and skills to perform a certain role. Professional role development means acquiring the skills and knowledge that are needed to function within a particular role. Growth and development within the role are influenced by previous experiences and the expectations for that role by

members of the profession and those who interface with such individuals. As stated by Thomas et al. (2016, p. 40):

A true profession has, at a minimum, these elements:

- A unique body of knowledge
- A code of ethics
- Autonomy
- Academic education and preparation
- Self-regulation

The role of the RN is a professional practice role, governed and guided by the profession in the elements stated above. As you enter this professional role, you will be held to expectations identified by the profession, and your development in the role will be guided by standards, regulations, and educational curricula central to the profession.

COHEN

Professional role development may also evolve in stages. Cohen (1981) identified four stages that relate to Erikson's developmental stages (Table 2.2). The first stage is called unilateral dependence, in which a student professional begins to learn theoretical content and to practice in a limited way under the supervision of an instructor. The second stage is negative independence, which provides the student professional more opportunities to apply theory to practice and to internalize some of the professional role behaviors that fit with their own values and self-concepts. Cohen identifies the third stage as dependence/mutuality, in which the student professional begins to recognize role limitations to be acceptable to other professionals and to society in general. The last stage is called interdependence, in which the professional role seems more real. The individual is able to accept more responsibility and to believe that the professional role is part of their identity. The comfort level is much higher because the person generally believes that the professional role is not in conflict with other roles.

Your professional role development has already begun. Your decision to become an RN initiated the process. As you progress in your academic program, you will acquire the knowledge, skills, and abilities needed to be a professional nurse.

TABLE 2.2 Professional Role Development—Cohen

Stage I	Unilateral dependence	Inexperienced student learns theoretical concepts for role development; applies theory to practice in a limited and supervised way.
Stage II	Negative independence	Student has increased opportunities to apply theory to practice and assumes more responsibility; develops confidence and takes on some of the role values; also is more willing to question traditional patterns and ways of knowing.
Stage III	Dependence/mutuality	Student is able to be more realistic about role expectations, and questions reflect a higher understanding of theoretical concepts; recognizes role limitations.
Stage IV	Interdependence	Student is able to make independent judgments and to take on the professional role; student's professional identity is more secure and not in opposition with other roles.

Adapted from Cohen, H. A. (1981). *The nurse's quest for a professional identity*. Addison-Wesley.

BENNER

Patricia Benner's (2001) Novice to Expert theory is a model that describes the nurse's development of skills, comprehension of patient needs, and clinical competence. This five-step model (novice, advanced beginner, competent, proficient, and expert) theorizes that nursing skills and competence develop over time through education, background, and experiences (Table 2.3). Each step builds on the previous step as the nurse develops and refines clinical performance. In each step, the nurse acquires greater capability through observation and clinical experience. Over time, the nurse develops relevant skills in a given step, then moves to the next, more advanced step. In the progression, the experiences impart the nurse with further development of insight into patient needs.

This model can be applied to several nursing roles. As nurses move from one discipline or specialty to another, this model illustrates the process of developing the skills needed for the new role. In your work as an LPN/LVN, you have already developed skills that will be applied to your new role as an RN; however, because of the role change and greater responsibilities, you will begin a new process of developing clinical expertise. This model serves as a means of assessment in professional growth and supports continuous development of skills that lead to supportive behaviors and the ability to teach and to mentor new nurses. Because developing expertise is learned over time, understanding the process of nursing development helps nurses support one another in new roles.

Today, new graduate RNs practice in highly complex environments and must quickly develop clinical reasoning and clinical judgment to meet complex patient needs. To help students prepare for patient care, many schools partner with clinical facilities to provide student internships or preceptorships. Internships may be a requirement of your nursing school and are usually completed during the last semester of the program. During an internship, under the guidance of a licensed RN, students are introduced to the responsibility of caring for full patient assignments. Similarly, many hospitals and clinical agencies offer student nurse externships. Externships are not affiliated with nursing

TABLE 2.3 Novice to Expert Theory—Benner

Novice	Beginner/no experience	The nursing student in first year of clinical education. Limited ability to predict patient needs.
Advanced Beginner	Demonstrates acceptable performance	New graduate nurse in first clinical job. Some experience recognizing meaningful elements of patient needs. Have knowledge but no in-depth experience.
Competent	A nurse with 2–3 years of experience	Two or three years of experience. Organized and efficient in planning and setting goals. Recognizes patient needs quickly, but lacks speed and flexibility.
Proficient	A nurse with 3–5 years of experience	Capable of seeing situations as "wholes" rather than parts. Has learned from experience what is likely to occur and is able to modify plan in response to events.
Expert	A nurse with 5 years of experience and on	Grasps situations and understands needs. Recognizes needs and resources for care. Does not rely on preplanning to guide their actions. Have intuitive grasp of situations based on knowledge and experience. Serves as a mentor and resource to less experienced nurses.

Adapted from Benner, P. (2001). *From novice to expert: Excellence and power in clinical nursing practice* (Commemorative Ed.). Prentice Hall.

schools; the student arranges these with hospitals or clinical agencies. Externships offer students the opportunity to provide basic hands-on care to patients in the hospital setting. Although externships generally do not allow students to administer medications or perform invasive procedures, the experience provides students with the opportunity to become familiar with a given hospital unit and to develop patient care routines.

As an LPN/LVN, you already have many strengths in organizing and providing patient care; however, internships and externships will give you the opportunity to become more familiar with the RN role in planning, organizing, and providing patient care. They will also benefit you by building your decision-making skills, allowing you to interact in the RN role with other professionals, developing your confidence, and helping you transition to your new role as an RN.

THINKING CRITICALLY

How has your role as an LPN/LVN affected your professional role development? Thinking of your experience as an LPN/LVN, what stage of Benner's theory do you feel you are in? Explore positive and negative effects and your present stage of professional role development. What will help or hinder you in reaching the next stage?

PROFESSIONAL DEVELOPMENT

Your education will not end after you are licensed as an RN. In your new role, you will continue the journey of lifelong learning and professional development. Learning resources include adult education courses, workshops, peer-reviewed academic journals, seminars, webinars, and conferences.

Continuing Education

In your role as an LPN/LVN, you are probably familiar with Continuing Education Units (CEUs) that are required by many licensing boards. Continuing education for nurses provides training for best practices in nursing to provide safe patient care. CEUs must be accredited by an approved provider such as select professional organizations. It is important to note that some of the CEU courses and sources from which you were previously able to submit CEUs may not apply to the registered nurse role. After you are licensed as an RN, you will want to ensure you are taking appropriate courses. Costs for CEU courses vary. Some employers offer free classes or reimburse for training. You may also find free or low-cost CEU courses through professional associations and universities.

Diversity, Equity, and Inclusion

Implicit (unconscious) biases are attitudes and stereotypes that occur unintentionally and influence judgments and decisions. Implicit biases impact how we see the world, collaborate with peers, and provide care to patients. Those biases can contribute to health disparities, quality and safety of care, and poor patient outcomes. There is a strong correlation between a diverse nursing staff and the ability to provide quality, culturally competent patient care to diverse populations. Ensuring that you are equipped to provide culturally competent care will enhance your relationships as a student, a healthcare provider, and a member of the larger community (American Association of Colleges of Nursing, 2023). Your school may include diversity, equity, and inclusion training in the curriculum; however, you may choose a more in-depth plan of self-reflection and insight. Some strategies to reduce implicit bias are as follows:

- Be aware of your own thoughts and feelings.
- Imagine what it would be like to be a person whose skills and abilities are discounted or questioned because of background or social identity.
- Identify when you are influenced by biased thoughts and interrupt those thoughts with mindful counteraction.
- Join workshops or other groups in your community that work to raise awareness about implicit bias.

THINKING CRITICALLY

What implicit bias have you identified within yourself? What bias have you witnessed in your personal life? What bias have you witnessed in your professional life? In what ways can you reduce implicit bias and build cultural competence when working with patients and coworkers?

PROFESSIONAL ROLE SOCIALIZATION

Professional role socialization is a complicated process during which an individual not only learns the necessary cognitive, attitudinal, and technical skills for a particular role but also gains an identity with that profession, adopting the values and norms of that profession. According to Cohen (1981), four goals are associated with such role socialization. The student will:

- Acquire technical and theoretical skills
- Take on the values of the profession
- Modify the professional role to one that is personally and professionally acceptable
- Balance the professional role with other roles

Several models have been developed to define the process of professional role socialization. The model developed by Hinshaw (1986) depicts three core stages for socialization or resocialization for a professional role (Table 2.4). In the first stage, students change their concepts of role expectations from those they had anticipated to those being taught by professional role models. The second stage is a time of attachment to role models within the educational and clinical settings. It is also a time when students have conflicts about incongruences of role behaviors that were not anticipated or expected. During this time, it is essential that role models assist students to cope with these incongruences. The last stage is the internalization of the values and standards of the new role.

In your socialization to the RN role, you will take on the values and standards for that role. As an LPN/LVN, you may not recognize all the differences that exist between the two roles, other than the technical/procedural tasks. However, you will be assuming new values and attitudes that will take a while to be internalized. This slow change and

TABLE 2.4 Model of Professional Role Socialization—Hinshaw

Stage I	Transition from anticipated role expectations to those that are taught	Adults who are new to a profession are committed to learning the expected role behaviors.
Stage II	Attachment to important role models; identification of inconsistencies	Attachments are made with significant faculty or staff members. Role models are important and essential. At this time, questions also arise regarding situations that are incongruent with those presented by role models.
Stage III	Internalization of role values and standards	The individual takes on the values and standards of the professional role. If the incongruences have been significant in the second stage, the internalization of values may be affected.

Adapted from Hinshaw, A. S. (1986). Socialization and resocialization of nurses for professional nursing practice. In E. C. Hein & M. J. Nicholson (Eds.), *Contemporary leadership behavior: Selected readings* (2nd ed.). Little, Brown and Company.

internalization process was noted in the mid-1900s by Kelman (1958), who identified three processes of attitudinal change:

- *Compliance:* An individual demonstrates appropriate behaviors to receive positive feedback but has not internalized the values.
- *Identification:* The individual is selective about the particular behaviors that are personally acceptable; this often depends on particular role models.
- *Internalization:* The individual believes and accepts the new standards of behavior as part of their own value system.

These processes of attitudinal change still apply today, and you will experience them as an LPN/LVN as you transition to the professional nursing role.

At this point in your career, you may see the difference between the LPN/LVN and RN roles as merely a matter of broadened technical skills, care plan development, and supervision of other licensed and nonlicensed personnel. However, the professional nurse role is much greater and more complex than this. Practice at the professional level involves working autonomously as a nursing diagnostician and within an interprofessional collaborative team. As you enter the registered nursing program, you may find your instructor has planned classroom and/or clinical learning activities that expose you to opportunities to engage in interpersonal collaborative teams with other health professionals. These experiences are designed to support your socialization into your new professional role (Wei et al., 2022).

Practice at the professional nursing level also involves exercising critical thinking for nursing diagnoses and the application of knowledge and research from a breadth of subject areas to formulate comprehensive client care planning. You may find your instructor incorporates case studies and other innovative teaching strategies to help you develop these critical thinking skills and, again, to socialize you into this more advanced professional role. Critical thinking skills will be covered in more depth in subsequent chapters.

Lastly, your new professional role will involve more extensive use of the nursing process, including clinical reasoning and nursing diagnostics, as described by Gonzalez et al. (2021), and engaging in evidence-based nursing practice, as described by Nowak and Colsch (2024). These are all examples of new skills you will develop as you move to this new professional role. Being a nurse professional brings with it responsibilities of the profession beyond the vocation and practice of nursing care in which you have operated as an LPN/LVN. Your education to become a professional nurse will change the way you think and who you are and that internalization will take some time.

ROLE TRANSITION

Role transition means the passage or shifts from one role to another and involves changing the way one thinks and acts. Bridges and Bridges (2016, 2019) differentiated between change and transition. They defined change as *situational* (getting a new boss, having a child, or returning to school) and described transition as *psychological*—a three-phase process that people go through as they internalize and come to terms with the details of the new situation that the change brings about. When people or organizations (which are made up of people) encounter a situational change, they experience the transition based on that change. This transition process involves the adoption of a new identity and the socialization of individuals into new attitudes, values, and beliefs. Bridges and Bridges identify three phases of transition: ending, the neutral zone, and the new beginning. A summary of Bridges and Bridges' three phases of transition is shown in Box 2.4.

ENDING

Bridges and Bridges (2016, 2019) call the first phase of transition *Ending*. Every transition begins with an ending—a loss, a letting go—to make room for the new. We have to let go of the old before we can pick up the new—not just outwardly but inwardly, where we keep our connections to the people and places that act as definitions of who we are. As you return to school, you will experience a sense of "ending" what was a comfortable, confident practice level as an LPN/LVN. You knew what to do and how to do it and were even likely to train others new to your assigned area. Now you are in new surroundings with a new protocol and may be feeling like everyone thinks you "know nothing." This ending brings with it a mixture of feelings. Bridges and Bridges describe four aspects of endings:

- *Disengagement:* separation from a familiar place within the social order. At various times, a person voluntarily or involuntarily is disengaged from activities, relationships, places, or roles that have been important.

BOX 2.4 Bridges and Bridges' Three Phases of Transition

Phase I: Ending, Losing, Letting Go	Letting go of the old ways and the old identity. This first step of transition is an ending and is a time when you need to help people to deal with their losses.	
Phase II: The Neutral Zone	Going through an in-between time when the old is gone but the new isn't fully operational. We call this time the "neutral zone": it is when the critical psychological realignments and repatternings take place.	
Phase III: The New Beginning	Coming out of the transition and making a new beginning. This is when people develop the new identity, experience the new energy, and discover the new sense of purpose that makes the change begin to work.	

Adapted from Bridges, W., & Bridges, S. (2016). *Managing transitions: Making the most of change* (4th ed.). Hachette Book Group.

- *Disidentification:* loss of self-definition; a process of not being quite sure of who you are. Often, the old identity can interfere with transition because it is hard to let go of what you were.
- *Disenchantment:* the realization that the beliefs and views in the past are no longer real. Life is a series of disenchantments in the many transitions; disenchantment may be related to the loss of a relationship or a change in career. The disenchanted person recognizes the old view as sufficient in its time but insufficient now.
- *Disorientation:* the lost and confused feeling that a person experiences when in transition. There is a sense of unreality about even ordinary events; nothing feels the same.

When you first entered the LPN/LVN program, the transition may not have been that difficult if you were moving from high school to another educational site. However, as a practicing LPN/LVN now returning to school, you may find a greater challenge with the transition, especially if you have been away from the educational environment for a number of years. This is due to several factors. First, you are transitioning back to a student role from that as a practicing, licensed healthcare provider. You will be viewed by some as a "new nursing student, without clinical expertise." Even in those areas where you have knowledge and experience, you may find that new knowledge, nursing care techniques, and medical/pharmacologic advances have taken place of which you are unaware. There are not only new procedures to learn but also adjustments to procedures you may have been doing for a long time or have done differently in another clinical setting. Some clinical settings will be new to you, and if you have been out of LPN/LVN training for a number of years, all the clinical sites other than those where you have been working have all changed as practice has advanced.

In addition to your transition to the student role, you will find yourself experiencing the transition from a practical nursing role to a professional nursing role. At this point, you may not see much difference between the two, but as you progress this next year, you will begin to see a whole new "world view" of nursing, healthcare, and research-informed and evidence-based practice, to name a few. You will be employing more advanced critical thinking and clinical reasoning skills and will be engaged in a new world of interprofessional collaborative practice with other professionals in the healthcare industry and beyond. With this transition will come the loss of comfort and familiarity with the directed patient care role you have held since licensure as a practical/vocational nurse. However, letting go of this role will allow you to practice at an expanded level that will be very gratifying.

THE NEUTRAL ZONE

The second phase of transition described by Bridges and Bridges is called *The Neutral Zone*. During this phase, a person is "in limbo," a temporary state of emptiness or loss or an in-between state of affairs. It is a time when a person appears to be in a void but is actually contemplating important inner thoughts. The first function of this phase is one of surrender, in which a person gives in to the emptiness and does not try to escape it. A second function is one of renewal, recharging, and possibly redirecting. The last function is a change in perspective about what a person has always known and learning how to view it differently. As you progress through the curriculum of the registered nursing program, you will experience this emptiness, yet an emerging new world as a nurse professional. You, your values, and your outlook on healthcare and the nursing profession will change as you move to new beginnings.

THE NEW BEGINNING

The last phase of transition identified by Bridges and Bridges is called *The New Beginning*. There is no clear path that can tell a person that a new beginning is at hand. Instead, there is just an initial hint that something is different. It occurs within the person, although the transition may be the result of changing jobs, changing relationships, or continuing an education. The beginning in the transition process is part of a continuum; it is a new chapter of one's life that is beginning. As the beginning becomes part of the whole, the person reintegrates the new identity with the old identity. None of us are the same as a result of a transition; rather, we are changed in many ways. Box 2.5 shows the transitions and new beginnings of one nurse over time.

THINKING CRITICALLY

As you read through role socialization and transition, where do you see yourself? What "endings" are you experiencing as Bridges and Bridges describe? Talk with a former LPN/LVN who experienced such transitions as those described in this section. Did they notice these three phases of transition? What were the catalysts for each, the coping mechanisms employed, and what values changed?

Role Conflict, Role Stress, and Role Strain

Role conflict develops when an individual is faced with expectations that are incompatible with each other. This can be *intra*personal or *inter*personal. *Intrapersonal role conflict* occurs within one's self when an individual struggles with multiple personal role expectations. For example, in your role as a student nurse, you may face conflict with the necessity of having to study as opposed to spending time with significant others in your life or enjoying a talent you have in the arts. *Interpersonal role conflict* occurs between two individuals when each has different expectations about the same role. An example of

---

BOX 2.5 | **Transitions and New Beginnings of a Nurse Over Time**

"When I worked as a nurse's aide, I was happy providing basic care to my patients, bathing them, assisting with activities of daily living, and alerting others when I noticed a change in vital signs or someone needed pain medication, etc. When I an RN encouraged me to go to school to become licensed, I didn't know if I wanted to do that. It appeared to me that all nurses did was give shots and do paperwork—neither of which appealed to me. The RN was very persuasive, and I did pursue my RN, and later my MSN, and a doctoral degree and became a nursing faculty member, program director, and then College dean, etc. I experienced a loss with each transition, but was pleasantly surprised with the opportunities in new beginnings as they emerged. I am grateful now to have allowed myself to let go of old roles to make room for new ones throughout my life. These new beginnings changed me in many ways, and I am a much deeper and broader thinker than I was in those early days because of these life transitions."

—From interview of a college president who started her 25-year career in nursing at age 18 as a nurse assistant, prior to moving on to licensed practice, nursing education, and college administration.

this type of conflict might occur in relation to others' expectations of you in your role as a nurse. You may think that your role is to spend time with a client with newly diagnosed diabetes so that you can begin teaching the process of self-care, whereas your supervisor may think that it is more important that you complete your written documentation.

Role conflict is a component of **role stress**, in which a person realizes that role obligations are conflicting or that role demands are overwhelming and seem impossible to fulfill. Feelings of discomfort, frustration, and anxiety can occur; this is referred to as **role strain**. Returning adult students who are trying to balance school, work, and home responsibilities may experience role strain and role stress. In addition to dealing with concerns about work while at home and those of home while at work, many women (and in today's world men as well) invest mental energy into reflecting on these two roles. They are continually assessing how well they are balancing home and work roles, which one is being compromised, and whether they are exercising good judgment in the choices they make each day (Freeman & Dodson, 2021). As individuals try to meet the expectations and deadlines in their professional, familial, and academic spheres simultaneously, the quality of their work and personal relationships may suffer. The constant struggle to balance these aspects of life can contribute to a sense of exhaustion, affecting mental health and overall well-being. The limited time available for personal and social activities can strain connections, leading to feelings of isolation and detachment (Mostafa, 2022).

With the increase in single-caregiver households and multigenerational households following the COVID-19 pandemic and the subsequent period of slow economic recovery, role strain and role stress for people of all genders has become even more prevalent than in the past. Role overload has also been exacerbated. The economic downturn has caused families to experience increased financial constraints, with family members assuming multiple roles to "make ends meet." Assuming additional employment and caretaking roles has become common, as extended family members rely on limited family workers for income, housing, and caretaking. The unemployed, underemployed, and those displaced from business and home foreclosures have placed additional burdens and role expectations on remaining family members.

Those who are veterans may experience an even greater than normal anxiety in transitioning both to civilian life and to the student role. Veterans often face unique academic and social hurdles when integrating into higher education. Balancing the demands of coursework, adapting to a different learning environment, and navigating the diverse student culture can be daunting. Veterans bring valuable skills such as discipline and leadership, but they may also encounter difficulties in relating to peers. Specialized support services such as counseling, mentorship, and veteran-specific resources can facilitate a successful transition from military service to academic life (Reyes & Cross, 2023). Such services can be found through your college advisor, student services personnel, and veterans affairs staff.

As a returning student, you may be experiencing a greater than normal amount of role overload and/or challenges in role transition. If this is the case, it is imperative at the early onset of such difficulties that you seek assistance from your nursing advisor or college counselor to access resources that can assist you.

Unfortunately, role conflict cannot be avoided, so it is important to develop methods of coping with conflict constructively. The following methods can be used to resolve conflict:

- **Avoidance:** This is also called withdrawing from or denying conflict. When this method is used, conflict is generally not resolved and may actually be perpetuated. Example: You checked a book out of the library and then loaned it to a fellow

student. They returned it to the library late, and you were billed for the fine. You decide to pay it rather than asking the student to do so.
- **Compromise:** This approach uses the techniques of bargaining or negotiating. It is recognized that there must be a give and take for the solution to be determined. Generally, compromise works well, although the conflict issue may recur. Example: You and your partner arrange to accomplish household chores based on time limitations and abilities. Both of you agree that it is a good plan that will satisfy the need for a clean house and mutual responsibilities.
- **Accommodation:** In this method, a person attempts to smooth over the conflict or to suppress the problems. Often, a peaceful environment will be maintained, but one person may feel as though they have made a tremendous sacrifice and is inwardly angry and frustrated. Example: In the compromise example above, one partner may not follow through on the predetermined tasks, and so the other partner says that they understand and helps the partner finish the undone household chores.
- **Competition:** In this strategy, one person decides to force the issue and to place personal goals or desires over those of others. This sets up a conflict of power. Example: A group of students meet to plan for an end-of-the-year banquet and select a leader. One student spends 10 minutes describing their experience in the LPN program chairing the banquet committee, the success of the banquet, and how grateful the classmates were for their leadership. The group agrees to let this student have primary responsibility for planning this banquet.
- **Collaboration:** This strategy requires participants to be willing to problem solve and confront the issues with the intent of setting mutual goals. All participants are involved in the decision-making process. Example: A group of student nurses is concerned about the volume of paperwork required by clinical instructors. The instructors recognize that there is a lot of work, but they believe it is necessary to ensure that each student is prepared for each clinical assignment. The program chairperson arranges a meeting with the students and instructors to develop methods that validate student preparation without being overly burdensome.

THINKING CRITICALLY

Consider each method of conflict resolution. Think of an example of your own for each method. Would another method have been more satisfactory? If so, what method and why?

The NCLEX-RN *Might Ask* 2.2

A client asks a nursing student what the changes to her role have been as she has gone from LPN to RN. The nurse would be incorrect by stating the following:
a. "I have acquired more advanced technical and theoretical skills."
b. "I have learned to balance my roles as wife and mother with my professional ones."
c. "I have interwoven new professional values into my existing ones."
d. "I have changed my professional roles to only what is acceptable to me personally."

• See Appendix A for correct answer and rationale.

CONCLUSION

Role development and transition are complex processes that involve individual and universal concepts. In this chapter, personal development is presented in relation to the work of theorists who perceive development in terms of stages and critical tasks that occur in a sequential pattern. Adult development is described as an ongoing and dynamic process. Family and professional role development is explained in terms of stages of development.

Concepts related to role socialization, role transition, and role conflict are presented with an emphasis on the meanings these concepts have for the LPN/LVN returning to school. Understanding the theories and concepts of role development and transition enhances a person's ability to examine their own experiences and to better assess client experiences. The impacts of role changes and health status changes are varied and yet more predictable when all concepts are considered. You will find many opportunities to apply this information in your personal and work experiences, including your transition to the RN role.

STUDENT *Exercises*

Exercise 2.1

Review the case study of Juan Martinez at the beginning of this chapter and answer the following:

1. Identify some of Juan's acquired and ascribed roles. Will any of these change as he returns to school?
2. In what stage of personal growth and development is Juan?
3. In what stage of role development is Juan?
4. What adjustments in role choice might Juan need to make as he returns to school?
5. Apply Bridges and Bridges' role transition theory to Juan's situation. What endings may be in store for Juan?
6. If you were paired with Juan for a group project, what unique considerations would you have in ensuring an effective working relationship together?

Exercise 2.2

1. Interview a student in your class.
2. Identify the various roles for this student.
3. Differentiate the individual's ascribed and acquired roles.
4. Ask the student to describe their experience with bias.
5. Explore with the student similarities and differences you have experienced related to bias.
6. Explore with the student what role changes are forthcoming.
7. Determine whether there is role strain, role stress, role conflict, or role overload involved, and explore what methods are being used or could be used for coping.

REFERENCES

American Association of Colleges of Nursing. (2023, April). *Fact sheet: Enhancing diversity in the nursing workforce*. https://www.aacnnursing.org/Portals/0/PDFs/Fact-Sheets/Enhancing-Diversity-Factsheet.pdf

Benner, P. (2001). *From novice to expert: Excellence and power in clinical nursing practice* (Commemorative ed.). Prentice Hall.

Bowen, M. (1985). *Family therapy in clinical practice*. Rowman & Littlefield Publishers.

Bridges, W., & Bridges, S. (2016). *Managing transitions: Making the most of change* (4th ed.). Hachette Book Group.

Bridges, W., & Bridges, S. (2019). *Transitions: Making sense of life's changes* (40th Anniversary ed.). Hachette Book Group.

Cohen, H. A. (1981). *The nurse's quest for a professional identity*. Addison-Wesley.

Covey, S. R. (2004). *The 8th habit: From effectiveness to greatness*. Free Press.

Covey, S. R. (2013). *The seven habits of highly effective people* (25th Anniversary ed.). Simon & Schuster.

Duvall, E. M., & Miller, B. C. (1985). *Marriage and family development* (6th ed.). Harper Collins Publisher.

Erikson, E. (1963). *Childhood and society*. Norton.

Freeman, A., & Dodson, L. (2021). Triple role overload: Working, parenting, and navigating public benefits. *Journal of Family Issues, 42*(8), 1737–1761. https://doi.org/10.1177/0192513X20949599

Gilligan, C. (1982). *In a different voice: Psychological theory and women's development*. Harvard University Press.

Gonzalez, L., Nielsen, A., & Lasater, K. (2021). Developing students' clinical reasoning skills: A faculty guide. *Journal of Nursing Education, 60*(9), 485–493. https://doi.org/10.3928/01484834-20210708-01

Hinshaw, A. S. (1986). Socialization and resocialization of nurses for professional nursing practice. In E. C. Hein & M. J. Nicholson (Eds.), *Contemporary leadership behavior: Selected readings* (2nd ed.). Little, Brown and Company.

Kelman, H. C. (1958). Compliance, identification, and internalization: Three processes of attitude change. *Journal of Conflict Resolution, 2*(1), 51–60. https://doi.org/10.1177/002200275800200106

Kohlberg, L. (1981). *The philosophy of moral development: Moral stages and the idea of justice*. Harper & Row.

Longworth, N. (2003). *Lifelong learning in action: Transforming education in the 21st century*. Routledge/Falmer.

Mostafa, A. M. S. (2022). The moderating role of self-sacrificing disposition and work meaningfulness on the relationship between work-family conflict and emotional exhaustion. *Journal of Happiness Studies, 23*(4), 1579–1597. https://doi.org/10.1007/s10902-021-00463-5

Nowak, E. W., & Colsch, R. (2024). *Brown's evidence-based nursing: The research-practice connection* (5th ed.). Jones & Bartlett Learning.

Piaget, J., & Inhelder, B. (1972). *The psychology of the child* (2nd ed.). Basic Books.

Potter, P., Perry, A., Stockert, P., & Hall, A. (2023). Developmental theories. In *Fundamentals of nursing* (11th ed., pp. 144–151). Elsevier.

Reyes, A. T., & Cross, C. L. (2023). Relationships among rumination, resilience, mindfulness, and perceived PTSD symptoms in military veterans returning to college: A cross-sectional study. *Journal of Psychosocial Nursing & Mental Health Services, 61*(6), 43–50. https://doi.org/10.3928/02793695-20221027-05

Taylor, C., Lynn, P., & Bartlett, J. L. (2023). *Fundamentals of nursing: The art and science of nursing care* (10th ed.). Wolters Kluwer.

Thomas, C. M., McIntosh, C. E., & Mensik, J. S. (2016). *A nurse's step by step guide to transitioning to the professional role*. Sigma Theta Tau International.

Wei, H., Horns, P., Sears, S. F., Huang, K., Smith, C. M., & Wei, T. L. (2022). A systematic meta-review of systematic reviews about interprofessional collaboration: Facilitators, barriers, and outcomes. *Journal of Interprofessional Care, 36*(5), 735–749. https://doi.org/10.1080/13561820.2021.1973975

On the WEB

For more information on Adult Development Theory, go to any search engine and type "Adult Development Theorists" or the specific theorist you wish to learn more about.

Association for Nursing Professional Development. https://www.anpd.org/

American Nurses Association—*Career and professional development.* https://www.nursingworld.org/resources/individual/

Adapting to Change

CHAPTER 3

LEARNING OUTCOMES

By the end of this chapter, the student will be able to:
1. Explore the paradoxes of change.
2. Differentiate individual and organizational change.
3. Summarize factors that motivate change.
4. Compare and contrast types of change.
5. Describe the process of planned change.
6. Outline Lewin's process of change.
7. Discuss the effects of change on individuals and systems.
8. Apply theoretical effects of change.
9. Describe the methods for adjusting to change.
10. Give examples of positive outcomes of change.
11. Compare and contrast Lewin's change theory with Bridges' phases of transition.
12. Evaluate effective strategies for managing the three-phase transition experienced by an individual or organization undergoing transformational change.

KEY TERMS

ambivalence	eustress	resonance
autonomy	flexibility	restraining forces
biotechnology	general adaptation	self-actualization
change	syndrome	stakeholders
change agent	individual change	stress
conflict	loss	transactional change
crisis	organizational change	transformational change
distress	paradox	
driving forces	resistance	

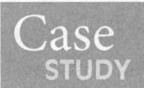

Case STUDY

Deborah Washington is a 46-year-old LPN who has worked in the mental health unit for the past 25 years. She is taking her first clinical nursing course in the LPN to ADN Bridge Program. After having difficulty with the clinical component in a hospital setting, she is meeting with her nursing adviser, John Tercha, to discuss her problems adjusting to change.

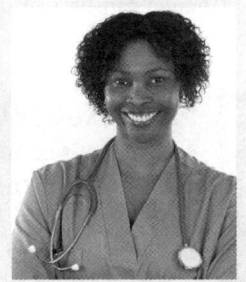

DEBORAH: I feel so inadequate! I remember being in the hospital setting years ago, but why do I need to go through all this again when there is a job opening where I have worked for 25 years? I just need to upgrade my license to the RN level. I'm not even going to work in a medical-surgical area, and I don't see why I should have to repeat all these basic procedures again. What "RN level work" am I learning by doing total care for a bedridden congestive heart failure patient? I just feel like I'm jumping through hoops!

ADVISOR TERCHA: I hear what you're saying, and I understand. It is often very uncomfortable for returning adult students to be in a new environment, and returning to school and being in the student role again is a big change. It sounds as if you feel frustrated and you're not seeing how your clinical rotation is applicable to your future professional work.

DEBORAH: Exactly! Do I really have to do all of this? I feel like I'm starting over. I already learned all this many years ago in LPN training, and I don't even use it where I work.

ADVISOR TERCHA: Yes, you will have to complete the clinical rotations of the Bridge Program, but the student learning outcomes you will be achieving are at a different practice level. I can assure you that others feel this way too and the change is uncomfortable. However, in time, you will become more at ease, and even though you cannot see the relevance of what you are learning, it is part of the bigger picture of not only bringing currency to your practice but also helping you to develop a lens for professional nursing practice. This includes helping you see the larger context of your clients, applying new theoretical concepts, and thinking critically to diagnose and design comprehensive care plans as a registered nurse, licensed to practice in a variety of settings. Change is difficult, and you are experiencing a necessary step in your development as a professional nurse. Let's discuss what specific difficulties you are having and apply the change theory you are learning in class to your own situation to help you through the transition process in this first clinical rotation.

CHANGE DEFINED

Merriam-Webster (n.d.) defines **change** as "to undergo transformation, transition, or substitution." William Bridges (2001, 2009, 2016), a leading author on change and transitions whose concepts were presented in the previous chapter, identified several change paradoxes that define its dynamic state (Box 3.1). A **paradox** is a statement that seems absurd or contradictory but is based on fact (Box 3.1).

Change can be planned or unplanned, but it is ever present in our daily lives. With change, each person, group, or organization has the opportunity to develop, grow, and

---

BOX 3.1

Paradoxes of Change

- To achieve continuity, we have to be willing to change.
- Change is the only way to protect whatever exists; without continuous readjustments, the present cannot continue.
- The very things we now wish that we could hold onto and keep safe from change were themselves originally produced by change.

adapt. Change is inevitable and dynamic. Each of us copes with change in unique ways. Our responses to change are affected by our past experiences, our current situations, our family dynamics and social context, and our comfort level with change. Huston (2023) notes that one of the challenges for nurse professionals is to assist clients and colleagues with developing comfort with the change process inherent in the healthcare industry today. She emphasizes that in order to foster an environment of innovation and change, leaders must first recognize, embrace, and demonstrate participation in innovation and change in their own leadership practices. For professional nurses to lead and provide support for those they supervise who are experiencing change in the healthcare setting, they must first understand the concept and process of change, factors influencing one's ability to adapt to change, motivational strategies, and approaches for successful, productive change.

PROCESS OF CHANGE

Examining the process of change is particularly important for the LPN/LVN to RN student for several reasons. First, you are experiencing personal change by returning to school. Second, you will be presented with many aspects of change within the nursing curriculum. For instance, in issues related to trends in healthcare, the faculty may present you with current methods of delivering care and have you explore how the future of healthcare delivery will be affected by advances in **biotechnology** or changes in healthcare policy or the economy. Third, as you prepare for your own role transition, you will learn about the new roles nurses have today and will have in the future, such as engaging in evidence-based practice and becoming an active and equal member of an interprofessional collaborative team. It is essential to understand that change is inevitable. Change occurs even when you think societal and work roles and values are stable or resistant to change, and the challenge for each individual is to learn to be more comfortable outside their "comfort zone."

INDIVIDUAL AND ORGANIZATIONAL CHANGE

When differentiating individual change from organizational change, one must remember that change always implies the alteration or modification of behaviors or functions. Within the individual, change may occur without any plan at all, or it may be the result of much planning. Later in this chapter, types of change are described. Organizational change also results in behavior or function alterations but has the potential to have a greater impact on parts of an organization and its individuals. Table 3.1 compares individual and organizational change.

TABLE 3.1 Individual and Organizational Change Compared

Type of Change	Description	Example
Individual change	The process of altering or modifying the current state in terms of behaviors or functions.	An LPN/LVN who has returned to school changes from full-time to part-time work to have more time to study.
Organizational change	The process of altering the structure or function of the whole or parts of the whole so that individuals or groups modify behaviors and functions.	A small hospital determines that it will move to a flexible staffing pattern with combinations of 4-, 8-, 10-, and 12-hour shifts. This affects staffing workloads, staffing mix, patient documentation systems, and functions of the various healthcare providers at the facility.

Change within an organization involves modifying working practices and procedures or causing individuals to work in different ways. This can produce a great deal of fear among employees. William Bridges (2016) offers many suggestions for assisting individuals in organizations experiencing loss and fear in such change processes, including honoring past history and culture, involving people in the transition, and establishing a "change manager" to monitor all the details of the change process and identify problems quickly as they arise.

FACTORS THAT MOTIVATE CHANGE

Many factors motivate change. If you were to examine your reasons for desiring a change from your role as an LPN/LVN to that of an RN, you may identify some aspects that are described in the following text. You may also recognize some factors that have played a part in other life changes.

CRISIS

One factor that can precipitate change is a **crisis**—a turning point or a critical time in the course of an event. A situational crisis involves an unexpected event, such as a natural disaster, loss of a loved one, illness, or divorce. This type of crisis can motivate an individual to make other changes. For example, a 40-year-old nurse who had recently been through a split from their partner recognized a need to further their education and develop a professional career. This may not have happened if they had remained with their partner.

CONFLICT

Another factor that can influence the process of change is conflict. There is always an implied sense of battle or opposition when the term **conflict** is used. In relation to change, it also denotes a struggle or variance with a particular situation or person. Conflict may result in change because an individual is frustrated with the current circumstances. An example is that of a person who has not been happy in their position as a nurse at a local hospital. They want to practice nursing in a more holistic way and believe that the fragmented care system is not adequate. Although the nurse has spoken to their boss about this many times, they have been unable to make any changes in the healthcare delivery system. Finally, the nurse decides that they can no longer deal with the conflict, and so they resign. They are subsequently hired by a community health agency that practices a more holistic approach. Conflict motivated this individual to make a change.

DISAPPOINTMENT

Everyone has experienced disappointment at some point. Disappointment is related to a sense of failure at not meeting expectations or fulfilling certain plans and can be another motivator for change. A nursing student who has done poorly in math has avoided working on math problems. After failing their first quiz, they meet with their advisor, spend time with a college tutor, and purchase a step-by-step nursing math review text. This student nurse has vowed to change their practice habits so that they will pass the next quiz and improve their clinical performance.

LACK OF REWARDS

Another stimulus for change is lack of rewards in the current circumstances. An individual may be in a position that affords little recognition or reward. For example, an LPN who has been working in a skilled nursing facility for 10 years has been passed over several times to move up to a charge nurse position, even though the LPN oriented the newly graduated RNs who have been hired and quickly promoted to the position the LPN has desired. This situation has caused disappointment and motivates the LPN to return to school to pursue an RN license.

DESIRE FOR AUTONOMY AND SELF-IMPROVEMENT
The desire for **autonomy** and self-improvement can also activate change. A person may feel stagnated and powerless in a particular position and thus may take appropriate steps to change the situation. For instance, a certified nursing assistant may enjoy their work but not feel able to influence policy or procedures. They may also want to learn more and take on additional responsibility. This sense of powerlessness and the need for self-improvement is a potent factor for change.

> **THINKING CRITICALLY**
> Identify factors that have motivated you to make a change in your life. Give examples of changes that you have made. Analyze the results of these changes and how certain behaviors or functions were affected.

TYPES OF CHANGE
There are various types of change that an individual or organization can face. Some are developmental; some are unplanned; and some are planned. From your own experiences, you can probably identify some of these. The following sections define three types of change that are generally encountered.

DEVELOPMENTAL CHANGE
Developmental change is change in which a person proceeds through stages in a fairly predictable order. Tasks are identified for each stage that must be accomplished to complete a stage. Examples of this type of change were described in the previous chapter. These stages of change can be due to age or changes in family structure.

UNPLANNED CHANGE
Unplanned change can refer to a positive or negative, desired or undesired change that was not planned. An example of positive unplanned change would be an unexpected promotion within an organization, whereas a negative unplanned stage might be unannounced layoffs at a place of employment. Two types of unplanned change are forced change and spontaneous change.

Forced Change
Forced change is a type of change that is imposed on an individual or organization that requires action, often of an immediate or emergent nature. An example would be a fire in a person's home, in which the entire home and its contents are lost. Family members are forced to consider rebuilding the home and replacing lost items, as well as realizing that everything is forever different.

Spontaneous Change

Spontaneous change refers to change that is impulsive or effortless and is often random or unpredictable. For example, when a person begins a new job, they may take on the characteristics of other coworkers. This may involve buying the same types of clothes or becoming interested in similar activities. In retrospect, it may seem like a planned response, but in reality, it occurred spontaneously and without forethought.

PLANNED CHANGE

Taylor et al. (2023) describe planned change as a deliberate, purposeful, methodical endeavor to effect change. Planned change involves advanced strategy by a **change agent** who serves as a "champion" to lead the change process. Members who are affected by the change are referred to as **stakeholders**. In an organization, anyone can become the change agent and present ideas to the stakeholders. For example, a planned change is your return to school; you probably made careful plans to achieve your goals. These plans may have included child care or other personal issues, revision of work schedules, or a change in daily activities. Other planned changes may have occurred in your workplace. Schedule changes are an example. Some healthcare settings have opted to have their employees work 12-hour shifts. To establish that schedule, an implementation plan is developed so that the transition to the new schedule is as smooth as possible. This is the process of planned change. There are several types of planned change.

Incremental Change

Incremental change involves a planned change that occurs gradually in steps or stages. This type of planning is often applied to long-term projects, such as hospital mergers or curriculum changes. You may have planned your return to school in increments. You may have taken your general education courses first at the initial stage of your education. The second part of the process involves completing the nursing courses. By doing this, you are able to continue working or have greater ability to care for a family or remain involved in other interests.

Rapid Change

Change that is planned quickly may or may not be successful. For instance, rapid plans may need to be developed in rescue situations to assist people quickly in precarious situations. Rapid change can also mean the implementation of an organizational plan without considering the ramifications. As an example, a nursing organization recognizes that staff positions need to be eliminated fairly quickly because of reduced census or revenue shortfalls. The plans are made to eliminate positions based on seniority, without considering what units have the highest staffing needs and how staff might need to be transferred and oriented. The plan is implemented quickly but without considering the fallout.

Transactional Change

Transactional change occurs for mutual benefit. For example, nursing faculty and students determine that a change is needed in clinical experiences so that all seniors have the opportunity for a leadership experience. Representatives of both groups meet to plan the best method to accomplish this goal. The plan is formed so that all parties are able to transact an appropriate and mutually agreeable plan.

Transformational Change

Transformational change can occur within the process of planned change. In your return to school, a change will occur as you progress through your ADN course work. With this process of change will come not only new knowledge and skills but also a new way of thinking and being. Transformational change can occur for an individual or an organization and implies that there is a radical difference as a result of change. This radical change results in the individual or organization experiencing a transition. Such a transition must be managed well, as described by Bridges and Bridges (2016), for there to be a positive outcome. As discussed in the previous chapter, attention must be given to managing each of the three phases of the transition—endings, the neutral zone, and the new beginning (see Chapter 2, Box 2.4).

THINKING CRITICALLY

Review the types of change that have been described. Think of experiences that have involved change in your life. Categorize these changes according to the previous descriptions. Consider these changes in terms of individual, group, and organizational changes. Are any of them transformational in nature? Why? In what ways were the three phases of the transition managed well? In what ways could they have been managed better?

The NCLEX-RN *Might Ask* 3.1

The nurse is taking care of a large group of clients in a community care setting. Because of the high influx of new clients, the nurse manager independently decides to make a radical change in the way clients are assessed and processed. This type of radical change would be most consistent with:

a. transactional change.
b. transformational change.
c. unplanned change.
d. spontaneous change.

• See Appendix A for correct answer and rationale.

STAGES OF PLANNED CHANGE

The process of change is complex because it involves the modification of behaviors. Unplanned change is, obviously, less structured and more haphazard than planned change. When change is planned, there will be a more systematic approach that entails problem-solving, decision-making, and deliberate steps. Kurt Lewin was a social scientist credited with doing the first work in change theory. The following text outlines his theory of planned change, which remains a core foundation of change theory today. You may see some similarities between Lewin and the more contemporary work done by William Bridges, discussed in the previous chapter. Lewin's (1951) theory remains applicable to nursing practice today, more than seven decades later. Box 3.2 summarizes this theory.

> **BOX 3.2**
>
> **Lewin's Stages of Planned Change**
>
> **Unfreezing:** An individual, group, or organization identifies the need for change and the need to change behaviors. It is necessary to identify restraining and driving forces for the planned change.
>
> **Moving:** Strategies for the planned change are developed. The individual, group, or organization gathers data, formulates plans, and enlists the support of all those involved with the change.
>
> **Refreezing:** The process of change is completed. The individual, group, or organization internalizes the behavior changes and attitudes that were identified as necessary for the change process.

Source: Lewin, K. (1951). *Field theory in social science.* Harper & Row.

UNFREEZING

The first stage that Lewin (1951) identified is referred to as the unfreezing stage, in which a person, group, or organization is motivated to bring about change. There is a need to learn new behaviors. This stage is one of imbalance and disequilibrium; it is very unsettling. During this stage, two types of forces are present: those against and those in support of the change.

Restraining Forces

Restraining forces are those that inhibit change. For example, as you have become motivated to return to school, you undoubtedly have encountered some restraining forces. Some of the restraining forces may have been related to family concerns, loss of income while in school, lack of confidence in your ability to succeed, or coworkers who fear you will be leaving.

Driving Forces

Opposing such restraining forces are **driving forces**. These are the forces that encourage and sustain change. For example, your motivation to return to school may have been supported by such forces as your desire for more decision-making, increased clinical skills, more recognition, or the encouragement and support of a family member, mentor, or friend.

MOVING

The second stage that Lewin identified is called moving. During this stage, plans are detailed and initiated. It is important to collect data and supplemental information from as many sources as possible. In addition, it is helpful when most, if not all, people involved in the change are in agreement that change is desirable. For example, you entered the moving stage after you began making plans to return to school. At this time, you formulated plans for child care or alternative work schedules. You may also have obtained information about financial aid and scholarships. You gathered as much information as possible to assist you in your plans. You may have enlisted the advice of a colleague who had been through this process. It may have been necessary for you to persuade those around you that this was an important move for you and that you needed their support and understanding. Use of "win/win agreements" as discussed in Chapter 1 can be helpful during this stage.

It is during this second stage of change that transitions occur, as described in Chapter 2. Letting go of the past (i.e., accomplishing endings) becomes essential to make room for new beginnings. Role conflict may increase as both you and others around you work to put old roles behind you to prepare for new ones. Often, there is a sense of loss for the role left behind.

REFREEZING

Lewin's last stage is called refreezing. The change has occurred and is now part of the individual, group, or organization. Refreezing requires a commitment to change and the stabilization of restraining and driving forces. There is a change of behaviors and attitudes within the change process. In continuing with the same example, as you reenter school, one change has already occurred: You are a student nurse again. You have internalized the value of continuing your education and have made the commitment to become an RN. This change is part of who you are. Your family, friends, and coworkers have also made adjustments to this change. You are now working through the internalization of this new identity that you will be assuming.

THINKING CRITICALLY

Recall a planned change with which you were recently involved. Critique your change as viewed through the three stages of planned change described by Lewin. What steps were taken to initiate the change? What were the restraining and driving forces? What was your role in the planned change? What role conflict did you experience? When did you become aware that the change was causing a major transition for you? How did you manage the three phases of the transition? What was the impact on those around you? What would you do differently if you could to better manage the transition?

EFFECTS OF CHANGE

Change can have many effects. Some are expected, and some are not. As previously stated, individuals cope with and adapt to change in unique ways.

STRESS, DISTRESS, AND EUSTRESS

Stress, distress, and eustress are terms defined by Hans Selye (1976) to describe various conditions that humans experience. **Stress** is a universal response to any situation or factor that disturbs a person's equilibrium. It has become a familiar term to all of us and may be a term that you will use frequently while in nursing school. Selye called the side effects of stress distress and eustress. **Distress** is the negative or maladaptive effects of change or stress, whereas **eustress** represents normal or moderate stress, which is more beneficial to the experiencer.

With any stress or change, nonspecific bodily changes occur. If a person is able to cope effectively with change, the side effects will be kept to a minimum, but poor adaptation to stress or change results in damaging side effects, or distress. Physical signs of distress can include prolonged elevated blood pressure, increased gastric acid secretions, and decreased urine output. Emotional signs may include insomnia and hyperexcitability. There also may be behavioral changes such as depression or anger. Selye (1976) believed that some conditions (e.g., hypertension, ulcers, certain emotional disturbances) represent diseases of adaptation. Although many researchers and providers argue differently, the concepts of distress and eustress provide a means for you to evaluate the typical coping patterns of your clients.

General Adaptation Syndrome

As just discussed, a common effect of any change, planned or unplanned, is stress, which disturbs an individual's equilibrium. Selye (1976) was the first to describe a nonspecific general response to stress, which he called **general adaptation syndrome**. He described stress as a condition of the body that is characterized by the changes that occur within the body and a stressor as any factor that upsets the equilibrium and results in stress. For example, a student may experience nausea before making a class presentation. The stressor is the impending presentation; the stress is the condition of nausea.

Selye delineated three stages that occur in the general adaptation syndrome: alarm reaction, resistance, and recovery or exhaustion. Table 3.2 shows these stages.

Alarm Reaction

The first stage of the general adaptation syndrome is the alarm reaction. The body responds to a particular stressor, such as an extreme in temperature, infection, verbal abuse, or other conscious and unconscious factors. With this process, the defense mechanisms of the mind and body are activated. The autonomic nervous system releases large amounts of hormones into the body. Blood volume is increased, and blood glucose levels rise to meet energy needs. Increased epinephrine results in a higher heart rate, more blood flow to muscles, better oxygen intake, and greater mental alertness. Norepinephrine is released in greater quantities to decrease blood flow to the kidneys. Increased rennin secretion will result in more angiotensin production, thus elevating blood pressure. This process initiates what is called the "fight-or-flight" response and may last for a short period to many hours. A person is ready for action during this phase.

Resistance

The second stage is called the resistance stage. During this stage, the alarm reactions stabilize. The hormone levels and cardiac functions return to previous levels. The person attempts to adapt to the stressor or to cope more effectively with its effects. For example,

TABLE 3.2 Stages of the General Adaptation Syndrome

Stage	Body Responses
Alarm reaction (fight-or-flight)	Increased release of hormones by the autonomic nervous system: • Increased heart rate • Increased oxygen intake • Increased blood sugar • Increased mental acuity • Increased blood flow to muscles • Increased blood pressure • Decreased flow to the kidneys • Decreased urine output
Resistance	Stabilization: • Hormone levels return to normal • Cardiac functions return to previous levels • Adaptation to stressor(s)
Recovery or exhaustion	Defense mechanisms described in the alarm reaction stage are exhausted Decreased energy levels Fatigue Decreased ability for adaptation Death

if a person has sustained a fracture, the body responds by beginning the process of healing at the site of the fracture. This would be considered recovery. If the stressor is more difficult, such as hemorrhage, adaptation may be impossible, and the outcome is exhaustion. In both cases, the individuals enter the next stage.

Recovery or Exhaustion

The third stage is referred to as the stage of recovery or exhaustion. The body will either recover or find it can no longer cope with the stressor, having exhausted its ability to defend itself. The effects of stress may involve the entire body. A person who experiences psychological trauma will enter a state of exhaustion and demonstrate physical and emotional symptoms, such as abdominal pain, insomnia, or depression. If the state of exhaustion is severe, such as the state that follows unchecked hemorrhage, death may occur.

The concepts of stress and adaptation should be familiar to you from your LPN/LVN program. One's ability to adapt to stress also describes the ability to adapt to change. Adaptation involves a person's capacity for change as they are faced with new experiences. Understanding how you adapt to change can assist you with some of the stress you may encounter as you return to the student role.

THINKING CRITICALLY

Recall a situation that has created stress for you. Review the stages of the general adaptation syndrome. Determine what physical, emotional, or behavioral changes occurred. What was the outcome of the change that took place? What is your general response to stressful situations? How do you adapt? What resources are available to you if you experience stress during the nursing program? What are some positive mechanisms you can employ to adapt to change?

The NCLEX-RN *Might Ask* 3.2

The nurse is caring for a client in the emergency room after an automobile accident. Although there are no visible signs of injury, the client's heart rate, blood pressure, and respirations are elevated. The client's peripheral oxygenation level is 100%, the blood glucose level is slightly elevated, and the client is answering questions appropriately. The nurse knows that this stage of the general adaptation syndrome is:

a. normal.
b. alarm reaction.
c. resistance.
d. exhaustion.

• See Appendix A for correct answer and rationale.

AMBIVALENCE

Another effect of change is **ambivalence**. This term pertains to concurrent opposing views an individual may have for a particular situation, person, or other factor. For instance, some claim to have experienced a love–hate relationship with a particular person. This means that within one's self are conflicting emotions of love and hate.

Feelings of ambivalence can occur when a person is experiencing change. During the change process, a person may have mixed feelings about what the change will involve. As an example, a nurse of a cultural background in which women assume subservient roles may be ambivalent about assuming the more autonomous role of a professional nurse, where the interprofessional team members of all genders are on an equal standing with other professionals and collaborate to determine diagnoses and care for a patient. Boyle et al. (2025) advocate for the profession of nursing to examine the impact of culture on all aspects of nursing. This applies to those newly entering the professional nurse level, such as yourself, to provide support for the ambivalence you may have about this change in your role based on your culture.

THINKING CRITICALLY

Consider changes that you have experienced, for example, a marriage, divorce, birth of a child, loss of a job, economic pressures, or change in a partner or living arrangements. Analyze ambivalent feelings you had about these changes. How did you resolve the ambivalence?

RESISTANCE

Resistance has been defined as conduct that tries to preserve the status quo. Buckway and Sowerby (2023) noted that most people are initially resistant to change, especially if the change requires new skills and new patterns of behavior or will take additional time to learn. There is always comfort in the way things are. Fear of the unknown or a lack of self-confidence can hinder a person's ability to welcome change. In a group, Taylor et al. (2023) note that change alters the balance of a group, and resistance is expected in any change process. Factors that may influence resistance to change include the following:

- Past experiences with change may not have been positive. Example: An employee who resists change states that previous job changes always meant loss of job, pay, or informal seniority standing with coworkers.
- People often see change in terms of how they personally will be affected. Example: If a hospital decides to change the mix of staffing at the facility, there may be fear that some will lose their jobs or that they will be reassigned to a different unit or shift.
- Resistance to change is higher if an individual or group has not participated in the decision to make the change. Example: The head nurse in an intensive care unit decides to implement the use of computerized standard care plans. The equipment that is purchased is labor intensive to learn and not nurse friendly. Many of the staff nurses are irate and refuse to comply with the change.
- Resistance can occur if people feel overwhelmed by the amount or speed of change. Example: If a new hospital administrator is hired and they implement multiple changes quickly and concurrently, there may be resistance even from those who are supportive of some or all of the changes.
- Lack of communication throughout the change process increases resistance. Example: Employees of a medical clinic are informed that there will be a change in the management structure to make the organization more efficient and less costly. They are told that more information will be coming soon. After several weeks of hearing nothing, some of the employees are disgruntled. Rumors are rampant, and many of the employees are now vehemently opposed to any change that may occur, although they initially recognized a need.
- Passive resistance may be manifested as inefficiency, lethargy, failure to complete tasks, increased errors in job performance, or poor attitudes. Example: A nurse at

a small hospital is unhappy about being floated to a similar medical-surgical unit. Although they go to the assigned unit, they barely speak to the other staff nurses and display a sullen attitude when they see the supervisor.

Resistance to change is important to consider not only from a personal or organizational point of view but also from the perspective of clients. Many of your clients will experience change, much of which may be undesirable and unwanted. These clients may resist the efforts of the healthcare system to accomplish the needed changes.

Cultural Resistance Factors
Predictability and linearity of change is basically a Western phenomenon. Looking at change from the Eastern perspective can be instructive. Taoist and Confucian philosophies view change as cyclic and ongoing rather than as having an end point. Life is a quest for balance and harmony within an ever-changing environment. Resistance may occur when needed changes are incompatible with cultural beliefs. For example, some people of some cultures may believe that illness is caused by diet imbalance and that certain foods in combination restore balance, even though some foods may be contraindicated in some medical conditions.

Social Resistance Factors
Resistance may also occur when needed changes are not seen as normal within a social group. For example, a person with chronic bronchitis does not change from their weekly social routine of playing bingo, even though the game is played in a smoke-filled room, which aggravates the bronchitis.

Psychological Resistance Factors
Finally, resistance to change may occur when needed changes produce anxiety secondary to fear of the unknown, lack of confidence, loss of control, and fear of being a burden. For example, a client with newly diagnosed diabetes is afraid to give themselves injections because they are fearful that poor technique will make the disease worse.

> **THINKING CRITICALLY**
> Consider a change that has occurred in your workplace or within another organization. Review the factors that increase resistance to change. What types of resistance did you observe? What strategies were used to overcome the resistance? Was the change a success or a failure? Why?

You must assess your clients' feelings and attitudes about a particular change. You must also not impose change without regard to a person's cultural, social, and psychological beliefs. Change is better perceived if a client/stakeholder is actively involved in the change process (Box 3.3).

> **BOX 3.3 Improving Reception to Change**
> Change will be better received if a person:
> - Perceives a need for change
> - Is open to change
> - Has choices regarding the change
> - Commits to the change process

LOSS

Change frequently involves some type of **loss**. The death of a spouse is an obvious example of loss. However, other changes can induce a sense of loss. Many recent graduates report a sadness or grief when they complete a program of study. This is often related to leaving school, being separated from friends, and beginning something new and unknown. The loss experienced with endings was discussed in the previous chapter.

Individual Loss and Change

Elisabeth Kübler-Ross (1969) developed a model of death and dying that describes stages when dealing with loss and change. You likely are familiar with this model from your LPN/LVN training:

1. The first stage is denial, in which an individual refuses to believe that anything has happened or is different. Others may believe that everything is under control.
2. In the second stage, the person experiences anger; they are mad at everyone and everything.
3. The third stage is the bargaining stage, in which a person attempts to barter or deal to make things better or to delay reality.
4. Depression is the fourth stage; it occurs when the person fully recognizes the impact of the loss. They frequently withdraw and are mournful and lonely.
5. The last stage is acceptance, in which the individual is more at peace with the loss and has come to terms with the situation.

Organizational Loss and Change

Perlman and Takacs (1990) developed a model based on Kübler-Ross' model to describe the phases that are seen within an organization that is involved with change. These phases can be used to depict the emotions that one may experience with any change. The following is a brief description of each stage:

1. Phase 1: Equilibrium—A person is happy with the current conditions, believes that everything is in balance, and experiences anxiety if the status quo is threatened.
2. Phase 2: Denial—When change becomes apparent, the person attempts to act as if nothing has changed or will change; they may choose to ignore what is happening or not participate in activities that help prepare for change.
3. Phase 3: Anger—Within this stage, the individual actively resists change by being visibly angry, disgruntled, and uncooperative. They typically blame others and want everything fixed.
4. Phase 4: Bargaining—A person tries to negotiate to keep things from changing. They are willing to make some concessions in an attempt to maintain as much of the status quo as possible.
5. Phase 5: Chaos—The person feels powerless to stop the change or to make it better. They feel insecure and disoriented because the change does not make sense.
6. Phase 6: Depression—The individual grieves and feels tremendous sorrow for the loss or change. They also experience self-pity and emptiness.
7. Phase 7: Resignation—The individual is lethargic and mechanical; the change is passively accepted.

TABLE 3.3 Comparison of Models of Stages of Individual Loss and Change (Kübler-Ross) and Phases of Organizational Change (Perlman and Takacs)

Stages of Individual Loss and Change (Kübler-Ross)	Phases of Organizational Change (Perlman and Takacs)
	Phase 1: Equilibrium
Stage 1: Denial	Phase 2: Denial
Stage 2: Anger	Phase 3: Anger
Stage 3: Bargaining	Phase 4: Bargaining
	Phase 5: Chaos
Stage 4: Depression	Phase 6: Depression
	Phase 7: Resignation
Stage 5: Acceptance	Phase 8: Openness
	Phase 9: Readiness
	Phase 10: Reemergence

Source: Kübler-Ross, E. (1969). *On death and dying*. Macmillan; Perlman, D., & Takacs, G. (1990). The ten stages of change. *Nursing Management, 21*(4), 33–38.

8. Phase 8: Openness—Within this stage, the individual becomes more engaged with the change and is more willing to be involved in the activities needed to complete the change.
9. Phase 9: Readiness—The individual continues to be more engaged and enthusiastic about the change; they are more willing to participate in necessary activities.
10. Phase 10: Reemergence—The person now values the change and is willing to make a personal investment in the change process.

The models by Kübler-Ross and Perlman and Takacs are compared in Table 3.3. These models will assist you in contemplating what change can mean for an individual or a group. It is helpful to consider these aspects when you are experiencing personal changes or when your clients are forced to adapt to a new situation. As with any stage theory, the phases may not be as clear or sequential as outlined, but the emotions that can accompany any change will be similar. The following critical thinking activity requires that you role-play the part of a client and imagine the stages of change that this client will experience.

THINKING CRITICALLY

Mr. Fleming is 40 years old. He is a lawyer in a prominent law firm. He is married and has two young sons. Last weekend, he was on a long bicycle ride and was hit by a truck. His injuries included a severe traumatic injury to his left foot, resulting in a below-the-knee amputation. His other injuries were not as severe. Consider the stages or phases of change shown in Table 3.3 and explain in each stage or phase what you might observe in terms of his behavior and emotions.

The NCLEX-RN *Might Ask* 3.3

The nurse is caring for a client who has had a radical mastectomy. The client refuses to look at the operative site and be involved in dressing changes. This client's behavior best describes which stage of grieving?
a. Depression
b. Denial
c. Bargaining
d. Acceptance

• See Appendix A for correct answer and rationale.

RESONANCE

The term **resonance** is generally used to define the reflection or reverberation of sound. However, it also describes the response of a system to changes from inside or outside the system. For example, if an individual has a cold, not only are the nasal passages affected but malaise, fever, and general discomfort also occur. Likewise, the individual who is depressed will also be fatigued and disengaged from day-to-day activities. An entire system is affected by what is happening to a part or parts.

General systems theory is often used to explain the interrelatedness of parts of a system and the resonance response. When one part of a system experiences change, the whole system responds. The system can be a human, a family, an organization, or a community. Although the parts may be defined as separate, each part has a function that contributes to the total function of the system. A change in one part resonates throughout the system.

The nursing profession has always held a holistic view of wellness and illness. Within this holistic view, change within one part affects the entire system. The whole is considered greater than and different from its parts. In using the holistic perspective, a person constantly experiences change internally and externally. These changes resonate within the entire system. An open system must be maintained for the exchange of energy, information, and matter to occur.

Following are examples of changes that occur to a part in which the entire system responds.

EXAMPLE 3.1 Juana dives into a cold pool. She experiences a sense of shock as she hits the cold water. She also feels other sensations related to internal changes, such as blood vessel constriction, an inability to focus on anything except the immediate sensations, and a feeling of discomfort. Juana will also experience other changes, depending on how long she remains in the pool. Her internal environment responds to the changing external environment.

EXAMPLE 3.2 There are four members of the Allen family. The parents work outside the home. Their two teenage daughters go to the local high school. The father has not been home from work on time for many weeks. When he arrives home, it is obvious that he has been drinking. The parents frequently fight about this situation. The oldest daughter frequently has headaches and stomachaches. Her grades at school have dropped. Her teachers are concerned about the change in her demeanor—she is withdrawn, quiet, and inattentive.

EXAMPLE 3.3 A respected resident of a small town dies suddenly as the result of a heart attack. Members of the community experience shock, dismay, and grief after this event.

In these examples, part of the system is affected by a change in the internal or external environment; the change resonates within the system, and the entire system responds in some way to the change that has occurred. The concepts related to general systems theory present a holistic approach to the effects of change. Nurses are able to intervene more effectively and holistically if they recognize how change in one part affects change of the whole.

THINKING CRITICALLY

Reflect on your own examples of resonance following change that have happened to you, within your family, work setting, or community. Consider how change to one part affected the whole. What changes did you note resonated throughout the whole system? How did the whole system also resonate refreezing, as Lewin described, after the change? Discuss this with another person in that system. How do the observations and perceptions of resonance by that individual compare with yours?

ADJUSTING TO CHANGE

In the process of adjusting to change, turmoil exists. Heath and Heath (2010) describe human beings as having two separate and sometimes competing "systems" in our brains—a rational system that plans and thinks logically and an emotional system that reacts intuitively and with instincts. When these two systems are in conflict during the change process, change can be quite arduous. Adjusting to change is not always an easy task. Emotions vary widely, from despair to joy, with much tension and doubt in between. Even experienced nurses can become overwhelmed by large amounts of change unless they approach it in an organized way and keep the ultimate goal in mind. This requires aligning the rational and emotional systems toward a greater goal.

You have probably learned through experience how to adjust more readily to change. For instance, when the COVID-19 pandemic caused widespread anxiety, fear, and panic, nurses needed to be rapidly adaptable and resilient. Senge et al. (2011) note that we must confront fear and anxiety. They describe the conflict that can exist between those who embrace and believe in the change and those who either do not believe in the change or resist it. As you embark on the registered nursing program of study, you may find yourself confronted at times with such challenges. Sometimes, it helps to read about others coping with change processes in order to view ourselves more objectively and thereby better cope and reach resolution. Two fun and easy-to-read books on change that describe how different people react and adjust to change may be helpful to you. In *Who Moved My Cheese?* author Spencer Johnson (1998) uses the analogy of a maze. Two mice, Sniff and Scurry, and two "little people," Hem and Haw, demonstrate differing reactions to change when a new cheese is introduced into the maze. In *Our Iceberg Is Melting: Changing and Succeeding Under Any Conditions*, authors John Kotter and Holger Rathgeber (2017) use the analogy of penguins who live on an Antarctic iceberg and describe their approaches in adjusting to change. When reading these two humorous but informative texts, you will likely see yourself and those close to you in various reactions and adjustments as you experience role transition and change in entering the registered nursing program.

THINKING CRITICALLY
Read the two books mentioned above. With which characters do you identify? What can you learn from other characters to help you adjust to the change you are experiencing in your role transition to a student nurse and then an RN?

ATTITUDE
The manner in which one approaches change can have a major effect on the ability to adapt. For instance, an employer informs a nurse who has been employed full time by a community health agency for 7 years that only full-time nurses will be taking emergency calls in the future. The nurse can approach this change in several ways. The first is to endorse the change as positive for continuity of care for the clients who are seen by the agency. The second approach would be to lament to the employer that this is not a fair system and that everyone should have to take calls. This nurse has some control over their adjustment to change, depending on which attitude they adopt.

In other changes that are more sudden, or in which an individual has less control, it may be more difficult to have the appropriate attitude. If a loved one dies suddenly, although a positive attitude will assist a person to adjust, other strategies are commonly used. For instance, one person may solicit the support of family members and friends. Others may benefit from joining a support group consisting of people who are experiencing a similar situation. Some people plunge into work or other activities so that they can get on with the business of living and avoid dwelling on the loss.

FLEXIBILITY
Maintaining an approach that incorporates **flexibility** also assists with successful adaptation to change. Especially during rapid or unplanned change, flexibility can help you shift priorities quickly to minimize negative results and move ahead. Flexibility allows you to discover unforeseen opportunities and to grow. In *The Reflective Life*, Tiberius (2008, 2010) advocates that one acquires self-knowledge in order to be more successful at what one attempts and to set future goals. She notes the need to know our values but to have the wisdom to be reflective, to question these values, and to be flexible to change as needed.

COPING STRATEGIES
Coping strategies vary and often depend on the circumstances and previous coping methods used. When faced with change, one person may try to avoid it, whereas another faces it directly. A third person may try to enlist the support of others or gather more information to deal with the change more effectively. All these methods may be effective in the adjustment to change.

In your return to school, you must identify what strategies will assist you in being successful. Obviously, a positive attitude is extremely beneficial, not only for you but also for your student colleagues. It is often useful to develop a support system within the student nurse group. A small group of colleagues will provide support and guidance for many issues that you encounter while in school. Some find that it helps to study together or to socialize away from school to adjust more effectively to the changes caused by returning to school.

> **THINKING CRITICALLY**
>
> In your return to school, consider the strategies that are useful for you as you adjust to the changes that school necessitates. Summarize methods that help you cope with change. Compare these methods with those of another nursing student and assess alternative methods you each could use.

Successful coping depends on our perception of change (i.e., how we approach it will determine the amount of stress it poses), our flexibility, and our ability to adapt to change. The degree to which we have support structures in place will also influence our ability to adapt to change. For example, the returning student who forms relationships with their peers will find that those same peers can be a support to some of the change that student is experiencing. Likewise, family and other social systems to which we belong can have a positive or negative effect on our ability to adapt to change. Consider the situation of Deborah, from the case study at the beginning of this chapter. As Deborah continues her employment at the mental health unit where she has worked for many years, and shares her frustration and concerns with her coworkers, their response(s) may influence her either positively or negatively in her ability to cope with the change she is confronting.

As discussed in previous chapters, there are also many support services at colleges today for students who are having difficulty with the return to school and the academic arena. Additionally, some nursing programs have established mentoring and "big brother/big sister" programs to support new students.

William Bridges (2009, 2016) describes how individuals manage transitions as they move through three stages. In the first stage, that of "ending, losing, and letting go," one lets go of the old ways and the old identity. In the second stage, which he describes as the "neutral zone," "critical psychological realignments and repatternings take place." In the third and final stage, "the new beginning" is established. He states, "This is when people develop the new identity, experience the new energy, and discover the new sense of purpose that make the change begin to work" (2009, pp. 4–5). It is at this time that you will experience positive outcomes of change. More information on Bridges' three phases of transition are presented in Chapter 2.

POSITIVE OUTCOMES OF CHANGE

Change has the possibility of many positive outcomes. Within any change process, the positive aspects of the change should be visualized as you embrace the change process. This will assist you in aligning rational and emotional systems toward common goals. In examining positive outcomes of change, the following relates to your process of returning to school and the changes that will occur.

The possible positive outcomes are as follows:

1. You will acquire more education and knowledge. Although the educational process can be overwhelming or frustrating at times, the benefit will be an

increased ability to integrate theory with practice and to be more informed regarding client care and healthcare issues.

2. One of the reasons that you returned to school may have been related to a desire to increase responsibilities and scope of practice. The RN role will provide more opportunities for career mobility, flexibility, and professional development.

3. Another positive outcome of change will be monetary rewards. Salaries for RNs have improved in the last decade. The potential for financial growth continues to be greater within the professional roles, even with the uncertainty of future healthcare reform.

4. With any additional education, there is a greater potential for increased prestige. Although such recognition may not seem important or may seem to have elitist overtones, being recognized for increased knowledge, skills, and associated achievements reaps the reward of educational changes. The ADN and the title of RN bestow a distinct and honorable recognition and provide opportunities for increased decision-making.

5. Along with increased prestige comes increased self-confidence and self-esteem. As you recall from your LPN/LVN training, Abraham Maslow identified a hierarchy of basic needs. According to his theory, after physiological, safety and security, and love and belonging needs are met, an individual has needs of esteem and self-esteem. Esteem needs include respect from others, recognition, prestige, and importance. Self-esteem needs encompass those related to achievement, competence and independence, and self-worth. Advanced education provides a greater means to achieve a belief in your own abilities and thus to have self-confidence and self-esteem.

6. A final positive outcome of change is self-actualization. Maslow theorized that the highest level of needs occurs when the other basic needs have been met. **Self-actualization** is the need to be all that you can be through self-fulfillment and reaching your potential. In your return to school, you are fulfilling a dream or a goal. You are also increasing your ability to solve problems, broadening your means to deal with various situations, and developing greater power to cope with stress. The positive outcomes of change are varied. Each change with which you are faced provides the opportunity for positive outcomes.

THINKING CRITICALLY

Critique an organizational change that has occurred in your workplace or within a community organization with which you are involved. Compare and contrast the positive outcomes experienced with that change, both for the organization and for yourself.

CONCLUSION

Change is a dynamic and ongoing process. Many of the changes that we face are not of our choosing. However, we also have the ability to effect our own change and to plan for and deal with the results. Nurses must understand the dynamics of the change process.

Not only do nurses face the challenges of personal changes but they also encounter the changes that their clients face. The processes of stress and adaptation, and the coping strategies that individuals use, are important to understand. Nurses are also involved with organizational changes, which can involve complex processes personally and collectively. The effects of change are varied and often depend on individual and group coping mechanisms.

Nursing and healthcare in general is ever changing. Although it is impossible to predict what changes will occur in the future, it is certain that change will be continuous. As you confront the changes occurring in your life as you return to school, you are in a unique position to develop new coping strategies to ease the transition process and experience the positive outcomes of change. Developing strengths during this transition will give you new knowledge of how to both be an effective change agent and assist clients and colleagues experiencing change.

STUDENT *Exercises*

Exercise 3.1

Recruit another student, peer, or friend to assist you with the following exercise:
Create a change situation that involves role-playing a client who is faced with a new diagnosis of heart disease.

1. Determine what factors may motivate this client to change their lifestyle.
2. Identify possible restraining and driving forces of the change.
3. Discuss the possible effects of change related to the impact of the diagnosis and the need for a change in lifestyle.
4. Develop a plan that will assist the client to move effectively through Bridges' three phases of the transition they will experience with the change.

Exercise 3.2

Given a case study of a planned organizational change in the healthcare industry:

1. Identify if the change is transactional or transformational.
2. Apply the three phases of Bridges' transition to the organization.
   a. What endings are in play and how well are they being managed? What else could be done?
   b. What characteristics of the neutral zone are in play?
   c. What new beginnings are evident in the case?
3. Apply concepts from one of the authors in the section *Adjusting to Change*. What characteristics are evident in the case? What strategies could the nurse manager use to assist those having difficulty with the change?

Exercise 3.3 (Optional but Fun Exercise)

Choose one of the following:

1. Read the short story *Our Iceberg Is Melting: Changing and Succeeding Under Any Conditions*, by John Kotter and Holger Rathgeber (2017). Evaluate the behavior of those in the above case study and which penguins are representative of which

individuals in the case. Compare your evaluation with those in your peer study group and discuss the differences in your evaluations.
2. Read the short story *Who Moved My Cheese?* by author Spencer Johnson (1998). Evaluate the behavior of those in the above case study and determine which individuals are represented by Sniff, Scurry, Hem, and Haw in Johnson's story by their differing reactions to change. Compare your evaluation with those in your peer study group, and discuss the differences in your evaluations.

REFERENCES

Boyle, J. C., Collins, J. W., Ludwig-Beymer, P., & Andrews, M. M. (2025). *Transcultural concepts in nursing care* (9th ed.). Wolters Kluwer.

Bridges, W. (2001). *The way of transition: Embracing life's most difficult moments.* Perseus.

Bridges, W. (2009). *Managing transitions: Making the most of change* (3rd ed.). Perseus.

Bridges, W., & Bridges, S. (2016). *Managing transitions: Making the most of change* (4th ed.). Hachette Book Group.

Buckway, A. J., & Sowerby, H. (2023). *Nursing in today's world: Trends, issues, & management* (12th ed.). Wolters Kluwer.

Heath, C., & Heath, D. (2010). *Switch: How to change things when change is hard.* Broadway Books.

Huston, C. J. (2023). *Professional issues in nursing: Challenges and opportunities* (6th ed.). Wolters Kluwer.

Johnson, S. (1998). *Who moved my cheese?* G.P. Putnam's Sons.

Kotter, J., & Rathgeber, H. (2017). *Our iceberg is melting: Changing and succeeding under any conditions* (10th anniversary ed.). Penguin Random House LLC.

Kübler-Ross, E. (1969). *On death and dying.* Macmillan.

Lewin, K. (1951). *Field theory in social science.* Harper & Row.

Merriam-Webster. (n.d.). Change. In *Merriam-Webster.com dictionary*. Retrieved from https://www.merriam-webster.com/dictionary/change

Perlman, D., & Takacs, G. (1990). The ten stages of change. *Nursing Management, 21*(4), 33–38.

Selye, H. (1976). *The stress of life* (rev. ed.). McGraw-Hill.

Senge, P., Kleiner, A., Roberts, C., Rose, R., Roth, G., & Smith, B. (2011). *The dance of change: The challenges of sustaining momentum in a learning organization.* Nicholas Bradley Publishing.

Taylor, C., Lynn, P., & Bartlett, J. L. (2023). *Fundamentals of nursing: The art and science of nursing care* (10th ed.). Wolters Kluwer.

Tiberius, V. (2008). *The reflective life.* Oxford University Press.

Tiberius, V. (2010). *The reflective life: Living wisely with our limits.* University Press.

On the WEB

For more information on change theory, go to http://www.google.com and enter "Lewin's change theory" or "change management"; see also http://www.elisabethkublerross.com (Kübler-Ross's website).

Transitions Throughout Nursing's History

CHAPTER 4

LEARNING OUTCOMES

By the end of this chapter, the student will be able to:
1. Describe the characteristics of a professional nurse.
2. Examine the significant historic events in nursing that influenced its development.
3. Outline benchmarks of the evolution of nursing as a profession.
4. Summarize the various educational programs in nursing.
5. Analyze the effects of societal trends on the profession and on the practice of nursing.
6. Give examples of the impact of changes in healthcare on the nursing profession.

KEY TERMS

- articulation agreement
- assistive personnel
- autonomy
- baby boomers
- bioethics
- biomedical technology
- bioterrorism
- cloning
- continuous quality improvement (CQI)
- cost containment
- cryogenics
- cultural humility
- cultural proficiency
- diagnostic related groups (DRGs)
- ecological intelligence
- educational mobility
- emotional intelligence
- entrepreneur
- evidence-based practice (EBP)
- experiential wisdom
- external degree
- flexible spending accounts (FSAs)
- gender equity
- genetic engineering
- globalism
- Health Insurance Portability and Accountability Act (HIPAA)
- health maintenance organizations (HMOs)
- health savings accounts (HSAs)
- holistic nursing
- managed care
- metaparadigm
- Nurse Licensure Compact (NLC)
- nursing informatics (NI)
- outcomes assessment
- palliative care
- posttraumatic stress disorder (PTSD)
- preferred provider organizations (PPOs)
- quality assurance (QA)
- robotics
- service learning
- student learning outcomes (SLOs)
- total quality management (TQM)

85

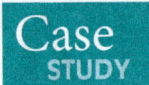 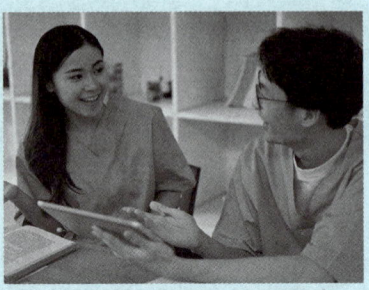

Case STUDY

Lucy Braveheart and Qian Chin are two students who have formed a study group. They are meeting in a library study room to discuss the upcoming lecture.

QIAN: Today, we're supposed to discuss the history of nursing. History is something I've never been really good at. I think it's because I find it boring.

LUCY: I think it all depends on how it's presented. I've heard that the professor has a unique way of presenting this topic. The fourth semester students say that she dresses up like Florence Nightingale and helps students learn about her thinking through a monologue. Some say you can imagine what it was like back then.

QIAN: I guess I'm remembering those dry history lessons in school where we were lectured to about historical battles and such.

LUCY: I've always been interested in history. Being Native American, my family has a lot of traditions, and I value the history of our customs. It's fun to imagine what it was like for my ancestors. I think it will be fun imagining what it was like for Florence.

QIAN: I'm Chinese, and I value my family's heritage and what the elders teach me. I guess it's important to learn history so we won't repeat the mistakes from the past and so that we can make the future better.

The history of nursing is rich and tumultuous. In many respects, the history of nursing is a general reflection of society, particularly regarding gender roles and the blurring of gender stereotypes. Knowing nursing history is crucial to understanding and appreciating today's world of nursing. Although nurses have existed in some form since there have been people on this earth, nursing as it is known today is a relatively young profession.

The workplace for nurses has changed radically in the past several decades, and nurses will continue to be challenged by changes in society, technology, and the healthcare industry. The issues that confronted nurses in the past are the foundation for the profession and practice of nursing today, just as those that exist today are the foundation for nursing tomorrow.

DEVELOPMENT OF NURSING

The history and origin of nursing are multifaceted. The evolution of nursing from ancient times through the ages was influenced by many factors, including Christianity, the military, and the Nightingale reform.

ANCIENT ORIGINS

People have always required care when they were sick, injured, pregnant, or dying. Women, as illustrated by cave drawings of women caring for sick children or preparing a brew of herbs and bark to aid an ill person, have generally done this work. Although little is known about nursing as a specific entity in ancient times, men and women caregivers can be found in early cultures.

In ancient Egypt, priests were usually identified as physicians or healers and were responsible for healing people who had diseases. The priests acted as the link between humans and the gods. It was believed that people had to keep the gods happy to have good health and peace of mind. The priests or physicians did not interfere with the process of childbirth and infant care; they left that work to midwives and wet nurses; these were women who had developed special skills and abilities to assist friends and neighbors.

The ancient Israelites formulated strict codes for personal hygiene and cleanliness. They instituted careful handwashing techniques, boiling of water, meat inspection, and other sanitation measures. Their practices were important in the development of hygiene practices in modern medicine.

Ancient Hindus in India had a team approach to the care of the sick. The team consisted of a patient, a healer (physician), and a nurse (who was a man). Each person had specific duties and functions. The Hindus employed the use of various instruments and surgical techniques. Many of the treatments that used herbs, plants, or animal parts were discovered by accident or trial and error.

Ancient China is known for the use of acupuncture, drug therapy, massage, hydrotherapy, and exercise to treat and prevent illness. Many of these same procedures and techniques are used today. Practitioners believed that a balance between Yang (which was defined as the male elements of light, life, and optimism) and Yin (which was defined as the female elements of dark, lifelessness, and cold) kept the body in harmony and health.

In other ancient cultures, such as those in South America, there is evidence that hygiene, diet, and herbal medicine practices were important. Not much is known about nursing care specifically, although it appears that women were esteemed for their knowledge of medicines. As with other ancient cultures, the emphasis was usually on the balance between good and evil spirits, and the appeasement of the gods.

CHRISTIAN ORIGINS

In early Christianity, there was a renewed focus on the value and dignity of human life. Bishops of the church were charged with caring for those in need, but the services were actually rendered by deacons and deaconesses. Women—in particular, deaconesses, matrons, widows, and virgins—took care of the sick in their homes.

To serve as deaconesses of the early Eastern Christian Church, women were required to be unmarried or widowed only once. The deaconesses were often wealthy women of culture and education from fine homes and backgrounds, were ordained, and worked on an equal basis with the deacon. Early counterparts to the community health nurses of today, the deaconesses carried medicine and food in baskets to people's homes.

As Christian churches were established, orders were formed that provided care for the sick, injured, poor, orphaned, widowed, and older adults. In early Christian times, men and women were considered equal, and there were more opportunities for single women to serve within these orders than had ever been available before. Within the religious orders, there was an established hierarchy of rank. This hierarchy demanded that there be absolute discipline and adherence to maintaining the rank and order. Some of the doctrines of faith, charity, servitude, and discipline of the early religious orders have continued to be part of modern nursing, serving to influence today's healthcare arena.

During the rise of Christianity, there was tremendous turmoil and chaos as battles and wars raged. Many men were killed, leaving many widows. Survival of widows during these troubled times was not a priority of society. For this reason, many of these women became interested in the various religious orders as a means of survival. Eventually, the Order of the Widows was formed. These women no longer had home responsibilities and were able to devote themselves to the care of the poor. As the church placed more value on purity of the body, the Order of the Virgins evolved. They were later called nuns nonnuptaeor, meaning "not married." Convents were built to provide safe shelter for women, and the nuns continued to care for the poor and the sick within these shelters. Deaconesses also existed in Western Europe, where they were called "matrons," but the Western church suppressed the deaconess movement, which became nearly extinct (Nutting & Dock, 1907).

The Middle Ages (c. 500–1500 AD) occurred after the fall of the Roman Empire. The development of medical science and nursing care halted because the focus of the Christian Church shifted to preparing for the afterlife. Europe was divided into many kingdoms, which were continually at war with each other; poverty, illness, and starvation were widespread. Religious orders grew even stronger, particularly as deaconesses lost favor and decreased in great numbers. Monks and nuns of various religious orders assumed control of hospitals. However, they were more concerned with spiritual, rather than physical, care of the ill.

MILITARY ORIGINS

The Crusades in the late Middle Ages lasted for about 200 years (c. 1090–1290 AD). The Crusaders were generally men of religious and military orders: priests, brothers, and knights. Their mission was to reclaim the Holy Land for the Christian faithful. As they traveled throughout Europe and the Near East, they gathered new information, learned new ways of doing things, and obtained different products and goods. The Crusaders were particularly interested in the organized facilities for the sick used by Muslims. As a result, similar hospitals were built near battlefields; the men were sometimes assigned to fighting and sometimes to caring for the sick and the injured. Eventually, military nursing orders evolved.

An example of a military nursing order was the Knights Hospitallers of St. John, located outside Jerusalem. These men staffed two hospitals and, in addition to caring for patients, frequently had to defend the hospital and the patients. They wore habits with a Maltese cross and a suit of armor underneath. Many nurses today wear pins that designate the school from which they graduated. One of the symbols used by some schools, such as the Nightingale School, is the Maltese cross, whereas other schools use another form of a cross. Additional symbols are also used, with many representing the military origins of earlier centuries. Military nursing orders advocated strict discipline and hierarchical lines of authority that emphasized devotion and obedience.

As the Crusaders returned to their homes, they brought with them a vision of improvement. Religious and secular groups developed hospitals and clinics that were better able to meet the needs of the sick and the injured. The organizations became structured and ordered. The caregivers, or nurses, wore white robes and were given a hood on completion of a novitiate period. They remained responsible to a director or maitresse. During this time, nursing care was valued, although advances in medical science were not. Nursing care generally involved providing comfort measures and hygiene. There was no scientific basis for nursing care. Toward the end of the Middle

Ages, many countries were faced with rampant diseases and plague. The need for advancements in medicine was acute.

PROTESTANT REFORMATION

Beginning in 1517, various Protestant churches were created as church leaders took issue with the Roman Catholic Church. In countries where the reformation was widespread, the care of the sick suffered because there were not enough nuns to provide that care. Deaconesses were urged to take on this work. However, the standards that had marked military and nursing orders previously were not maintained; thus, the quality of care greatly diminished. In addition, Protestant women had religious freedom, but they did not have other freedoms, such as being able to work outside the home. Society expected them to remain at home to provide care for children and older family members and to assume other domestic responsibilities. As a result, the caliber of nurses was diminished. In countries such as England, nurses in the 1800s were generally considered to be drunkards or thieves because many women chose to do their jail time serving within a hospital setting. Conditions in hospitals were deplorable, and mortality rates escalated greatly.

In the 15th to 19th centuries, medical progress was more profound. Many advances were made in the knowledge of anatomy and physiology, as well as in the use of pharmaceutical agents and surgical techniques. For example, the vaccination for smallpox was developed, the microscope was invented, and pasteurization was developed. However, the practice of nursing did not advance until after the mid-1800s.

THE NIGHTINGALE REFORM

In 1836, in Kaiserswerth, Germany, a young Protestant minister named Theodor Fliedner strove to revitalize the deaconess movement by starting a training institute for deaconesses. As part of this institute, he and his wife started a nursing course that included hands-on training and some lectures by physicians. Fliedner's work and the formation of other secular and religious groups once again laid the foundation for the growth of nursing.

Florence Nightingale was born in 1820 to a family of wealth and social standing. With her culture and education, she was expected to marry and continue the traditions of English society women. However, she had a strong desire to be a nurse. Her family considered this ambition absurd, but she nonetheless managed to learn about hospital reforms and public health issues and became an expert in these areas. In her travels and through information from friends, she learned about the institute at Kaiserswerth. Because it was a church-sponsored institution, she was allowed to attend the nursing program. She spent 3 months in the program learning as much as she could about nursing.

After returning to England, Nightingale continued her own studies and served on a committee that oversaw the Establishment for Gentlewomen During Illness. Although her family was not happy about her continued interest in nursing and in hospitals, Nightingale was later appointed superintendent of this organization. Her work in that capacity resulted in general acknowledgment of her expertise about hospitals and the need for educated nurses. Nightingale was asked to take a group of nurses to the Crimean War battlefields to improve the conditions there. Thirty-eight nurses who met Nightingale's standards accompanied her to Scutari. The work that was accomplished there was nothing short of miraculous. When they arrived, the conditions were filthy and unsafe. Through Nightingale's extraordinary efforts and with the assistance of powerful English friends, the situation improved dramatically. Sanitary and hygienic measures were instituted and maintained, nutritious food was provided, and conditions radically improved. Nightingale was especially concerned about the welfare of the soldiers and was able to obtain sick pay for them, along with other benefits that improved their health and well-being. The mortality rate was reduced from 50% to 60% to approximately 1% to 2%. Nightingale became known as a ministering angel and the "lady with the lamp" because of her late night rounds to ensure that all was well.

Improving conditions at the battlefields was not without its own conflicts. The physicians and military officers resented Nightingale's intrusion, and some of the nurses who were involved argued with each other and disagreed with Nightingale. She tended to be resolute in accomplishing her mission and was known to be stubborn, obstinate, and strong willed. During her service in the Crimean War, Nightingale became ill with what was called the Crimean fever and came close to death. However, she recovered and remained in service until the end of the war.

When Nightingale returned to England, she became somewhat of a recluse due to her health problems. However, she still was able to exert a powerful influence on the development of nursing because of the widespread fame that she attained as a result of her accomplishments in the Crimean War. She wrote many books and reports that demonstrated her ability to use research and statistics. Many refer to her as the first nurse researcher, drawing conclusions that today would be termed "evidence-based nursing research." Nightingale also continued to work to develop nursing education and to improve the conditions for soldiers, particularly those stationed abroad. She established the Nightingale Fund, which was later used to establish a training school for nurses, and was awarded the Cross of St. George by Queen Victoria.

Nightingale System of Education

Nightingale established a training school for nurses in 1860. It was founded at St. Thomas' Hospital as a 1-year program. Women between the ages of 25 and 35 years were selected based on qualifications relating to their character, conduct, and desire to be a nurse. The nursing program was highly structured and rigorous. Nightingale also recognized the need for both theory and practice in training nurses and saw that the educational program must stand alone so that students could focus on their training apart from hospital service. See Box 4.1 for Nightingale's principles for the education of nurses.

BOX 4.1

Nightingale's Principles for the Education of Nurses

1. Nursing is an art and a science.
2. The student must be taught to treat the patient as a human, not a disease, and there must be compassion and empathy for each individual.
3. The emphasis must be on education, not service. For this reason, a school of nursing should be independent from the hospital.
4. Graduate nurses should always continue their education.
5. Nurses must be taught to take care of the sick and must not do the laundry, clean, run errands, and other such chores that take them away from their nursing responsibilities.
6. Education for nurses should be a combination of theory and practice.

Source: Buckway, A. J., & Sowerby, H. (2023). *Nursing in today's world: Trends, issues, and management* (12th ed.). Wolters Kluwer.

The Nightingale system of education is considered to be the beginning of modern nursing education and the start of professional nursing. Nightingale's insistence on discipline and high moral character had a profound effect on the growth of modern nursing and the education of nurses—effects that continue to influence nursing education today. Within the first two decades after the Nightingale Training School opened, its graduates became superintendents in hospitals throughout Europe, Asia, and the United States. A whole new system of professional nursing was introduced throughout the world. For a more in-depth review of the history of nursing, refer to Buckway and Sowerby (2023).

THINKING CRITICALLY

Consider the following statement from the commemorative edition of Nightingale's first 1859 edition (Nightingale, 1992):

> I use the word nursing for want of a better. It has been limited to signify little more than the administration of medicines and the application of poultices.... It ought to signify the proper use of fresh air, light, warmth, cleanliness, quiet, and the proper selection and administration of diet—all at the least expense of vital power to the patient. (p. 6)

What is the relevance of this statement to nursing as you know it today? How does this philosophy relate to the expansion of holistic nursing and spiritual nursing? What would you add to this statement to reflect the current broader, more comprehensive scope of professional nursing?

NURSING IN THE UNITED STATES

The growth of nursing in the United States was stimulated in particular by the Civil War, which began in 1861. Prior to that, there was no organized method for caring for the sick, especially during times of war. Women were the primary caregivers in the home or in the homes of neighbors. There were few formal educational programs available, except those that were within Catholic sisterhoods, and nursing education was relatively unavailable to men and those from other religions and ethnicities.

The beginning of the Civil War uncovered an obvious need for nurses and prompted many women to volunteer to care for wounded soldiers. Although they were not trained as nurses, they demonstrated great compassion and concern. The Union Army appointed Dorothea Dix, a woman who had championed causes for people with mental illness, to be the superintendent for these nurses and to provide them with some training. Women from religious orders, assisted by other women who were not trained nurses, volunteered in the North and the South. In the South, fewer women volunteered because it was not socially acceptable. Many hospitals were built during the Civil War to house the large numbers of wounded soldiers. The nurses of this time experienced multiple difficulties: The working conditions were deplorable, the Army medical staff did not always think highly of them, and they were generally poorly treated. However, they persevered, and in some areas, their work was well received and respected.

After the Civil War in 1865, there was a recognized need for educated nurses. The popularity of Florence Nightingale in England and the proliferation of educated

Nightingale nurses also helped promote the growth of nursing in the United States. In 1869, the American Medical Society proposed that the issue of trained nurses should be investigated. As a result of that study, three schools for the training of nurses opened in 1873: the Bellevue Training School in New York City, the Connecticut Training School, and the Boston Training School. Although these training programs were theoretically modeled after the Nightingale system, the major thrust was service, as opposed to education. From around 1873 to 1883, several schools of nursing opened. Hospitals realized that there was economic value in having student nurses deliver the bulk of patient care and other tasks; essentially, the student nurses provided a free labor force for the hospitals. Despite the hardships, these programs were popular because they provided young women, who had limited choices during that time, with the eventual means to earn a living. Nursing was considered an acceptable role for women and provided a slightly higher income than any other occupation available to them (Jacob, 2023).

Uniforms and caps were not originally a traditional characteristic of training schools. In 1875, the first cap was used to cover long hair and particularly long, dirty hair. Its function was practical, not decorative. Later, a student at Bellevue Training School designed a student uniform. Eventually, caps, uniforms, and school pins came to signify a certain school or particular accomplishments within the school and have continued to be part of nursing heritage.

In the early 1900s, nurses were expected to be submissive within a hospital organization and to the dominance of physicians, similar to the general expectation for women in the patriarchal society. The woman was esteemed by her husband and had limited power within the confines of the home and society. She was expected to be hard working and able to maintain harmony while also being submissive to the demands of her husband. However, some women of this time worked hard for reform and laid the foundation for future societal changes for women in general and nurses in particular.

The first licensure laws for nursing did not exist until 1903, and even with the first law's passage, licensure was not mandatory or enforced. Hospitals continued to promote their own needs and not those of nurses or students. A few nursing programs moved to an educational setting, but the education continued to be practice driven and involved long hours. There were many objections to nurses being overeducated and overtrained. Physicians in particular did not perceive a need for nurses to have increased education. Two important factors in the development of nursing in the United States were the upgrading of The Johns Hopkins School of Nursing in 1918, in which the need for improved education of public health nurses was stressed, and the opening of the Yale School of Nursing in 1924, which was the first separate university department with its own dean.

Many of nursing's important leaders emerged from the late 1800s to the early 1900s. A few of the many leaders who helped change the course of nursing were:

- Lavinia Dock (1858–1956): She was an early graduate of Bellevue Training School and later an assistant to Isabelle Hampton Robb. She was an early organizer of what is now known as the National League for Nursing (NLN). She wrote *History of Nursing*, which remains a classic on that subject.
- Adelaide Nutting (1858–1948): She was a graduate of the Johns Hopkins program and later a principal of that school. She obtained funding to improve the education for public health nurses and was a strong advocate for reform in nursing education. Nutting later developed the nursing department at Teachers College, Columbia

University. She was able to establish a 3-year nursing program and to reduce a student nurse's workday to 8 hours.
- Linda Richards (1841–1930): Called American's first trained nurse, she moved from one hospital to another to establish new training programs and to upgrade the quality of nursing services.
- Isabelle Hampton Robb (1859–1910): She graduated from Bellevue Training School after having been a teacher. She was instrumental in improving conditions for student nurses and founded the program at Johns Hopkins. When she married and resigned her position, she still maintained an active interest in nursing. She authored nursing textbooks, helped in the formation of the first nursing organization, and was one of the founders of the *American Journal of Nursing*.
- Lillian Wald (1867–1940): She founded the Henry Street Settlement in New York in 1893. This marked the beginning of public health nursing in the United States. She was particularly interested in the ability of nursing graduates to provide high-quality care to people within their homes.

The changes that occurred in the 20th century reflect the hard work and dedication of women who were compelled to advocate reform in nursing. Although the women's movement sometimes ignored their work, their accomplishments did contribute to the advances women have experienced in general.

The presence of African Americans and men in nursing is not well documented. The first African American graduate of a training program was Mary Mahoney in 1879. She was dedicated to the promotion of excellence in the care of private duty patients and the acceptance of African Americans within the nursing profession. Although African American nurses were not accepted for military service until World War II, Adah Thomas fought for the acceptance of African American nurses in World War I and was effective in enabling African American nurses to work for the American Red Cross. The prejudice against men in nursing also was high, and men were not influential in nursing until after World War II. Today, however, nurses who are men and nurses from multiple ethnicities are common, although the nursing workforce is still not as diverse as the patients/clients in their care ("Nursing Workforce," 2023). Ongoing efforts in this area will continue to strengthen the profession of nursing, because multiple perspectives yield an enriched foundation upon which evidence-based practice (EBP) can be built.

The NCLEX-RN *Might Ask* 4.1

Which of the following social trends is most likely to impact the future supply and demand for nurses?
a. Aging population
b. Multiculturalism
c. Healthcare reform
d. Telecommunications

- See Appendix A for correct answer and rationale.

PROFESSIONAL NURSING ORGANIZATIONS

The formation of nursing organizations initiated the process of using cooperative efforts to achieve common goals and missions. Nurses found that a collective voice was much more likely to have an impact on the development of nursing.

NATIONAL LEAGUE FOR NURSING

The NLN focuses on nursing education. The first nursing organization in the United States, the NLN was established in 1893. The group was initially called the American Society of Superintendents of Training Schools for Nurses in the United States and Canada. These nurses gathered for the purpose of improving and standardizing the education of nurses. In 1912, they changed the organization's name to the National League of Nursing Education. Membership was originally limited to nurses, but in 1943, the League decided to open membership to lay members. There continue to be two levels of membership: individual and agency. Schools of nursing and other agencies that provide nursing services are eligible for membership as agency members.

In 1952, a major reorganization took place, along with another name change. The group became the NLN and actually merged seven organizations into one. These groups were the National League of Nursing Education (1893), the National Organization for Public Health Nursing (1912), the Association of Collegiate Schools of Nursing (1933), the Joint Committee on Practical Nurses and Auxiliary Workers in Nursing Services (1945), the Joint Committee on Careers in Nursing (1948), the National Committee for the Improvement of Nursing Services (1949), and the National Nursing Accrediting Service (1949). Although in some respects these were very diverse groups, they were able to formulate a common mission of promoting and providing for quality healthcare through effective nursing practice and education. The NLN supports nursing faculty and nursing education programs through its publications, newsletters, professional development activities, and accreditation processes. The NLN's (n.d.-a) focus on nursing education is reflected in its mission statement: "The National League for Nursing promotes excellence in nursing education to build a strong and diverse nursing workforce to advance the health of our nation and the global community." The NLN (n.d.-a) operates under a set of four core values:

- *CARING:* promoting health, healing, and hope in response to the human condition
- *INTEGRITY:* respecting the dignity and moral wholeness of every person without conditions or limitation
- *DIVERSITY:* affirming the uniqueness of and differences among persons, ideas, values, and ethnicities
- *EXCELLENCE:* cocreating and implementing transformative strategies with daring ingenuity

The NLN is associated with two nursing program accreditation entities. In 1996, the NLN Board of Directors approved the establishment of The National League for Nursing Accreditation Commission (NLNAC) to provide accreditation processes to schools that choose to participate. In 2013, the NLNAC was renamed the Accreditation Commission for Education in Nursing (ACEN) and became a subsidiary wholly owned by the NLN. The NLN then established the Commission for Nursing Education Accreditation (CNEA) as a programmatic accrediting body that is an autonomous accreditation division of the NLN. The NLN CNEA and ACEN are separate accrediting agencies, each with their own standards and policies. Accreditation via the CNEA process and through ACEN is voluntary for schools of nursing, involving the writing of a self-study report according to established criteria. Representatives of the Commission then visit the school to assess and evaluate the nursing program according to the established standards. These visitors make recommendations regarding accreditation of the program. Graduation from the NLN-accredited program provides for national recognition and the acceptance of credits from another NLN-accredited program if a graduate chooses to continue their education.

Not all schools of nursing participate in the labor-intensive and costly process. However, every nursing school participates in the accreditation/approval process conducted by its own state board of nursing. For those located in institutions of higher education, the institution's accreditation by a regional accrediting commission, recognized by the U.S. Department of Education, provides students and graduates portability and transfer of credit for ongoing education at another such institution within the same state or in a different state. The official research journal of the NLN is *Nursing Education Perspectives*. This peer-reviewed, bimonthly journal provides evidence for best practices in nursing education. Through the publication of rigorously designed studies, the journal contributes to the advancement of the science of nursing education. It serves as a forum for research and innovation regarding teaching and learning, curricula, technology, and other issues important to nursing education.

In addition, the NLN produces many books, monographs, and multimedia, and maintains a website. In an effort to make available vital statistics on nursing programs, nursing faculty, and nursing students, in 2008, the NLN began publishing all its data on the web (NLN, n.d.-c) under Nursing Education Statistics.

Since its inception in 1893 for the purpose of improving and standardizing the education of nurses, the NLN has maintained as its central theme a commitment to nursing education and has continued to be the leading professional association for nursing education. Its focus on nursing education includes all levels of nursing education. One of its most important publications is its *Outcomes and Competencies for Graduates of Practical/Vocational, Diploma, Associate Degree, Baccalaureate, Master's, Practice Doctorate, and Research Doctorate Programs in Nursing*, last updated in 2012. This document provides a set of outcomes and competencies for all program types. It helps nurse educators build curricula for their programs, further the science of nursing education, and explore and refine teaching, learning, and evaluation.

AMERICAN NURSES ASSOCIATION

The Nurses' Associated Alumnae of the United States and Canada was organized in 1896 by a group of nurses who believed that group action by nurses would be beneficial. In 1903, Canada's name had to be removed from the name of the organization to be able to incorporate, according to the laws of New York. The name of the organization was changed to the American Nurses Association (ANA) in 1911, and Canadian nurses formed their own national organization. The ANA is known as the professional organization for RNs) and limits its membership to RNs. There have been numerous changes throughout ANA's history, but it has always maintained a commitment to individual nurses, and in turn to the public, as recipients of the work nurses do. The ANA's (n.d.) mission statement is: "Lead the profession to shape the future of nursing and health care."

A significant change occurred in 1982, when the ANA adopted a federation model of membership. With this model, individual members join state nurses associations (SNAs), and the SNAs are members of the ANA. This was done in hopes of strengthening the state organizations and possibly increasing membership. Unfortunately, only a small percentage of employed nurses belong to their state organization. However, despite the relatively low membership, the ANA has been a powerful voice in nursing issues.

The official journal of the ANA is *American Nurse Today*. As a fresh, evidence-based voice of nursing, *American Nurse Today* covers cutting-edge issues in nursing practice and keeps nurses abreast of the ANA's advocacy on behalf of the profession. The journal also provides practical, clinical, and career management information that nurses can use to stay up to date on best practices, enhance patient outcomes, and advance their professional careers. ANA maintains a website, and an online publication named *The Online Journal of Issues in Nursing*, a peer-reviewed publication that provides a forum for discussion of the issues inherent in current topics of interest to nurses and other healthcare professionals. The intent of this journal is to present different views on issues that affect nursing research, education, and practice, thus enabling readers to understand the full complexity of a topic. The interactive format of the journal encourages a dynamic dialogue resulting in a comprehensive discussion of the topic, thereby building up the body of nursing knowledge and suggesting policy implications that enhance the health of the public.

The ANA encompasses a number of councils that represent specialty areas. Standards of practice have been developed by each council, whose function is to be a forum for discourse related to continuing education, consultation, and other issues that pertain to that council's interests. There are also two congresses, one for nursing practice and the other for nursing economics, whose function consists of setting policies, standards, new programs, and other related responsibilities. Other activities of the ANA include the following:

- Advanced certification of RNs
- Accreditation of continuing education programs
- Participation in public policy issues
- Development of an economic and general welfare program
- Promotion and support of research activities
- Publication of journals, pamphlets, and multimedia

Several areas of controversy have been prevalent throughout ANA's history and may be the reason that some nurses choose not to belong to this organization. One issue is ANA's position on entry into practice. In 1965, an ANA position paper advocated that the entry level for professional nursing should be the baccalaureate nurse. This issue has caused, and continues to cause, a great deal of conflict within nursing. Another area of conflict began in 1974 with the passage of the Taft–Hartley Act. This act legislated that professional nursing organizations could also be labor unions. Nurses in management positions or nurses who disagree with nurse professionals being represented by a bargaining unit frequently choose not to support the ANA. Other areas of conflict relate to ANA's support of various issues proposed for legislation. The ANA's active involvement in national and state health policy issues, although important, contributes to controversy over the positions and direction of the ANA by professional nurses. ANA's position statements on a wide array of issues can be found on its website.

NATIONAL COUNCIL OF STATE BOARDS OF NURSING

The National Council of State Boards of Nursing (NCSBN) comprises the boards of nursing from all 50 states in the United States and its five territories: American Samoa, Guam, Northern Mariana Islands, Puerto Rico, and the Virgin Islands. The mission of the NCSBN is to provide leadership to advance regulatory excellence for public protection. To that end, the NCSBN conducts studies of nursing practice to develop current, relevant test plans for the NCLEX-RN and the NCLEX-PN. These test plans are revised every 3 years, following a comprehensive workplace analysis, to ensure that they are up-to-date with current practice. In conjunction with the revision of the test plan, the

NCSBN also reviews and updates the passing score of the NCLEX. The most recent update to NCLEX testing in 2023 introduced Next Generation NCLEX (NGN) style questions. NGN questions are constructed to evaluate critical thinking, clinical reasoning, and clinical judgment in various patient scenarios that simulate real-life clinical settings ("Next Gen," n.d.).

Another effort by the NCSBN is to ensure that RNs and LPN/LVNs maintain continued competence in nursing following initial entry into the profession. The NCSBN has also taken a lead role in examining certification requirements for advanced practice registered nurses (APRNs). Each state's Nurse Practice Act outlines the scope of practice for APRNs. Similar to RN and LPN/LVN licensure, this often presents a barrier to nurses practicing in multiple states, and/or moving from one state to another, when the scope of practice for APRNs differ between states. In order to support licensure, certification, and practice portability, the NCSBN recommends APRN certification examinations as a basis for licensure decisions, advocates the APRN compact for mutual recognition of licensure to promote quality advanced practice nursing care within states and across state lines, and endorses the 2008 *Consensus Model for APRN Regulation: Licensure, Accreditation, Certification & Education*. The ANA's new *Nursing: Scope and Standards of Practice for Nursing* (2021) outlines standards also for APRNs. However, because practice is regulated at the state level under each state's Nurse Practice Act, efforts have been ongoing to gain support for this Consensus Model for APRNs. More than 40 nursing organizations thus far have endorsed the model.

OTHER NURSING ORGANIZATIONS

There are more than 60 organizations for and about nursing, including Sigma Theta Tau, nursing's professional honor society. Many clinical nursing specialties have their own organizations, and there are also organizations for nurses that are related to educational, religious, ethnic, and other special interests. All of these groups have recognized the importance and value of sharing ideas, research, and experiential knowledge, as well as collective effort and advocacy. In the area of nursing education, two organizations represent entry-level educational programs at the associate degree and baccalaureate degree levels. And one organization is responsible for creating the taxonomy of nursing diagnoses in use in many facilities.

Organization for Associate Degree Nursing

The Organization for Associate Degree Nursing (OADN), founded in 1984, is recognized nationally as the voice for Associate Degree Nursing. OADN is dedicated to enhancing the quality of Associate Degree Nursing education, strengthening the professional role of the Associate Degree Nurse, and promoting the future of Associate Degree Nursing as an entry point into registered nursing in the midst of healthcare changes. OADN's (n.d.) mission statement is: "OADN is the national voice and a pivotal resource for community college nursing education and the associate degree pathway."

OADN's official publication is *Teaching and Learning in Nursing*. It also publishes a variety of Position Statements and provides professional development opportunities for nursing faculty and practicing RNs.

OADN is a strong advocate for promoting the academic progression of ADN graduates in furthering education to reach their maximum professional potential. OADN also believes in collaboration with and among other nursing organizations to facilitate unity of the nursing profession.

American Association of Colleges of Nursing

The American Association of Colleges of Nursing (AACN) is the national voice for America's baccalaureate and higher degree nursing education institutions. Formed in 1969, it represents over 800 member schools of nursing at public and private universities nationwide. These schools offer a mix of baccalaureate, graduate, and postgraduate programs. AACN's mission is: "As the collective voice for academic nursing, AACN serves as the catalyst for excellence and innovation in nursing education, research, and practice."

The organization has a number of publications, white papers, and position statements on the profession of nursing. AACN works with other nursing organizations for advocacy and to promote the profession of nursing.

BUILDING A COALITION OF ORGANIZATIONS WITHIN NURSING

Increased economic pressures of the 21st century, healthcare reform, and a looming severe nursing shortage have together been a catalyst for even further collaboration among nursing organizations and led to the formation of The Nursing Community in 2009. The Nursing Community is a coalition of national professional nursing associations that builds consensus and advocates on a wide spectrum of healthcare and nursing issues, including practice, education, and research. The Nursing Community is committed to improving the health and healthcare of our nation by collaborating to support the education and practice of RNs and APRNs. Collectively, the Nursing Community is comprised of 63 national nursing organizations that represent nearly one million practicing nurses, nurse executives, and nursing students, faculty, and researchers. You can view the Nursing Community's core principles at http://www.thenursingcommunity.org/core-principle.

INTERNATIONAL COUNCIL OF NURSES

In addition to the many organizations for nursing in the United States and other countries, there is also an international organization where many of these organizations convene for an even broader collective effort. Founded in 1899, the International Council of Nurses (ICN) is a federation of more than 130 national nurses associations representing the millions of nurses worldwide. Operated by nurses, and leading nursing internationally, ICN works to ensure quality care for all and sound health policies globally. The ICN meets regularly and has produced such publications as *The ICN Code of Ethics for Nurses*, last updated in 2021. ICN commemorates International Nurses Day each year on May 12th—Florence Nightingale's birthday. (Visit https://www.icn.ch/sites/default/files/2023-04/Strategic%20plan.pdf to view the ICN strategic plan.)

> ## THINKING CRITICALLY
> As an LPN/LVN, do you currently belong to any nursing organization? As you enter professional nursing practice, your role will include advancing the profession. What areas of nursing do you feel need collective effort for redesigning or advancing the profession of nursing? Which nursing organization do you believe has an interest in this area or similar areas? What are the advantages of collective effort?

> **The NCLEX-RN** *Might Ask* 4.2
>
> Which of the following factors increased the need for cultural proficiency in nursing practice in the United States?
> a. The baby boom of 1946
> b. Demographic changes of patient populations
> c. A decrease in access to healthcare
> d. A decreasing rate of immigration
>
> • See Appendix A for correct answer and rationale.

EVOLUTION OF NURSING AS A PROFESSION

In the development of nursing as a profession and nurses as professionals, it is necessary to assure the public that the title of nurse represents a defined scope of responsibility and obligation to professional criteria and standards of practice. These are documented and updated regularly by the profession, as will be discussed later in this chapter, and licensure assures the public of the RN's practice within these parameters.

As a profession, nursing has a unique, distinct role and autonomy. RNs are professional, independent thinkers who observe, assess, think critically, perform evidence-based nursing diagnoses, and exercise clinical judgment in planning care for their patients/clients. Professional nurses also belong to organizations of the profession and advocate for advancement of the profession and its beliefs. These are examples of qualities necessary for the RN to be considered a professional and are inherent in the licensure process.

QUALITIES OF PROFESSIONAL NURSES

Professional nurses possess three intellectual characteristics: a body of knowledge on which professional nursing is based, a specialized education to transmit this body of knowledge to others, and the ability to use their knowledge in critical and creative thinking. Professional nurses use information and research from other professional disciplines and through their own evidence-based research and reflective practice contribute to the ongoing growth of knowledge in the discipline of nursing (Hood, 2022).

Professional nurses perform a service to society and as such have ethical obligations defined by the profession's code of ethics. The *Code of Ethics for Nurses with Interpretive Statements* (ANA, 2015) is discussed later in this chapter. This ethical and legal obligation to the public is guaranteed through a self-regulating licensure and credentialing system. Many nurses also reap intrinsic rewards from their professional practice, another characteristic common among professionals within a defined discipline.

A defining characteristic of a professional is one's **autonomy**, or self-determination over practice. Through the nursing process, the professional nurse is able to diagnose and design a plan of care for their clients, and supervise other healthcare providers who will assist in carrying out that plan of care. Additionally, the professional nurse's intellectual characteristics and discrete body of knowledge is used within collaborative healthcare teams to provide holistic care to the client/patient.

THINKING CRITICALLY

Which of the characteristics of a professional described above have most contributed to your motivation and desire to become an RN? Why are these qualities important? Beyond the additional technical skills you will gain, how do you see your nursing practice changing as you transition from the LPN/LVN role to the professional nurse role?

The move toward mandatory licensure; the development of nursing diagnoses, separate from medical diagnoses; the development of a social policy statement and a code of ethics for nurses; the growth of nursing theory, nursing conceptual models, and the establishment of doctoral degrees in nursing; the advances in nursing science and nursing research; and the formalization of EBP have all promoted nursing as an independent profession. Hood (2022) describes the profession of nursing as one that has gained many of the characteristics of a profession but is still an "emerging profession" because it has yet to adopt a standardized education for entry into the profession. Currently, there are three levels of education that qualify persons to take the licensing exam for professional nurse registration: diploma, associate degree, and baccalaureate degree nursing programs. These will be discussed later in this chapter.

LICENSURE

In the late 1800s, there was a move in the United States to license nurses. Nursing leaders of that time believed that a mechanism should exist to assure the public that nurses were competent to practice nursing according to defined standards. Licensed nurses would be designated as RNs. These early leaders recognized that the great variance in nursing education programs did not guarantee adherence to any standards. The organizations that preceded the NLN and the ANA supported the licensure of nurses. Although it was a difficult battle, licensure was eventually achieved, and a national examination called the NCLEX-RN was instituted. It is interesting to note that Florence Nightingale did not support nursing licensure. She advocated instead for ongoing education for nurses. Today, we call this "lifelong learning," and RNs participate in continuing education after initial licensure. It is common for a state to require a certain amount of continuing education for license renewal each year. See Box 4.2 for more information about the history of nursing licensure.

The early licensure laws granted permissive licensure, which means that the person was "permitted" to be licensed if requirements were met. Licensure was not required for a person to practice nursing. For that reason, employers made a distinction between RNs and nurses. North Carolina, New Jersey, New York, and Virginia first granted permissive licensure in 1903. Mandatory licensure was later advocated as an additional assurance to the public that all nurses were registered and thus met specific criteria and standards. In 1938, the first mandatory licensure law was passed in New York, and today, all 50 states require nurses to pass the NCLEX-RN examination and to be licensed and registered as professional nurses. Some states distinguish between "active" and "inactive" licensure status, requiring continuing education to maintain active status.

BOX 4.2 The History of Nursing Licensure

Date	Event
1867	Dr. Henry Wentworth Acland first suggests licensure for nurses in England.
1892	American Society of Superintendents of Training Schools for Nurses organized and supported licensure in the United States.
1901	New Zealand initiates first nursing licensure in the world.
1903	United States initiates nursing licensure (NC, NJ, NY, and VA—in that order).
1915	ANA drafts its first model nurse practice act.
1919	England initiates nursing licensure.
1923	United States completes nursing licensure in all 48 states.
1935	First mandatory licensure act in the United States: New York (effective 1947).
1946	Ten states include definitions of nursing in the licensing act.
1950	State Board Test Pool Examination in use in all U.S. states and territories.
1965	Twenty-one states include definitions of nursing in the licensing act.
1971	Idaho becomes the first state to recognize expanded practice in its nursing practice act.
1976	California becomes the first state to institute mandatory continuing education for relicensure.
1982	National Council Licensing Examination for Registered Nurses (NCLEX-RN) initiates use of nursing process as its organizing framework.
1987	North Dakota requires baccalaureate degree for RN licensure (rescinded 2003).
1994	Computer-adapted testing (CAT) is adopted nationwide for licensure.
1998	Mutual Recognition Nurse Licensure Compact (NLC) finalized; Utah is the first to become part of the Compact.
2000	Nursing Licensure Compact Administrators (NLCA) formed; NUR *SYS* completed, housing licensure and disciplinary data on nurses from more than 30 states.
2006	Twenty-three states complete adopted legislation to implement the NLC.
2007	NCLEX-RN begins new "integrated client needs" format; interactive CAT individualizes testing for each candidate.
2008	NCSBN adopts *Advanced Practice Registered Nurse (APRN) Model Act/Rules and Regulations* for licensure/certification of APRNs.
2011	APRN Compact: Utah, Iowa, and Texas join the APRN Compact.
2015	Twenty-five states have adopted NLC.
2015	APRN Compact: New Compact language allows an advanced practice registered nurse to hold one multistate license with a privilege to practice in other compact states.

Source: Buckway, A., & Sowerby, H. (2022). N*ursing in today's world: Trends, issues and management* (12th ed.). Wolters Kluwer; NCSBN, https://timeline.ncsbn.org/

Nurse practice acts evolved as licensure laws were enacted. Their purpose is to:
- Define nursing
- Stipulate the qualifications to practice nursing
- Outline the methods of obtaining licensure, licensure renewal, and interstate endorsement or reciprocity
- Establish and maintain rules and regulations of nursing
- Delineate unlawful acts, misconduct, or disciplinary actions
- Name the state agency (and its functions) that will oversee the nurse practice act (usually the state board of nursing comprising nurses, other professionals, and consumers)

By 1923, all states had some form of a nurse practice act. Since then, nurse practice acts have changed to reflect changes in nursing, the advent of the national examination and mandatory licensure. Licensure of APRNs is also covered in many states' nurse practice acts. It is imperative that licensed nurses are familiar with the nurse practice act for the state in which they practice, not only for current practice regulations but also to keep informed of changes and requirements for licensure renewal.

As of July 2023, 41 states or jurisdictions have adopted the **Nurse Licensure Compact (NLC)** for mutual recognition of RN licensure between and among states (National Council of State Boards of Nursing, 2023). In more recent years, many boards of nursing have adopted regulations for APRN in specialty areas, and many states are also considering the APRN Compact for mutual recognition of licensure for APRNs as well.

THE DISCIPLINE OF NURSING

Essential to any profession is an articulated definition of the discipline, its scope, practice standards, and beliefs. The ANA publishes three foundational documents, which are regularly reviewed and revised by members of the profession of nursing. These three, with their current revision dates, are as follows:

- *American Nurse's Association (2010)*
- *Code of Ethics for Nurses with Interpretive Statements (2015)*
- *Nursing: Scope and Standards of Practice (2021)*

Although the ANA publishes many other single-topic documents and policy statements regarding the profession of nursing, these three serve as the foundation for the discipline of nursing. They not only provide a unifying structure and guide for practicing nurse professionals but also serve to define the discipline of nursing and its scope, practice standards, and beliefs for other healthcare professions and the public to view. More information on these three documents (and the actual documents for purchase) can be found on ANA's website.

NURSING'S SOCIAL POLICY STATEMENT

Defining nursing has historically been problematic for the nursing profession. There are many viewpoints related to philosophical and practice perspectives. To address this issue, the ANA formulated and published *Nursing's Social Policy Statement*. First adopted in 1980, the *Social Policy Statement* was developed to assist nurses in conceptualizing their practice; to provide direction to educators, administrators, and researchers within nursing; and to inform other health professionals, legislators, funding bodies, and the public about nursing's contribution to healthcare. It is reviewed and revised as needed every several years to remain current with the profession.

Within this policy statement, the ANA incorporated the use of the nursing process and the diagnosis and treatment of human responses. This defined the autonomous and unique practice of nursing. The statement also stipulated that nurses are responsible and accountable to society for their actions, which may be in a variety of settings for clients of all ages. The ANA asserts that nurses must include preventive health measures in their practice. The policy statement also included a section about specialization in nursing practice, spearheading the move toward advanced nursing practice.

The statement has been important to the development of the nursing profession in that responsibility and professional accountability are viewed as essential elements of professional nursing practice. As new knowledge is gained, and as nurses' roles evolve, changes must also be made in the responsibilities. However, the accountability to the public remains unchanged; nurses accept defined responsibilities for providing care at a particular level. They are always accountable and must practice according to state licensure, rules and regulations, standards of practice, and the policy statement. The *Nursing's Social Policy Statement* has been revised several times since its initial 1980 adoption, with the most recent revision in 2010. As noted previously, *Nursing's Social Policy Statement* and two other documents, *Nursing: Scope and Standards of Practice* and *Code of Ethics for Nurses with Interpretive Statements*, serve as an ongoing core foundational trio for guiding the profession of nursing.

NURSING'S CODE OF ETHICS

A professional code of ethics is a guide for ethical behavior of practitioners in that professional field. A professional code does not have any legal authority, but it does advocate ethical and moral behavior for the profession's practitioners.

To address ethical issues in nursing, the ANA developed the first *Code for Nurses* in 1985. The ANA has reviewed and revised the code since its initial adoption, with extensive review and input from practicing nurses and nursing organizations. The most recent document, *Code of Ethics for Nurses with Interpretive Statements (Code of Ethics)*, was adopted in 2015 and can be viewed at https://www.nursingworld.org/practice-policy/nursing-excellence/ethics/code-of-ethics-for-nurses/. The *Code of Ethics* clearly expresses nursing's own understanding of its ethical standards, commitment to society, and the ethical obligations and duties of every individual entering the profession.

As noted previously, the ICN maintains an international code of ethics for nurses, *The ICN Code of Ethics for Nurses*, which was last updated in 2021. More information about this code and its four principal elements that outline the standards of ethical conduct can be found on the ICN website at https://www.icn.ch/sites/default/files/2023-06/ICN_Code-of-Ethics_EN_Web.pdf.

THINKING CRITICALLY

Compare and contrast the *Code of Ethics for Nurses with Interpretive Statements (Code of Ethics)* and *The ICN Code of Ethics for Nurses*. How are they similar? How do they differ? Which ethics statements are most meaningful to you? Are there areas you believe should be added to the ethics code(s)?

NURSING'S SCOPE AND STANDARDS OF PRACTICE

Important to any profession is an understanding of the scope and standards of practice expected of practitioners in that profession. However, fundamental to the scope and standards of practice of any profession is first and foremost a definition of the profession itself. The third important foundational document, *Nursing Scope and Standards of Practice* (2021), includes the most contemporary definition of nursing as follows:

> Nursing is the protection, promotion, and optimization of health and abilities, prevention of illness and injury, facilitation of healing, alleviation of suffering through the diagnosis and treatment of human response, and advocacy in the care of individuals, families, groups, communities, and populations.

The document also provides the "who," "what," "where," "when," "why," and "how" of nursing practice. It outlines and describes the tenets characteristic of nursing practice, the art and science of nursing, standards of practice, and standards of professional performance. Used in conjunction with *Nursing's Social Policy Statement* and the *Code of Ethics for Nurses with Interpretive Statements*, the definition, scope, practice standards, and beliefs of the discipline of nursing have been articulated for professional nurses, other healthcare providers, other professions, and the public at large.

TAXONOMIES FOR NURSING DIAGNOSIS

Since the mid-1960s, the concepts related to the nursing process have become more common in the nursing world. In most all educational and practice settings, some form of the nursing process is used. This involves assessing the client, making nursing diagnoses, formulating and implementing plans of care, and evaluating the client to determine the effectiveness of the care plan. Later in this text, in-depth information about this process is presented, as well as its role in providing the foundation for the nurse's application of critical thinking and clinical judgment. It is mentioned here because one component of nursing as an independent profession has been the development of a nursing diagnostic taxonomy, separate from medical diagnoses and those of other professions. This means that diagnoses are classified and ordered based on a set of principles in the discipline of nursing.

The first organization to tackle the taxonomy of nursing diagnoses was formed in 1982, after the 1973 First National Conference on the Classification of Nursing Diagnoses. Its members were from the United States and Canada, and its purpose was to provide a forum to discuss information and issues related to nursing diagnoses and to develop uniform language for nursing diagnoses. A formal taxonomy of nursing diagnoses was adopted, which has been regularly and continually updated over time. In 2002, NANDA International (NANDA-I) was formed (and while the title "North American Nursing Diagnosis Association" was formally dropped at that time, the term "NANDA" was retained due to its familiarity to nurses). NANDA-I has continued to provide overall leadership and approval authority for nursing diagnoses worldwide. Since its inception, NANDA (now NANDA-I) has approved over 200 nursing diagnoses.

NANDA nursing diagnoses and nursing diagnoses established by other organizations (such as the International Classification for Nursing Practice [ICNP]) represent the domain of the nursing profession, distinct from medicine and other professions. These diagnoses are used in the autonomous practice of professional registered nursing in developing comprehensive individualized nursing care plans for patients and clients and directing the work of LPN/LVNs, certified nurse assistants (CNAs), and nonlicensed **assistive personnel**.

EVOLUTION OF NURSING SCIENCE

As nursing developed as a profession, with its social policy statement, code for nurses, standards of practice, taxonomy of nursing diagnoses, licensure, and registration, the science of nursing was also developing. Doctoral degrees in nursing were initiated, and research was undertaken to identify nursing theory, construct conceptual models of nursing, and articulate the key constructs of nursing.

As described by Hood (2022), most all nursing theories and conceptual models are based on the same metaparadigm of nursing. A **metaparadigm** is an overarching concept above the paradigm, or overall concept of the relationship among ideas, common to all within a discipline or field of study. For many years, the accepted metaparadigm of nursing comprises the concepts of four key phenomena, or constructs, with which the discipline of nursing concerns itself. These are person, environment, health, and nursing.

Nurse theorists have studied each of these metaparadigm constructs to develop nursing conceptual models upon which curricula in nursing education programs are built. Each construct, however, has undergone study and research, and the definition of each construct has evolved. For example, the World Health Organization (n.d.) describes health as, "a state of complete physical, mental and social well-being and not merely the absence of disease or infirmity." (para. 1). As a result, nursing conceptual models and therefore nursing curricula continue to evolve and be revised.

The evolution of the science of nursing has resulted in an increasing emphasis on **evidence-based practice (EBP)**, to be discussed later in this chapter. Theory guides practice, and practice informs theory. It is through EBP, for example, that new nursing diagnoses are approved and used by nurse professionals in their practice. To strengthen the support for EBP, nursing identified the need to have doctoral degrees, whereby quality research could be conducted, and a journal for nursing where such research could be published and shared among nursing professionals. In the mid-1970s, the *Journal of Advanced Nursing* (JAN) began to accomplish this purpose. Three types of doctoral programs are now in place for nursing:

- Two research-based degrees:
  - The doctor of philosophy (PhD)
  - The doctor of nursing science (DNS)
- A practice-focused degree: The doctor of nursing practice (DNP)

On an international level, the International Network for Doctoral Education in Nursing (INDEN) began out of efforts from the University of Michigan, when it hosted the 1995 Doctoral Forum in Nursing titled "Generating Nursing Science in a Global Community." In 1999, INDEN was formed to advance quality doctoral nursing education globally and to create an international network for dialogue and global collaboration among doctoral-prepared nurses.

TRANSITIONS IN NURSING EDUCATION

As mentioned earlier in this chapter, Florence Nightingale believed that the education of nurses should be a function separate from service to patients. However, in the United States, hospitals and physicians advocated having nurses educated within a hospital setting, which essentially provide an inexpensive labor force. It took many years and hard effort to change this mentality in order to support nursing education as a collegiate experience, in which students attain theoretical knowledge as a foundation for not only technical skills but also for client assessment and higher-order thinking and problem-solving. Most nursing education programs are now located in collegiate settings. Even those that are based in a hospital or other healthcare setting usually have an affiliation with a college or university. All graduates in the United States and its territories take the same NCLEX-RN for licensure and entry into practice as a professional RN.

Another important transition in nursing education has been the educational preparation of nursing faculty. Most states now require a master's degree for nurse educators, and many faculty possess a doctoral degree.

TYPES OF NURSING EDUCATION PROGRAMS

In nursing education programs, the student bodies generally have a large variance in age, with the average age often being around 25 to 35 years. Many students are married or have partners. Many have children, and single caregivers and multigenerational families are also common. An increasing number of men and individuals of various gender identities are entering nursing, and the profession comprises a wide array of ethnicities. Students often enter professional nursing as a second or third career. For some, it is their first time in higher education, and for others, it is a return to school after having earned other certificates, diplomas, or degrees. Most students work at least part time to pay the rising costs of tuition, fees, books, and uniforms and to support themselves and those in their support system.

To meet the needs of working adult students and those with family and other responsibilities, evening, weekend, part-time, and distributive education (including online) programs are available. A challenge for nursing programs has been the increased cost of nursing education and how to provide quality education at a reduced cost in nontraditional formats. Nursing education programs are among the most costly programs on college campuses and often struggle for adequate funding to provide high-quality, relevant, technologically advanced instruction.

In each state, the state board of nursing or other designated state agency must approve all programs. Some schools also seek accreditation from ACEN, CNEA, or the Commission on Collegiate Nursing Education (CCNE), a division of the AACN. Most programs require that faculty possess or are seeking graduate degrees. Both theoretical and clinical components are required in all registered nursing programs, and students participate in practicum assignments in a variety of laboratory and clinical settings. Many programs also use practicing RN mentors and/or preceptors, especially in the more advanced clinical components of the program.

There are five basic modes of entry to the profession of registered nursing. Each mode of entry is discussed in the sections that follow. There are many similarities and some differences among the five educational pathways to registered nursing. Most programs are built on the metaparadigm of nursing, comprising nursing's four constructs of person, environment, health, and nursing. Each program has an adopted philosophy and conceptual model that directs curricula for the program. Although these vary from one program to the next, most are based on the aforementioned nursing metaparadigm, and most use the nursing process and nursing diagnoses for designing patient care plans.

It is also important to note that for all modes of entry into professional nursing, the same national exam is used for RN licensure—the NCLEX-RN. This exam is differentiated from the national exam for practical/vocational nurse licensure—the NCLEX-PN. There are approximately 1900 registered nursing education programs in the United States and many internationally as well.

Diploma Programs

The oldest form of nursing education is the diploma program. These programs began in 1873 and were initially similar to on-the-job training programs. Traditionally, they were strict and structured modes of instruction, practice, and conduct. Most diploma programs continue to be located in hospitals, require 3 years to complete, and include basic theory courses along with structured clinical experiences. Many diploma programs are now affiliated with local colleges, so students may receive college credit for general education courses. Graduates of diploma programs are prepared to function as primary caregivers in hospital and ambulatory care settings; they are not educationally prepared for administrative, school nursing, or public health nursing positions.

There has always been a fierce loyalty to diploma education; however, the number of diploma programs has declined since the 1980s, partly because of the increased costs for the programs and partly because of the growing number of ADN programs, which are 2 years in duration, and confer the associate degree on completion. Diploma programs now comprise less than 4% of all entry-level RN programs nationally.

Associate Degree Nursing Programs

ADN programs were instituted in the 1950s as a result of Mildred Montag's published doctoral dissertation in 1952 titled *"Education for Nursing Technicians."* She proposed that technical nurses could be educated in 2 years within a community or technical college and work as RNs. Although there was much opposition to this mode of education, the postwar need for nurses was an impetus for the start of these programs as an additional mode of entry to registered nursing practice. Initially, seven programs were started. They were so successful that many community colleges started similar programs.

This mode of entry has become very popular, with approximately 1,100 ADN programs in place nationally today. ADN programs provide an accessible and affordable mode of entry into professional nursing, and research has shown that NCLEX-RN pass rates and job performance as an RN are comparable to other modes of entry into practice.

ADN education was designed to have a balance between general education and nursing courses, without affiliation to a particular hospital, but rather clinical nursing experiences in one or more agencies for "hands-on" practicums to accompany collegiate theoretical classes. These programs are generally 2 years in duration and are usually located in community and technical colleges. However, some programs are found in 4-year colleges or within hospitals. ADN programs provide college credit and are regionally accredited higher education institutions, so coursework also applies toward the baccalaureate degree. Many ADN programs have articulation agreements with partner 4-year universities for this purpose. An **articulation agreement** is an agreement between the two institutions that courses from the ADN program will transfer to the 4-year institution and count as equal to its coursework so that students do not need to repeat course content they have already completed. A written articulation agreement guarantees the student of this credit even if there are personnel changes at one or the other institutions.

ADN graduates are prepared to be direct caregivers in hospitals, long-term care facilities, and ambulatory care settings. They are not prepared educationally for nursing administration, school nursing, public health nursing, or nurse educator positions, although some may work in these settings as part of a "tiered, team approach" to healthcare delivery. ADN programs comprise approximately 58% of all entry-level RN programs nationally.

Baccalaureate Degree Nursing Programs

Baccalaureate of Science in Nursing (BSN) programs were first established in 1909 at the University of Minnesota. Early programs took 5 years to complete; however, most programs are now 4 to 5 years. The early programs were greatly opposed by most nurses and physicians, who did not see the need for women and nurses to have higher education. BSN programs today generally begin with 2 years of liberal arts and science education. Nursing courses may begin in the second year but are largely concentrated into the last 2 years. Clinical practicums are similar to that of ADN programs, with additional public health practicums, and also include the use of research in the practice setting. BSN graduates are prepared to care for clients in a variety of settings, including administrative, school, and public health settings. BSN programs comprise approximately 38% of all entry-level RN programs nationally.

Master's Degree Programs

Another option available to prospective registered nursing students is the master's degree program that leads to an initial degree in nursing at the master's level. Such programs are designed for the student who already holds a bachelor's degree in another major and decides to pursue registered nursing as a career. Generally, the programs last 2 to 3 years and involve a combination of undergraduate- and graduate-level courses. Graduates of these programs can practice in all the same settings as ADN and BSN graduates but can additionally, with the graduate course preparation of the advanced degree, engage in research-related nursing activities, case management, and teaching in a nursing education program.

Nurses Immigrating to the United States

The last mode of entry into registered nursing is designed for nurses immigrating to the United States, many of whom are non-English or limited English–speaking adults who practiced nursing in their native country. Each state's board of nursing establishes requirements for such nurses who desire to become licensed RNs in the United States.

EDUCATIONAL MOBILITY AND CAREER ADVANCEMENT

An increasing number and variety of options are available today for nursing **educational mobility** and career advancement. Stacked credential and career ladder programs provide multiple entry and exit points in nursing programs. For example, CNAs may find they can "advance-place" into a registered nursing program for a shorter time-to-degree pathway. Likewise, a person who is already an LPN/LVN may enter the second year of an ADN program after completing prerequisite general education courses and an LPN/LVN transition course. Alternatively, a person may enter a 2-year ADN program and exit at the end of the first year to year and a half after completing a practical/vocational nursing program option. These types of educational mobility programs are popular because a student can better meet their needs in terms of education and work.

Additionally, some ADN and BSN programs offer students the opportunity to take challenge examinations for credit in lieu of some of the coursework.

Career advancement opportunities are available to those who are already RNs but are seeking a bachelor's or master's degree for career advancement. Many ADN programs have direct "2 + 2" articulation agreements with 4-year university BSN programs. Likewise, 2 + 2 + 2, 2 + 1 + 3, and 4 + 2 options are available to those wishing to pursue a master's degree for career advancement. Essentially, this means that units or credits from the associate degree and/or bachelor's degree transfer directly to the university offering the advanced degree the nurse desires. Relatively new to the educational arena are bachelor degrees offered by community colleges in an effort to bring education closer to the student nurse, thereby reducing travel and avoiding work and child care barriers to their pursuit of a BSN.

A final option is the availability of **external degree** programs, in which courses that are required for a BSN or MSN may be taken online, as independent study, or at a local community college that hosts the university program on site. Often, a student will have a preceptor or advisor for this process. There are benefits in that the student has more flexibility and can eliminate some of the problems related to traveling, child care, and work schedules. Drawbacks are that students do not always have the benefit of learning from other students' experiences and must be self-disciplined to complete reading, paper writing, and other learning activities in an online and/or independent study mode.

The choice for initial entry into practice as an RN is important, regardless of which route is taken. The availability of educational mobility and career advancement opportunities give both prospective and licensed nurses more options to pursue their present and future career goals.

Professional nurses never stop learning. Through both continuing education courses, and advanced degrees, professional nurses maintain their commitment to lifelong learning. Continuing education in nursing is essential for remaining current in the practice of nursing, and as mentioned previously, continuing education units (CEUs) are now mandatory for license renewal in most states. Many CEU courses are available to nurses through work, professional organizations, or local community and technical colleges. CEUs are also awarded for some coursework taken by those working on a higher level nursing degree.

Many nurses desire to attain advanced certification in a specific practice area through the ANA or other professional organizations. Advanced practice roles require a master's or doctoral degree, as do many jobs in specialty areas and in schools of nursing as a nurse educator. The increasing variety of educational mobility and career advancement options supports vitality and ongoing growth of the nurse and the profession as a whole.

FACTORS THAT HAVE INFLUENCED TRENDS AND TRANSITIONS IN NURSING

Throughout history and continuing today, influences outside the realm of nursing have had a major impact on the growth and development of nursing. Nursing does not exist in a vacuum. As technology and communication advance, so does the influence of society on the profession and practice of nursing. This section briefly examines some of the historic and societal trends that influence nursing.

WAR

The impact of war has been mentioned several times in this chapter. Nursing education was born in the United States as a result of the Civil War. When the Spanish American War occurred in 1898, injured soldiers required the services of nurses from training schools, although the military physicians were greatly opposed. There was less opposition after the war, but it was 1901 before the Army Nurse Corps was created. The Navy Nurse Corps was founded in 1908.

World War I initiated a new dimension for military nurses; injuries caused by shrapnel and gas were now evident, and there were massive numbers of casualties. This war also created a great demand for nurses, which prompted quicker training programs to satisfy some of the demand. After this war, with the return to longer training programs, a nursing shortage continued.

World War II created more demand for nurses and more need for them to be at the battlefront. Educational programs were not providing the necessary numbers of nurses, so the Cadet Nurse Corps was created, in which students received tuition and living costs in exchange for serving as a military or civilian nurse for the duration of the war. The curriculum for these programs was shortened, which prompted all nursing programs to reevaluate the duration of programs. Eventually, nurses in the military were able to achieve officer status, although it took longer for men and African American nurses to gain equal status.

The Korean War initiated the use of mobile army surgical hospital units. Nurses were in greater demand than ever. The Vietnam War and the Persian Gulf War emphasized the important role that nurses continue to have in wartime. However, by this time, ADN programs were plentiful, providing a low-cost, high-quality educational program in a shortened time frame.

An additional impact of war on nursing is the challenge nurses face in meeting the needs of veterans suffering from **posttraumatic stress disorder (PTSD)** and difficulties encountered entering and adjusting to civilian life. The nature of war has changed in today's era of Middle Eastern war and fighting acts of terrorism. Today's veterans have experienced not only the carnage of war itself but also the use of suicide bombers, terrorism, and bombings injuring and killing civilians, including children. These have had lasting psychological impacts on veterans and have caused an increase in the number of cases of veterans with PTSD (U.S. Department of Veterans Affairs, n.d.).

GENDER ROLES

Throughout time, nursing has been, and continues to be, a profession dominated by women. Today, men are widely accepted in the nursing profession and make up a little over 12% of the nursing workforce (U.S. Bureau of Labor Statistics, 2024). Changes in gender roles in society have had an impact on nursing over the years.

Traditionally, the women's role included raising children, housekeeping, and caregiving, and these were mostly unpaid. Research done predominantly by men, about men, yielded results that were then incorrectly generalized to women. Various works such as Kohlberg's stages of moral development did not portray the "different voice" of women. Although women were not included in his study, Kohlberg generalized his results to include women, concluding that women were not able to reach the higher level of moral development and were in some way deficient (see Chapter 2).

The women's movement, which began in the 1960s as a component of the "Sixties Revolution" (which consisted of the concepts of free love, antiestablishment, zero population growth, civil rights, gay rights, peace, and talk of the upcoming "Age of Aquarius"), brought with it a new emphasis on the role of women and equal rights. *The Second Sex* (1949) by Simone De Beauvoir and *The Feminine Mystique* (1963) by Betty Friedan were already in print, and bookstores carried dozens of books on women's roles. Reaching perhaps a peak in the late 1970s and early 1980s with Title IX (gender equity), and affirmative action legislation, researchers began to study the development of women, and nurse theorists began to study the profession of nursing.

Carol Gilligan, a student of Kohlberg who conducted research on women, produced the seminal text, *In a Different Voice* (1982), in which she contrasted men's ethos of "justice and rights" with women's ethos of "care and connectedness." She concluded that women's moral reasoning, based on the latter, was not inferior, just "different." Women's roles in general, and more specifically in nursing, began to be valued. The development of nursing as a profession—with advanced degrees, research, and an independent taxonomy of diagnoses—contributed not only to the valuing of nursing but also to the valuing of women.

Concurrent with, and subsequent to, the women's movement, men were also questioning their traditional roles. With the onset of more "career moms" came more "stay-at-home dads." Men were no longer viewed as inadequate when choosing to assume caregiver roles, and such phrases as "the sensitive man," "it's okay to cry," and "you're okay, I'm okay" were coined. **Gender equity** began to apply to all people, and nursing became a more acceptable, feasible career for men, as did other caregiver professions.

Over the past four decades, there has been an explosion of research on the psychology of women, gender, and roles. Most notable is the recognition and appreciation of diversity, the impact of social context, and the influence of ethnicity, class, sexual orientation, gender identity, and so forth. All these research findings continue to shape nursing today. As more men enter the profession, and as gender roles in society continue to evolve, so too must the profession of nursing.

SOCIETAL TRENDS AND THE CHANGING ROLE OF NURSING

Societal trends have had, and continue to have, an impact on nursing. Several of these are described in the following sections and listed in Box 4.3.

Aging Population

As the population ages, there are increasingly greater numbers of older adults who require healthcare services. This is partly due to the **baby boomers** entering their 60s and partly due to advances in healthcare that detect disease early and thus prolong life. The inclusion of older adult care and gerontologic concepts in nursing curricula increased in the 1990s. Emphasis began to be placed on individualizing care for three distinct groups of older adults—the young old (65 to 74 years), the middle old (75 to 84 years), and the old-old (85 years and older) (Yoost & Crawford, 2023). Emerging concepts in caring for the well but frail older adult, as well as concepts of family-centered care for four- and five-generational families, are now included in nursing curricula.

Shortened Lengths of Stay in Hospitals

Acute care settings have seen a shift to clients who are more critically ill than in the past, yet are staying in the hospital for shorter periods of time. Fewer hospitalized patients are ambulatory. There is also a greater need for high-tech and highly skilled care in long-term and home care settings. Many surgeries and procedures previously performed on clients as inpatients have shifted to the outpatient setting, creating a greater demand for outpatient nursing services and increased acuity in inpatient settings. For nurses working in inpatient settings, the ability to prioritize care to more acute patients, think critically, and watch for complications is imperative, as are increased technological skills. Nurse–patient ratios also need to be addressed because nurses can only safely care for a smaller number of patients than in the past. Many states are passing legislation to

> **BOX 4.3** **Societal Trends That Have Influenced the Profession of Nursing**
> - Aging population
> - Shortened lengths of hospital stay
> - Nursing shortage
> - Diversity, multiculturalism, and emotional intelligence
> - Immigration issues for nurses
> - HIV/AIDS and pandemic flu
> - Disaster preparedness, bioterrorism, and homeland security
> - Cyberterrorism
> - Advancing technology, bioethics, and globalism
> - Healthcare reform
> - Managed care and collaborative practice
> - Quality outcomes
> - Medical benefits, social security, and reimbursement programs
> - Changes in family structures
> - Nursing informatics
> - Telehealth and Health Insurance Portability and Accountability Act (HIPAA)
> - Experiential wisdom and EBP
> - Holistic and spiritual care
> - Nursing entrepreneurism
> - Service learning
> - Social and healthcare advocacy
> - Social/political policies

limit the nurse-to-patient ratio to ensure safety to the public. Nursing education has to continue to be vigilant and creative in preparing graduates for this new environment.

Nursing Shortage

Throughout history, there have been numerous times when there was a nursing shortage, especially in times of war. However, today, several societal trends are contributing to an exacerbated nursing shortage, and that shortage is expected to worsen over time.

The population is aging due to the baby boomers entering retirement, and life expectancy is increasing due to advances in medical and nursing science. This means that many nurses in the current workforce are also retiring at a time when there is an increased need for care. These retirees include both nursing faculty and those in clinical practice. Also, because many students entering registered nursing programs are working adults and those choosing nursing as a second career, these new entering nurses will remain in active practice a shorter length of time than their earlier counterparts, requiring more entrants to nursing education program form the higher turnover.

Increased patient acuity and shortened lengths of stay also mean that nurses cannot care safely for as many patients as in the past, thereby further increasing the demand for nurses. Nurses may experience more stress from this increased level of patient acuity, finding themselves working overtime and taking fewer rest breaks throughout the shift. Additionally, many facilities have designed the workweek into shift schedules of four 10-hour shifts ("4 tens") or three 12-hour shifts ("3 twelves"), which can lead to further fatigue. Nursing organizations concerned about patient loads, nurse fatigue, and "burnout" have written position papers on these subjects in recent years. Such challenges in nursing may cause prospective students to choose other professions and practicing nurses to leave the profession earlier than expected, further contributing to the nursing shortage.

Because the nursing shortage continues to be of such grave concern, nurses and nursing organizations have joined to seek solutions. Many healthcare facilities schedule hiring events around nursing school graduation dates, when numerous graduate nurses are entering the job market. Hiring decreases during the periods when fewer graduates are available to enter the job market. Although peaks and valleys in usual working staffing are cyclical, the projected nursing shortage has been described as a "tsunami," or tidal wave. To address the impending severe shortage, the ANA and participants from 60 other national nursing organizations joined a summit in 2001 to address the nursing shortage. A steering committee of 19 national nursing organizations including ANA, NLN, and NSNA identified 10 domains, or areas of focus, for their work, with the goal of achieving *Nursing's Agenda for the Future* by the year 2010. As Cherry and Jacob (2022) noted, these efforts generated many positive results. An unexpected number of young people entered the workforce from 2002 to 2009; the number of full-time RNs aged 23 to 26 years increased by 62%—a rate of growth not seen since the 1970s. However, although this influx of new nurses reduced the nurse shortage, more RN jobs (more than 200,000) remained available (through 2022) than for any other profession. With more than 1 million seasoned RNs anticipated to retire by 2030, the U.S. Bureau of Labor Statistics projects the need to produce 1.1 million new RNs for expansion and replacement of retirees to avoid a severe nursing shortage (AACN, 2022).

Compounding this problem are changes in the nursing educational system and economic pressures. Nursing programs are requiring higher qualifications among nursing faculty, yet the number of nurses with master's and doctoral degrees remains inadequate to fill this need, and salaries for these positions are not competitive with those in the clinical workplace (Mazinga, 2023). Several strategies have been introduced to combat the nursing faculty shortage. In response to a call for public and private initiatives, the Health Resources and Services Administration (HRSA) has implemented nursing faculty loan repayment programs; however, the process is limited to specific application dates, and application completion can be complicated. Lacking both faculty and clinical placement sites, coupled with economic pressures due to the high cost of nursing programs, many colleges and universities are increasing student–teacher ratios, reducing the frequency of cohort start-ups and overall incoming class sizes, "capping" enrollments, and shifting educational dollars to other disciplines. This, of course, runs counter to the goal of producing more nurses. Nursing faculties are finding creative ways to provide high-quality experiences for students, including the use of high-tech clinical simulations to build clinical experiences and develop critical thinking skills via laboratory simulations but that will be insufficient to address the shortage.

As Benner et al. (2010) note, many graduate-prepared nurses come from clinical specialties without requisite teaching knowledge to blend nursing science with pedagogy for strong instruction of nursing students. Using Benner's terms, while perhaps an "expert" in the art and science of nursing, these new faculty are often a "novice" in the art and science of teaching. With huge turnovers in faculty due to retirements and recruitment from the workplace, where salaries are often higher, these new nursing faculty have few seasoned nursing professors to mentor them, and educational institutions have a paucity of professional development funds at their disposal for such support. Yet, such mentoring and development is critical for these new faculty for them to develop teaching expertise and employ the teaching pedagogies necessary to foster problem-solving, critical thinking, and the application of theory to complex client situations in their students.

Economic pressures exist in the workplace as well. Competition for experienced nurses, and those with a BSN, has increased. The rising cost of healthcare in general has challenged healthcare providers to reduce costs by reducing RNs in preference to lower paid healthcare professionals and assistive personnel. Healthcare providers vacillate between such "tiered" approaches to reduce costs and "all-BSN" staffing patterns to support holistic care models, in an effort to enhance quality of care. Lastly, healthcare reform has further exacerbated the nursing shortage as the impact of the Affordable Care Act, enacted in 2010, continues to bring millions of new people into the healthcare system, requiring more services and more RNs to care for these individuals.

Diversity, Multiculturalism, and Emotional Intelligence

Ethnic diversity has increased greatly in the United States, resulting in a growing need for nurses who are multiculturally sensitive and who value diverse perspectives and cultural views. Lindsey et al. (2013) encourage the development of "**cultural proficiency**" across all levels of education. The cultural proficiency continuum, as well as the six stages of development for individuals, leaders, and organizations to become culturally proficient (Table 4.1), are a framework for building cultural competence in nursing schools. Although cultural proficiency emphasizes the acquisition of knowledge needed to provide culturally competent care, application to practice can sometimes lead to stereotyping and assumptions about an individual based solely on their cultural background (Smith & Foronda, 2021).

TABLE 4.1 Lindsey and Roberts' Cultural Proficiency Continuum

Stage of Social Competence	Behaviors
Cultural destructiveness	Negating, disparaging, or purging cultures that are different from your own.
Cultural incapacity	Elevating the superiority of your own cultural values and beliefs and suppressing cultures that are different from your own.
Cultural blindness	Acting as if differences among cultures do not exist and refusing to recognize any differences.
Cultural precompetence	Recognizing that lack of knowledge, experience, and understanding of other cultures limits your ability to effectively interact with them.
Cultural competence	Employing any policy, practice, or behavior that uses the essential elements of cultural proficiency on behalf of the school or district. Cultural competence is interacting with other cultural groups in ways that recognize and value their differences, motivate you to assess your own skills, expand your knowledge and resources, and, ultimately, cause you to adapt your relational behavior.
Cultural proficiency	Advocating in ways that honor the differences among cultures, seeing diversity as a benefit, and interacting knowledgeably and respectfully among a variety of cultural groups.

Source: Lindsey, R. B., Roberts, L. M., & Campbelljones, F. (2013). *The culturally proficient school: An implementation guide for school leaders* (2nd ed.). Corwin Press, Sage.

To foster a deeper connection with patients, nurses are encouraged to develop **cultural humility**, which focuses on self-awareness and a willingness to engage in lifelong learning about diverse cultural perspectives (So et al., 2024). In developing cultural humility, nurses engage in introspection and acknowledge their own cultural biases and limitations. Approaching each patient with openness and respect and actively seeking to understand the unique cultural context and values that influence patients' health beliefs and practices enhances communication and promotes more meaningful and equitable care for individuals from diverse backgrounds (Rebar & Heimgartner, 2021).

The standard of professional nursing practice is to provide care to all individuals. The ANA's (2015) *Code of Ethics* addresses equity in patient care in provision eight, which states that nurses must protect human rights, promote health diplomacy, and reduce disparities. As an RN, you will be expected to both model and provide leadership for the development of cultural proficiency and cultural humility in healthcare settings and among those you supervise.

Nursing school recruitment, admission, and retention practices need to address this challenge of increasing the ethnic diversity of incoming student classes, as well as their retention, persistence, and graduation rates. Nursing faculty must prepare nurses to think and act from a multicultural perspective and to develop cultural competence. Boyle et al. (2025) describe cultural competence not as a destination but as an ever-evolving journey that requires continuous self-reflection, motivation, and dedication. To achieve cultural competence, nurses must value, respect, and refrain from judging the beliefs, languages, and culturally based health practices of individuals and families for whom they provide care.

Although developing and refining cultural competence is also important for nursing faculty, strategies to diversify faculty are also needed, to attract and retain men, those of other genders, and individuals who are ethnically diverse. Cherry and Jacob (2022) note that although the annual survey done by AACN shows an increase in these areas, as of 2022, only 7.8% of nursing faculty were men, and only 13.1% were from underrepresented groups.

The NLN supports diversity, equity, and inclusion in nursing education by advocating for inclusive admissions processes, promoting culturally sensitive curriculum development, offering resources and support for faculty cultural competence training, and providing scholarships and grants to underrepresented students. The NLN's (n.d.-b) Diversity and Inclusion Statement can be viewed at https://www.nln.org/public-policy/nursing-education-issues/diversity.

Likewise, the AACN (2017) recognizes the importance of diverse life experiences, perspectives, and backgrounds in nursing education to enhance learning opportunities and experiences for both students and faculty. As part of their Diversity, Equity and Inclusion statement, the AACN is working to reduce healthcare disparities by ensuring that nurses are trained to meet the needs of all individuals in an increasingly diverse society. The AACN (2017) Diversity, Equity and Inclusion in Academic Nursing Position Statement can be viewed at https://www.aacnnursing.org/Portals/0/PDFs/Position-Statements/Diversity-Inclusion.pdf.

Another aspect of cultural proficiency is the need to be aware of one's own and others' emotions. Goleman (1998) stated that leaders must be attentive to **emotional intelligence**. He emphasized the need for those who want to be successful, especially as leaders, to learn more about their own and others' emotions and what motivates them to inspire, work collaboratively, and adapt to change. As our society becomes more diverse, nurses must develop emotional intelligence. Moss (2005) described the emotionally intelligent nurse as one who is better equipped to provide leadership in issues of day-to-day patient care and ethical dilemmas. Moss also pointed out that emotions become even more important in our ever-increasing technological world, and the emotionally intelligent nurse will be a stronger member of the collaborative healthcare team.

Immigration Issues for Nurses

Another societal trend is the public debate over issues of immigration. The nursing shortage and the overall shrinking workforce compared to the overall population have placed an increased emphasis on immigration issues. Nurses from outside the United States are being relied on by the healthcare industry in greater numbers, and state boards of nursing are challenged to adopt appropriate regulations for nurse licensure. This comes at a time when mutual recognition of RN licensure between and among states, through the NLC, is also being adopted, thereby complicating decisions on legislation and regulations.

The ANA has noted that creating a positive environment for all RNs, whether educated in the United States or another country, will result in better patient outcomes, improved retention of nursing staff, and optimal performance by the healthcare facility. Federal legislation to relax nurse immigration standards in response to the U.S. nursing shortage, however, is being met with opposition by the ANA and others who are concerned about a possible decrease in standards and other ethical implications of the proposals.

Healthcare Reform

Today's political agenda surrounding healthcare reform emphasizes access, medical record portability, primary preventive care, **cost containment**, and choice in caregivers. There is also more emphasis on primary preventive care that is more community based. The primary care provider will serve as a gatekeeper in the continuum of healthcare needs. The role of acute care centers is changing to one of providing only acute intensive care. Simple surgeries, procedures, and treatment of illness are provided in community-based settings whenever possible. Cost containment efforts emphasize quality care in more reduced and efficient ways, and insurance carriers are funding only limited inpatient stays. Restorative and rehabilitative services are required to be conducted in ambulatory care settings. Communities must ensure that services are integrated and consolidated so that costly duplication is eliminated. The work that nurses, especially advanced practice nurses, do now is held in high esteem because of nursing's holistic and preventive tradition. The quality of care and the reduced cost of that care will be greatly influenced by the work that nurses do.

Grossman and Valiga (2020) posited that the new leadership challenge for nursing is to create its future. To continue to successfully provide healthcare, the nursing profession must find ways to use resources efficiently, validate the benefits of nursing interventions on patient outcomes, and create innovative ways to deliver high-quality and cost-effective care. Grossman and Valiga (2020) note that meeting this challenge will require not only incremental change but also transformational change in healthcare.

Managed Care and Collaborative Practice

The expansion of healthcare systems and **health maintenance organizations (HMOs)** caused by mergers and cost-saving strategies has affected nursing and how clients receive care. The use of **preferred provider organizations (PPOs)** and **diagnostic** related groups (DRGs)** in an effort to contain skyrocketing inflation in healthcare costs has had some impact. However, the use of unlicensed assistive personnel to defray costs is causing the profession of nursing to be concerned with the quality of care being given. Nurses are aware that many "tasks" they perform are also accompanied by skilled assessment, critical thinking, and clinical judgment not possessed by untrained and unlicensed personnel. For example, while taking vital signs, the nurse may also notice early signs or symptoms of sepsis, which likely will not be noticed by unlicensed assistive personnel, who are merely taking vital signs.

The initiation and expansion of managed care approaches, compared to the traditional primary care approach, has raised concerns for nurses who want to ensure illness prevention and health promotion for their patients, in addition to medical treatment. In **managed care** settings, a patient often sees different physicians and other providers at each visit and/or each day during a hospitalization. This is not only confusing to patients but can also lead to missed secondary complications not passed on from one provider to another or not observed when subtleties are only seen with consistent observation over several days.

Two trends have developed in nursing as a result of managed care approaches and the increased use of electronic devices (rather than human senses) to monitor patients' conditions. First, nursing has returned to its "roots," focusing on "holistic healthcare," viewing the patient as a complex biologic system, where all components interface and have an impact on each other: biologic, psychological, sociologic, emotional, and spiritual. Eastern healing philosophies are becoming more apparent, blended with Western medicine, and healthcare reimbursement is examining the cost–benefit of reimbursement of preventative medicine, which was previously excluded. Whole fields of holistic and spiritual nursing and other nursing specialties have emerged. These are discussed in a later section in this chapter.

Second, a "team approach" has become critical in managed care settings, and today's RN must engage as a "collaborative practitioner." When nurses collaborate, they work with other members of the healthcare team to think critically, drawing on the expertise of various team members to analyze and solve complex problems in patient care. Collaboration by all members of the healthcare team is essential for creativity and for developing the best strategies for quality outcomes.

Nurses must organize information about the patient to provide a comprehensive picture of the patient's situation, to prevent miscommunication with the healthcare team, and to promote patient safety. A widely used tool that enhances communication is the SBAR (Situation, Background, Assessment, Recommendation) framework, which provides a structure for conveying critical patient information efficiently and accurately and reduces the risk of miscommunication or misunderstanding among team members. Using the SBAR framework ensures that all relevant details are communicated, including the patient's current condition (Situation), pertinent medical history and context (Background), the healthcare provider's assessment of the situation (Assessment), and proposed actions or recommendations (Recommendation). The SBAR framework not only presents a comprehensive description of the patient's condition but it also allows nurses to exercise and demonstrate critical thinking and judgment skills, learn more about the patient themselves, and strengthen collaboration among members of the healthcare team (Yoost & Crawford, 2023).

The Institute of Medicine (IOM) also noted the need for collaborative practice and better information systems. In its publication *The Future of Nursing: Leading Change,*

Advancing Health (2011), the IOM noted the need for nurses and doctors to be full partners, along with other healthcare professionals in redesigning healthcare in the United States, and engaging in effective workforce planning and policymaking that requires better data collection and an improved information infrastructure.

Quality Outcomes

Efforts to incorporate **quality assurance (QA)**, **total quality management (TQM)**, and **continuous quality improvement (CQI)** practices are adding work to already overworked nurses. Although these initiatives are designed to ensure accountability for quality-based outcomes, the increased management of patient/client care is removing nurses from the "soft skill" side of promoting health, patient education, and meeting psychosocial needs.

Accrediting associations for nursing programs, higher education, and healthcare agencies are all monitoring for quality outcomes. Colleges and universities are being held accountable for **student learning outcomes (SLOs)** in order to be regionally accredited. **Outcomes assessment**, evaluation, performance indicators, organizational "scorecards," and accountability measures are prominent in society today as policy makers determine allocation of limited resources. This is impacting healthcare agencies, nursing programs, and nurses themselves. For nursing, such information not only drives finances but also, even more importantly, is necessary for nursing research, continuous improvement of quality patient care, and the expansion of EBP (discussed later in this chapter). In 2007, the ANA hosted its first annual National Database of Nursing Quality Indicators (NDNQI) data use conference. The conference focused on such topics as how hospitals use NDNQI reports to improve the quality of nursing care, how nurse staffing affects patient outcomes, mandates for public reporting initiatives, data collection practices, and cost savings achieved with quality improvement. This is consistent with the growing emphasis on the science of nursing and EBP. Additionally, nursing informatics (NI) (discussed later in this chapter) has been added as a specialty area in nursing.

Medical Benefits, Social Security, and Reimbursement Programs

Perhaps the greatest challenge for older persons today is the change in medical benefits, social security, and reimbursement programs. Not only are such changes confusing but also they raise fears for both patients and healthcare providers. What costs will be covered by insurance providers, Medicare, and social security programs? How will noncovered costs be paid?

For nurses and other healthcare providers, both employment and retirement planning must take into account such programs as **health savings accounts (HSAs)**, **flexible spending accounts (FSAs)**, prescription plans, long-term care insurance, and the ever-changing national healthcare agenda. As healthcare agencies struggle with rising costs and cost containment strategies, reductions in benefit packages can drive nurses to other professions, contributing to the nursing shortage and, ultimately, further compounding cost escalation. In addition, issues of guardianship and who is covered on benefit plans arise with the increase in same-sex couples, multigenerational families, and other living arrangements. These all impact the nurse's role both in planning care and legal compliance.

Changes in Family Structures

Another societal trend effecting nursing is the diversification and change in family structures. As discussed previously, the aging population has resulted in multigenerational families. Also, an increase in same-sex couples has caused a growth in public policy debate regarding same-sex marriage and individual rights. For nursing, this raises ethical dilemmas related to patient confidentiality, legal guardianship, authorization for surgery, medical procedures, organ donation, and end-of-life decisions.

HIV/AIDS and Pandemic Flus (Such as COVID-19)

The AIDS epidemic greatly influenced the world of nursing. Implementation and maintenance of standard precautions can minimize the danger of AIDS and other bloodborne pathogens, and the workplace is a much safer environment for healthcare workers if universal precautions are practiced. But healthcare workers continue to have increased risks. The fear of an impending pandemic flu became a reality during COVID-19. Detailed plans for such a disaster were needed in all healthcare settings; however, the swift surge of the virus caught most healthcare agencies worldwide off guard. Nurses played a lead role in the event and, although preparation for this type of challenge had been practiced, nurses were stretched to their limits physically and emotionally. Many had to oversee surges in patient volume, provide patient care with equipment and PPE shortages, and provide comfort not only to patients but also to patient families who were unable to be at the bedside with their loved ones (Pearman et al., 2020). The full impact of the pandemic on the nursing profession is still unknown. Many nurses reported high levels of anxiety, depression, concerns about their own health, and the need to examine COVID-19–related stress and response so that these aspects can be improved during future pandemics (Pearman et al., 2020). These issues have prompted some nurses to leave the profession and have possibly deterred others from seeking a nursing education.

Disaster Preparedness, Bioterrorism, and Homeland Security

Disaster preparedness is vital in the 21st century. In just the first two decades of this century, the United States experienced the terrorist attacks of September 11, 2001; disasters such as Hurricane Katrina on the Gulf Coast, the Asian Tsunami in the Pacific Ocean, and Hurricane Sandy off the East Coast; **bioterrorism** and multiple terrorist attacks; and numerous floods and fires across the country. These have caused the healthcare industry, and nursing in particular, to respond to this need. Communities and countries are vulnerable to these disasters and are often ill prepared to cope with the nature and extent of the disaster.

Both the ANA and ICN have established web pages devoted to terrorism, bioterrorism, and disaster response, with information for nurses on how to care for patients, how to cope and protect themselves, and how to prepare for disaster. Many articles have been written on these topics, healthcare agencies have adopted new policies and procedures in the event of such emergencies, and nursing programs have added curricula focused on preparing nurses adequately to face such challenges.

The NCSBN and individual state boards of nursing have also responded to issues of disaster preparedness and homeland security. Additionally, a number of states have implemented criminal background checks for nurse licensure applicants.

Advancing Technology, Bioethics, and the Global Economy

Technological changes and the growing trend toward specialization have changed the educational needs and practice of nurses. In most settings, nurses must be highly skilled technicians who are well trained to manage highly advanced technology. Computer-based documentation and high-tech caregiving equipment are now common, demanding new skills from all RNs. As advances continue in medical care, the need for highly specialized nurses will increase. Like technology advances in acute care settings, the technology in home care and long-term care settings has also escalated. This has an obvious impact on families and healthcare providers in those settings. Along with this "high-tech" environment, the "high-touch" skills of nurses will be of even greater importance because clients and their families require more patient teaching and communication to allay fears and care for themselves at home.

Bioethics and societal trends such as organ replacement, life-prolonging procedures, **cryogenics**, euthanasia, genetic reengineering, **cloning**, and stem cell research pose ethical dilemmas for healthcare professionals. Nurses, in collaboration with other healthcare professionals, must think critically about these issues to examine their secondary effects on patients, their families, and society as a whole. Nursing organizations must study and engage in critical dialogue about these controversial issues. As an example, the ANA announced its support for the Stem Cell Research Enactment Act of 2007, which promotes the ethical use of stem cells for research and therapeutic purposes that impact health. Today's nurses need to be knowledgeable about these issues not only to be politically active but also to engage in patient education on a daily basis.

Technological advances in telecommunications have provided greater opportunities for medical consultation and the portability of medical records. However, this has placed patient confidentiality at greater risk, and it challenges today's nurse to be especially mindful of privacy issues. This is discussed in more depth later in this chapter.

Another challenge of the societal trend toward overuse of information technology and digital devices (Arenas-Escaso et al., 2024) is that people have become dependent on cell phones, tablets, and other technological devices. Rarely is one free from these assistive devices, and the distractions they can pose cause increasing social disconnects. An often-stated observation is that never throughout history have we been so connected and yet as socially disconnected as today. In nursing, "connecting" with patients has become more difficult, and patient teaching that "sticks" has become a challenge. Goleman (2007) describes the need for practitioners today to develop not only personal "emotional intelligence" but also interpersonal "social intelligence," citing the emerging field of social neuroscience whereby decreased neuronal activity has been found in social situations where certain neurons are activated by the body.

Another societal trend impacting nurses is **globalism** and the global economy. The NLN's Hallmarks of Excellence in Nursing Education emphasized the need for curriculum to reflect local and global perspectives of societal and healthcare trends. The NLN's definition of global perspective is included in the Hallmarks of Excellence in Nursing Education, which can be viewed at https://www.nln.org/education/teaching-resources/professional-development-programsteaching-resources/hallmarks-of-excellence-%C2%A9-dffbb05c-7836-6c70-9642-ff00005f0421.

The world has "become smaller" as transcontinental travel has become faster and more common and because telecommunications allow for increased competition and contribute to an expanding global economy. The poor recovery from the 2007-2010 mortgage crisis followed by the COVID-19 pandemic is fueling a global economic crisis. Because the healthcare industry is part of the global economy, the impact on nursing has been great.

The need to develop more energy efficient, clean energy (nonfossil fuel) systems, and sustainable, "green" products are impacting nursing and decisions in the healthcare field globally. Goleman (2009) described the need for **"ecological intelligence"**—to be aware of the hidden impact of foods and products on health and ecological systems.

Nurses who are multilingual, culturally proficient, and sociologically and ecologically intelligent will play an active role in this new economy and make wise decisions for political advocacy. The 1960s phase "Think globally, act locally" has taken on another whole tier of meaning in this new high-tech global economy.

THINKING CRITICALLY

Select three of the societal trends presented. How do you think each will affect your practice as an RN in the future? How will clients be affected? What role can nursing organizations play in the advancement of nursing related to these societal trends? What collaborative practice will assist in the challenges faced by nursing?

NURSING INFORMATICS AND HIPAA

Nursing informatics (NI) is a relatively new area of practice that emerged from the developing information society in which we now live. In 1992, the ANA's Congress of Nursing Practice established NI as a specialty practice. Like other specialty areas, standards of practice are developed, published, and regularly updated by the ANA.

The ANA (2022) describes NI as a specialty that integrates nursing science with multiple information management and analytical sciences to identify, define, manage, and communicate data, information, knowledge, and wisdom in nursing practice. ANA's *Nursing Informatics: Scope and Standards of Practice, Third Edition* (2022) covers the full scope of NI and outlines the competency level of nursing practice and professional performance expected from all informatics nurses and nurse specialists. Outlined are 17 standards, along with specific competencies for each, for which all informatics nurses are held accountable. The American Nurses Credentialing Center offers nurses board certification by examination in Nursing Informatics. Nurses who specialize in Informatics and meet eligibility requirements may apply for the examination. The competency-based certification credential is recognized by the Accreditation Board for Specialty Nursing Certification and is valid for 5 years, upon which time nurses must renew their certification (ANA, 2022).

Automation in healthcare and health information technology have grown tremendously over the past 25 years, and the specialty of NI has grown with it. However, today, even the general practice of professional nursing now requires some competencies in NI. The ANA standards also outline competencies needed by any RN, spanning all nursing careers and roles, and reflecting the impact of informatics in any healthcare practice environment. McGonigle and Mastrian (2022) provide an overview of NI, including its origins, evolution, current state, and projected future.

Although younger nursing students and new RNs are generally more at ease with technology in general, practicing nurses, adult students, and those returning to school later in life may find new technology challenging. Computer literacy is imperative in today's healthcare industry, and NI is an extension of this societal trend. The ability to share patient data provides both advantages and challenges to nursing today. Shared healthcare records support a collaborative, holistic approach to patient care. The portability of such data and information gives new providers a more comprehensive view of the patient. One of the greatest challenges is ensuring the confidentiality and privacy of the patient, which becomes increasingly more difficult with today's technological advances. Another is the challenge of portability among noncompatible information systems across the healthcare industry.

The **Health Insurance Portability and Accountability Act (HIPAA)** was passed in 1996 with compliance required by 2003 to make healthcare more efficient. It has provided portability of medical coverage for preexisting conditions, defined the underwriting process for group medical coverage, and standardized electronic transmittal of billing and claims information. Because standardization and portability also means that access to patient information has been expanded, a key component of HIPAA has been its regulations to maintain confidentiality and security of health data. Nurses play an important role in guarding the privacy of patients and their confidential health information and records.

Another outcome of advanced technology, informatics, and HIPAA is the telehealth industry. The Department of Health and Human Services (n.d.) defines telehealth as "the use of electronic information and telecommunications technologies to support long distance clinical health care, patient and professional health-related education, public health, and health administration" (para. 1). This has been especially helpful to patients, nurses, physicians, and other healthcare professionals in rural areas who are seeking consultative advice from specialists, as well as patient education and professional development opportunities they might not otherwise be able to access.

EXPERIENTIAL WISDOM AND EVIDENCE-BASED PRACTICE

In her book titled *From Novice to Expert: Excellence and Power in Clinical Nursing Practice*, Benner (2001) argued that although a great deal was known about nursing from a sociological perspective, evidence of that learned through actual clinical practice had not been documented. She described how nurses gain experiential knowledge throughout their clinical practice, from novice beginnings until they become nurse "experts" with **experiential wisdom**. In the 21st century, the profession of nursing has broadened its body of knowledge by documenting such evidence-based outcomes of nursing practice since Benner's seminal book.

As you already know, you will spend more time at the bedside than any other healthcare provider. As an RN, you will be responsible for recognizing your patient's clinical deterioration and communicating and collaborating with other providers. Some barriers you may encounter are lack of confidence in your own clinical judgment, fear of being judged when alerting other providers, and intimidation by colleagues with more experience. Benner described experience and intuition as catalysts to expert patient care. Benner explained that nursing intuition—also referred to as intuitive suspicion—is more than just a "gut feeling"; is based on knowledge, experience, and research-based evidence. Developing intuitive suspicion to identify and interpret subtle changes in your patient's condition will be integral in clinical decision-making and providing safe quality patient care (Liu et al., 2022).

Documenting the effects of nursing practice, including evidential discovery, can then lead to empirical research on preventive, reparative, restorative, and palliative nursing care to improve quality outcomes. This provides rich information for both novice and experienced RNs and for nursing education reform.

With experience, the nurse has the ability to document the effects of care provided. Nurses are in the mode of "evidential discovery" every time they engage in the practice of nursing. Collecting evidence of "what works and what doesn't" by nurses every day is what leads to questions for research in order to change nursing practice for contemporary times. The nurse who uses such findings from research, rather than performing actions because "it's the way we've always done it" is what leads to sound clinical judgment, which will be discussed later in this text. Godshall (2020) defines EBP for nursing as, "Using the best available evidence to guide clinical practice so that patients receive the best possible nursing care" (p. 8).

Begun in 1998, the journal *Evidence-Based Nursing* is published quarterly and contains articles of international nursing research for application to the practice of nursing. Numerous articles and books are now published on EBP, ranging from an introduction to EBP for students and nurses who want to know more about EBP and how to collect and use evidence for efficient and effective care (McGonigle & Mastrian, 2022) to full summaries of best practices of nursing procedures organized by clinical specialties (Melnyk & Fineout-Overholt, 2023). It must also be noted, however, that when using EBP, the nurse must also employ clinical/professional judgment, consider patient/client preference, and be mindful of available resources.

HOLISTIC AND SPIRITUAL CARE

There has been increasing attention to holistic and spiritual care in nursing over the past few decades. Providing holistic and spiritual care amidst the increasing complexity of multiethnic client populations, however, poses new challenges for nurses. Although nurses have always cared for their patients' biologic, psychological, sociologic, spiritual, and other needs, the practice of **holistic nursing** has only become a distinct nursing specialty in recent years.

The American Holistic Nurses Association (AHNA) was formed in 1981 in an effort to bring the concepts of holism to every arena of nursing. Its mission is to "unite nurses in healing." Holistic nursing became officially recognized as a nursing specialty by the ANA in 2006. AHNA, working with the ANA, defined the scope and standards of practice of this specialty, publishing the foundational document *Holistic Nursing: Scope and Standards of Practice* in 2007. ANA and AHNA worked together on the standards of practice for holistic nurse specialists, and the text was updated in a third edition in (2019). The document articulates the essentials of holistic nursing, its activities, and its accountabilities at all practice levels and settings. For holistic nursing specialists, 16 standards and their associated competencies are provided. The book includes an overview and history of holistic nursing, core values of the profession, educational preparation necessary, standards of practice, and standards of professional performance as well as references and information about complementary and alternative modalities.

Holistic nurses honor each patient's subjective experience about health, health beliefs, and values. They integrate self-care, self-responsibility, spirituality, and reflection in their patients' lives (Yoost & Crawford, 2023). The emphasis is on the nurse facilitating the healing of others, and the AHNA views itself as a bridge between the traditional medical paradigm and universal complementary and alternative healing practices.

Spiritual nursing care is another nursing field that has received increased attention in the past couple decades. Yuksel et al. (2022) explored the meaning of spirituality among older adults in various stages of health and identified three themes: connection to God; spirituality's contribution to personal wholeness, health, and interpersonal relationships; and the sustainability of comfort in stressful situations.

Differences between the spirituality of the nurse and that of the patient can cause tension. Regardless, nurses can provide spiritual care for patients by supporting religious or spiritual practices and by creating a safe space where spiritual concerns can be expressed. Actively listening to patients' spiritual concerns without judgment, respecting patients' beliefs and values, and offering time for reflection, prayer, or meditation support spiritual well-being. Nurses can also offer to connect patients with spiritual resources, such as chaplains or religious leaders (Yoost & Crawford, 2023). The ability to address religious and spiritual preferences and concerns of patients by RNs has been enhanced with the increased diversity in culture, ethnicity, and religion among today's nurses and the inclusion of such concepts in today's nursing curricula, whereby nursing students engage in classroom discussions about this topic.

Spiritual nursing is recognized by the ICN as an important element of palliative care in caring for dying patients and their families. **Palliative care** is the holistic care of patients with advanced progressive illness who are not responsive to curative treatment. Palliative care includes pain management; symptom management; social, psychological, emotional, and spiritual support; and support for the patient's caregiver.

Hospice nursing is a specialty for nurses particularly interested in palliative care. Established in 1986, the Hospice and Palliative Nurses Association (HPNA) is the nation's largest and oldest professional nursing organization dedicated to promoting excellence in hospice and palliative nursing care. The ANA, working with the HPNA, developed the *Palliative Nursing: Scope and Standards of Practice—An Essential Resource for Hospice and Palliative Nurses* in (2014). Similar to other nursing specialties, standards and competencies were developed for palliative nurses, with additional standards established for APRNs.

Working with HPNA, the ANA adopted the *Call for Action: Nurses Lead and Transform Palliative Care* on March 13, 2017. The conclusion provided in the Call to Action was that seriously ill and injured patients, families, and communities should receive quality palliative care in all care settings and that this is achieved by the delivery of primary palliative nursing by every nurse, regardless of setting. Most recently, the HPNA convened the *Palliative Nursing Summit* on May 12, 2017. The ANA and Representatives from 26 specialty nursing organizations worked to develop a collaborative nursing agenda and action plan focused on three aspects of palliative nursing: communication and advance care planning, coordination/transitions of care, and pain and symptom management.

NURSING ENTREPRENEURISM

Entrepreneurism is somewhat new in the nursing profession. An **entrepreneur** is defined as one who organizes, manages, and assumes the risk of a business or enterprise. Nurse entrepreneurs are risk takers who use their nursing knowledge, expertise, networking, and business skills to assume an independent or collaborative role in a new business or enterprise. Nurses become entrepreneurs for many reasons. Changes in the healthcare setting, the desire for greater autonomy, and interest in a particular specialty where one wants to devote increased attention are all examples of catalysts that may cause a nurse to become an entrepreneur.

Although nurses are making important contributions to healthcare reform and quality care, the loss of nurses from clinical practice to entrepreneurism is contributing to the nursing shortage. Nurses are pursuing specialized interests in such areas as hospice and palliative nursing, spiritual nursing, and NI. They are also assuming such roles as legal nurses, insurance nurses, lobbyists, diabetes educators, salespersons of a wide array of products, consultants, business owners, and travel and travel agency nurses. As described previously, bioterrorism preparedness and internet-based entrepreneurial opportunities are also growing.

The Nurse Entrepreneur Network (NeN) was founded by Lea Rae Keyes, RN, to help nurse entrepreneurs start, manage, and grow their businesses. Launched in 2004, NeN is an online network that also helps members form collaborative alliances and promote their businesses. For more information on nurse entrepreneurism, visit the NeN website.

SERVICE LEARNING, ADVOCACY, AND POLICY MAKING

The need for social healthcare reform (i.e., prevention of obesity, diabetes, cancer, AIDS, teenage pregnancy, chemical dependency, etc.) poses new roles and challenges for nursing. In an effort to build awareness of social issues causing increased healthcare needs, many nursing programs have added service learning strands to their curricula. **Service learning** experiences are those experiences that provide an opportunity for students to develop civic responsibility by working with individuals and agencies in the community to improve quality of life, assist veterans, serve senior citizens, work with chemical dependency and battered women's shelters, and provide services following disasters (e.g., floods, hurricanes, fires) or acts of terrorism, to name a few. The "fit" of this curriculum with nursing's need for more community-based learning experiences is evident. Through such experiences, the nursing student is exposed to healthcare reform issues and develops an appreciation for the important nursing roles in advocacy and policy making.

Nursing involvement is also needed to address policy needed in such areas as **biomedical technology**, informatics, cyberterrorism, **genetic engineering** (e.g., foods, cloning), **robotics**, ecologically green and sustainable technologies, and bioethical decision-making.

Nurses comprise the nation's largest healthcare profession. Acting individually and collectively through their organizations, nurses can shape and refine public policy. The ANA website provides useful information for nurses on how to become involved in important efforts for healthcare reform and the development of social policy, both as an individual and as members of national nursing organizations.

COLLABORATIVE PRACTICE AND NURSING'S FUTURE

Nursing has undergone many transitions throughout time and has grown as a profession. Many factors have influenced trends and transitions in nursing. As nursing has grown and changed, so have other health professions. One change that is apparent in all is the need to work more collaboratively to address the challenges faced by patients, clients, and the healthcare industry as a whole.

In 2010, an interdisciplinary committee, comprised professionals across the healthcare spectrum, examined the future of nursing. Both medical and nursing professionals acknowledged the need for more collaborative practice. In 2011, the IOM published a landmark study, *The Future of Nursing: Leading Change, Advancing Health*. The interdisciplinary committee recommended that nurses (1) should practice to the full extent of their education and training; (2) should achieve higher levels of education and training through an improved education system that promotes seamless academic progression;

(3) be full partners, with physicians and other healthcare professionals, in redesigning healthcare in the United States; and (4) engage in effective workforce planning and policy making that requires better data collection and an improved information infrastructure.

There is widespread support for this study, as nursing strives to fulfill its leadership role as a profession among healthcare professions. As you enter registered nursing, you will have the opportunity, as a member of the profession, to help create this future.

CONCLUSION

Nursing has experienced many transitions throughout history. It has evolved based on historical, political, and societal events and has been especially influenced by the changing roles of women, men, and minorities in society. Also important has been nursing's emergence and continuing growth as a profession, with licensure, regulations, standards of practice, ethics, and theories and research guiding the science of nursing distinct from other sciences.

The impact of societal trends on nursing cannot be underestimated. There will always be a cause and effect on and practice by what happens in the context of our society. The evolution of nursing is a reflection of society in general. Nurses must have an understanding of both their roots and ongoing societal trends to better understand the future, prepare for tomorrow's challenges, and provide leadership in advocating for quality healthcare in all settings.

In today's world, nursing and all health professionals face new challenges. Major changes are emerging in both society and the healthcare industry that will bring new transitions to the practice of nursing, medicine, and all the health professions. Today's professional nurse must be vigilant of the changes and transitions to help shape nursing's preferred future.

STUDENT *Exercises*

Exercise 4.1
Choose an event in the history of nursing that interests you. Research that event more thoroughly and then consider the following points:
   a. What was the general tone in society at that time?
   b. What was the role of both women and men at that time?
   c. What were the functions of nurses, even if not defined in a formal sense?
   d. What drew you to this particular event?
   e. What impact did this event have on the profession of nursing?

Exercise 4.2
As you enter the role of the professional RN today, reflect on the societal trends presented and how they may impact patients and their families in an area of nursing in which you intend to practice. How will you serve as an advocate for change? What organizations might have an impact, and what actions will you take to become involved in such organizations?

REFERENCES

American Association of Colleges of Nursing. (2017, March 20). *Diversity, equity, and inclusion in academic nursing.* https://www.aacnnursing.org/news-data/position-statements-white-papers/diversity-equity-and-inclusion-in-academic-nursing#:~:text=AACN%20recognizes%20diversity%2C%20inclusion%2C%20and,families%2C%20communities%2C%20and%20populations

American Association of Colleges of Nursing. (2022, October). *Fact sheet: Nursing shortage.* https://www.aacnnursing.org/Portals/0/PDFs/Fact-Sheets/Nursing-Shortage-Factsheet.pdf

American Nurses Association. (n.d.). *Welcome to the American Nurses Association.* https://www.nursingworld.org/ana/

American Nurses Association. (2010). *Nursing's social policy statement: The essence of the profession* (10th ed.).

American Nurses Association. (2014). *Palliative nursing: Scope and standards of practice—An essential resource for hospice and palliative nurses.*

American Nurses Association. (2015). *Code of ethics for nurses with interpretive statements* (2nd ed.).

American Nurses Association. (2019). *Holistic nursing: Scope and standards of practice* (3rd ed.).

American Nurses Association. (2021). *Nursing: Scope and standards of practice* (4th ed.).

American Nurses Association. (2022). *Nursing informatics: Scope and standards of practice* (3rd ed.).

Arenas-Escaso, J., Folgado-Fernández, J.A., & Palos-Sánchez, P.R. (2024). Internet interventions and therapies for addressing the negative impact of digital overuse: A focus on digital free tourism and economic sustainability. *BMC Public Health, 24,* 1–12. https://doi.org/10.1186/s12889-023-17584-6

Benner, P. (2001). *From novice to expert: Excellence and power in clinical nursing practice* (Commemorative ed.). Prentice-Hall.

Benner, P., Sutphen, M., Leonard, V., Day, L., & Schulman, L. S. (2010). *Educating nurses: A call for radical transformation.* Jossey-Bass.

Boyle, J. C., Collins, J. W., Ludwig-Beymer, P., & Andrews, M. M. (2025). *Transcultural concepts in nursing care* (9th ed.). Wolters Kluwer.

Buckway, A. J., & Sowerby, H. (2023). *Nursing in today's world: Trends, issues, and management* (12th ed.). Wolters Kluwer.

Cherry, B., & Jacob, S. R. (2022). *Contemporary nursing: Issues, trends, & management* (9th ed.). Elsevier.

Godshall, M. (2020). *Fast facts for evidence-based practice in nursing* (3rd ed.). Springer Publishing.

Goleman, D. (1998). *Working with emotional intelligence: Why it can matter more than IQ.* Bantam.

Goleman, D. (2007). *Social intelligence: The new science of human relationships.* Random House.

Goleman, D. (2009). *Ecological intelligence: How knowing the hidden impacts of what we buy can change everything.* Broadway Books.

Grossman, S. C., & Valiga, T. M. (2020). *The new leadership challenge: Creating the future of nursing* (6th ed.). F. A. Davis.

Hood, L. (2022). *Leddy & Pepper's professional nursing* (10th ed.). Wolters Kluwer.

Institute of Medicine. (2011). *The future of nursing: Leading change, advancing health.* National Academies Press.

International Council of Nurses. (n.d.). *ICN strategic plan.* https://www.icn.ch/sites/default/files/2023-04/Strategic%20plan.pdf

International Council of Nurses. (2021). *The ICN code of ethics for nurses.* https://www.icn.ch/sites/default/files/2023-06/ICN_Code-of-Ethics_EN_Web.pdf

Jacob, S. R. (2023). The evolution of professional nursing. In B. Cherry & S. R. Jacob (Eds.), *Contemporary nursing: Issues, trends, & management* (9th ed., pp. 1–20). Elsevier.

Lindsey, R. B., Roberts, L. M., & CampbellJones, F. (2013). *The culturally proficient school: An implementation guide for school leaders* (2nd ed.). Corwin Press, Sage.

Liu, S. I., Shikar, M., Gante, E., Prufeta, P., Ho, K., Barie, P. S., Winchell, R. J., & Lee, J. I. (2022). Improving communication and response to clinical deterioration to increase patient safety in the intensive care unit. *Critical Care Nurse, 42*(5), 33–43. https://doi.org/10.4037/ccn2022295

Mazinga, G. (2023). NLN annual survey of schools of nursing academic year 2021–2022: Executive summary. *Nursing Education Perspectives, 44*(5), 328–329. https://doi.org/10.1097/01.NEP.0000000000001187

McGonigle, D., & Mastrian, K. (2022). *Nursing informatics and the foundation of knowledge* (5th ed.). Jones & Bartlett Learning.

Melnyk, B., & Fineout-Overholt, E. (2023). *Evidence based practice in nursing and healthcare: A guide to best practice* (5th ed.). Wolters Kluwer.

Moss, M. T. (2005). *The emotionally intelligent nurse leader*. Jossey-Bass.

National Council of State Boards of Nursing. (2023). *NLC States*. https://www.ncsbn.org/public-files/NLC_Map.pdf

National League for Nursing. (n.d.-a). *Core values*. https://www.nln.org/about/about/core-values

National League for Nursing. (n.d.-b). *Diversity & inclusion*. https://www.nln.org/public-policy/nursing-education-issues/diversity

National League for Nursing. (n.d.-c). *Nursing education statistics*. https://www.nln.org/nlnNews/newsroom/nursing-education-statistics

Next Generation NCLEX. (n.d.). National Council of State Boards of Nursing, Inc. https://www.nclex.com/next-generation-nclex.page

Nightingale, F. (1992). *Notes on nursing: What it is and what it is not* (A commemorative edition of the first edition published in 1859.). Lippincott.

Nursing Workforce Diversity. (2023). *Nursing for Women's Health, 27*(4), e1–e5. https://doi.org/10.1016/j.nwh.2023.04.002

Nutting, M. A., & Dock, L. L. (1907). *A history of nursing: The evolution of nursing systems from the earliest times to the foundation of the first English and American training schools for nurses*. G. P. Putnam's Sons. https://archive.org/details/historyofnursing01nutt/page/n13/mode/2up

Organization for Associate Degree Nursing. (n.d.). *About*. https://oadn.org/about/

Pearman, A., Hughes, M. L., Smith, E. L., & Neupert, S. D. (2020). Mental health challenges of United States healthcare professionals during COVID-19. *Frontiers in Psychology, 11*(2065) https://doi.org/10.3389/fpsyg.2020.02165

Rebar, C. R., & Heimgartner, N. M. (2021). A renewed commitment to cultural humility. *Medsurg Nursing, 30*(2), 147–148.

Smith, A., & Foronda, C. (2021). Promoting cultural humility in nursing education through the use of ground rules. *Nursing Education Perspectives, 42*(2), 117–119. https://doi.org/10.1097/01.NEP.0000000000000594

So, N., Price, K., O'Mara, P., & Rodrigues, M. A. (2024). The importance of cultural humility and cultural safety in health care. *Medical Journal of Australia, 220*(1), 12–13. https://doi.org/10.5694/mja2.52182

U.S. Bureau of Labor Statistics. (2024, January 26). *Labor force statistics from the current population survey*. https://www.bls.gov/cps/cpsaat11.htm

U.S. Department of Health and Human Services. (n.d.) *What is telehealth?* https://www.hhs.gov/hipaa/for-professionals/faq/3015/what-is-telehealth/index.html#:~:text=The%20Health%20Resources%20and%20Services,professional%20health%2Drelated%20education%2C%20and

U.S. Department of Veterans Affairs. (n.d.). *How common is PTSD in veterans?* https://www.ptsd.va.gov/understand/common/common_veterans.asp

World Health Organization. (n.d.). *Constitution*. https://www.who.int/about/governance/constitution

Yoost, B. L., & Crawford, L. R. (2023). *Fundamentals of nursing: Active learning for collaborative practice* (3rd ed.). Elsevier.

Yuksel, C. O., Songul, D., & Kubra, D. (2022). The meaning and role of spirituality for older adults: A qualitative study. *Journal of Religion and Health, 61*(2), 1490–1504. https://doi.org/10.1007/s10943-021-01258-x

On the WEB

American Assembly for Men in Nursing: http://www.aamn.org

American Association for the History of Nursing: http://www.aahn.org

American Association of Colleges of Nursing: http://www.aacn.nche.edu

American Holistic Nurses Association: http://www.ahna.org

American Nurses Association: http://www.nursingworld.org

Florence Nightingale Museum: http://www.florence-nightingale.co.uk

Health Care Information and Management Systems Society: http://www.himss.org

Health Insurance Portability and Accountability Act of 1996: http://www.hipaa.com

Hospice and Palliative Nurses Association: http://www.hpna.org

Institute of Medicine: http://www.iom.edu

International Council of Nurses: https://www.icn.ch

International Network for Doctoral Education in Nursing: http://www.indenglobal.org

NANDA International, Inc.: http://www.nanda.org

National Council of State Boards of Nursing: http://www.ncsbn.org

National League for Nursing: http://www.nln.org

Nurse Entrepreneur Network: http://www.nurse-entrepreneur-network.com

Organization for Associate Degree Nursing: http://www.oadn.org

The Nursing Community: http://www.thenursingcommunity.org

CHAPTER 5

Learning at the ADN Level

LEARNING OUTCOMES

By the end of this chapter, the student will be able to:
1. Describe learning concepts related to the adult learner.
2. Apply adult learning concepts to oneself.
3. Describe the differences between medical and nursing conceptual models.
4. Give examples of learning activities in each of three learning domains: cognitive, affective, and psychomotor.
5. Compare and contrast the graduate competencies of LPN/LVNs and ADNs in the NLN's four broad program outcome areas.
6. Discuss the roles of LPN/LVNs and ADNs related to the nursing process and nursing diagnosis.
7. Differentiate among the six cognitive learning achievement levels: knowledge, comprehension, application, analysis, synthesis, and evaluation.
8. Differentiate between passive and active learning processes.
9. Analyze development needs you may have related to being successful in today's changing educational environment.
10. Identify learning strategies to maximize success in an ADN program.
11. Describe the similarities and differences in transition needs of LPN/LVNs entering ADN programs as advanced placement generic, straight-through LPN/LVN-to-ADN students, and time-out LPN/LVN-to-ADN students.
12. Differentiate between the ADN student and LPN/LVN practice roles, and evaluate areas that you anticipate may be challenging for you or that may cause role confusion.

KEY TERMS

active learning
conceptual model
experiential knowledge
learning achievement levels:
- knowledge
- comprehension
- application
- analysis
- synthesis
- evaluation
learning domains:
- affective
- cognitive
- psychomotor
Massive Open Online Courses (MOOCs)
nursing diagnosis
nursing process
Open Education Resources (OERs)
proxemics
self-actualization
transcultural literacy
virtual learning space

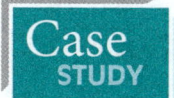

George Dobian is apprehensive about his first nursing course, which he will take in the fall. He has heard from others that nursing school is very different from when he attended LVN school 10 years ago. Because he has never been good at taking tests, test-taking anxiety has haunted him throughout his adult life. He is afraid of being embarrassed because his employer is paying for his education. He wonders if he has the wrong study skills or if he has a learning disability. He has talked about his concerns with his friend John Scott, a student in his anatomy and physiology class. John took a "Success Strategies for the Returning Student" seminar at the community college and speaks openly about his professor's introduction to skills in learning. George is impressed when John says that his test scores and overall recall of materials improved when he began rewriting his notes, discussing course content with others, experiencing problems firsthand during clinical sessions, and participating in teaching projects. George is on his way to sign up for the next instance of this seminar and has made an appointment to talk with a counselor about determining whether he has a learning disability.

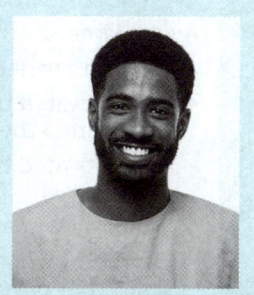

ADULT LEARNING THEORY

Much has been written about adult learning theory; adult learning styles were discussed briefly in Chapter 1. The knowledge and life experiences you brought to the ADN program are valuable assets as you return to school to pursue becoming an RN. Perhaps you find yourself in a situation like George's. George has a clear understanding of his goals and motivation mechanisms but really needs help with the transition process of returning to school. To aid you in the transition process as an adult learner, you need a clear understanding of your societal roles, goals, learning style(s), motivational mechanisms, strengths, and potential barriers.

Adult learners draw on a wide variety of life experiences as they pursue additional education. These experiences serve as a resource and support as you engage in your new educational pathway. Adults are generally self-motivated and self-directed and have developed a preferred learning style. Chapter 1 presented the work by Ellis (2022a, 2022b) on learning styles, and you were given an opportunity to reflect on your preferred learning style(s) as an adult learner. Unlike the child's learning environment, which is structured and directed by the teacher, the milieu for the adult learner must provide opportunities for self-established goals and learning techniques.

Additionally, adults are motivated to learn when they see the meaning and relevance of learning in fulfilling societal roles or solving daily problems faced at home or on the job. As Bradshaw et al. (2021) stress, adult learners assume responsibility for their own learning, especially when they see meaning and usefulness of that learning in their career advancement.

We each develop our own unique intrinsic motivation as we mature, based on emotions, and shaped through culture. Many variations exist among adult learners based on their learning styles, age, gender, ethnicity, and socioeconomic and cultural backgrounds. This intrinsic motivation influences the degree to which we engage

> **BOX 5.1 Characteristics of Adult Learners**
>
> Adult learners:
> - Draw on a variety of life experiences in the educational process.
> - Are motivated to learn when they see that such learning solves problems confronting them.
> - Are motivated to learn when such learning is needed to fulfill social roles.
> - Are self-motivated and self-directed, and seek learning to fulfill self-established goals.
> - Learn best when the program of learning addresses the individual learning styles they have developed with time.
> - Are motivated to learn for purposes of self-actualization and to make a meaningful contribution to society.

in and are motivated by various learning activities. The same learning activity that frustrates you may be enjoyed by another student, and vice versa, based on your social and cultural backgrounds and life experiences. Recognizing your emotional response, accepting it, and moving forward will minimize stress in the learning process. The key characteristics of adult learners are provided in Box 5.1.

EXPERIENTIAL KNOWLEDGE AND THE ADULT LEARNER

As an LPN/LVN and an adult with a wide variety of life experiences, you bring to the ADN program a great deal of knowledge, including expertise in specific content areas of the curriculum. This extensive **experiential knowledge** enhances the educational process in several ways.

First, having both theoretical and practical knowledge, skills, and abilities provides you with the self-confidence to tackle new areas of learning and venture into new clinical experiences. Your familiarity with the workplace, the variety of patients for whom you have provided care, and your life experiences as an adult all give you confidence.

In today's ADN program, the clinical learning begins in the nursing laboratory with high-tech simulations. Huston (2023) advocates the use of these advanced simulations to provide alternative scenarios of patient situations to challenge the nursing student to apply problem-solving and critical thinking skills in determining care needs. Additionally, many schools are now employing simulated experiences for interprofessional learning teams, composed of students from multiple professions, to challenge the students in each discipline to think holistically about patient care. Interprofessional team learning is a valuable strategy for enhancing communication and collaboration among health professionals (Poore & Cooper, 2020).

Second, your areas of expertise will be a rich resource to peers, as theirs will be to you, as you participate in learning activities and work in groups to fulfill course objectives and meet clinical competencies at the RN level.

Third, your rich experiential background provides a wealth of information for making connections between prior learning experiences and new ones, problem-solving, and analyzing and synthesizing new theoretical content and practical applications.

MEANING AND RELEVANCE OF NEW KNOWLEDGE

Adult learners are motivated to learn when their learning is relevant and useful in their work and home lives. The LPN/LVN who returns to school to pursue an ADN often does so for monetary reasons or for increased autonomy or career mobility. However, once in the transition process, this same nurse discovers the increased ability they have to plan and implement individualized care to clients. This increased ability may also provide motivation. The most effective motivational factor for adults is competence. Competence is a reality check because it identifies personal limits. Adults have a strong desire to be competent, and they frequently look to learning as a means of achieving this goal. This human urge for competence transcends cultural boundaries; it is an innate trait that can be reinforced or weakened through learning opportunities (Knowles et al., 2020).

The ability to make nursing diagnoses, solve problems, and work collaboratively with physicians and other healthcare professionals to provide comprehensive client care results in additional motivation and the incentive to continue pursuit of the increased scope of practice of professional nursing. The increased independence and ability to solve problems, use evidence-based research, think critically, and accept new challenges in their everyday world creates even greater motivation for LPN/LVNs to further their learning.

THINKING CRITICALLY

Reflect on an experience when some new knowledge had particular meaning and relevance to you in your personal or work life. How did this motivate you to learn even more?

PERSONAL AND PROFESSIONAL ACHIEVEMENT AND SELF-ACTUALIZATION

A parallel but different motivational force in adults pursuing further education is self-fulfillment or self-actualization. To **self-actualize** is to realize fully one's potential. Whether for personal or professional achievement, one motivation for LPN/LVNs to seek ADN education is to realize their potential as nurses and to acquire the knowledge, skills, and abilities to practice at the RN level. Covey (2004) noted that when one finds one's own voice, effectiveness is enhanced, and one is able to go from good to great. Perhaps your pursuit of a professional degree and professional practice is this desire to find your own voice for self-actualization.

THINKING CRITICALLY

Reflect on the factors that have motivated you to pursue an ADN. When things get tough from time to time throughout the program, how can you draw on these resources to maintain that motivation?

SELF-DIRECTED, INDIVIDUALIZED LEARNING

In addition to a wealth of experiential learning, the adult learner has gained insight into the means by which they learn best. Individualizing your approach to new content can offer many possibilities for maximizing the learning process.

The adult learner is self-directed and seeks learning to fulfill self-established goals. The LPN/LVN who sets personal goals related to the accomplishment of competencies and objectives of the ADN program is more likely to experience success than are those who are not self-directed.

PRACTICAL/VOCATIONAL AND ASSOCIATE DEGREE NURSING EDUCATION: A COMPARISON

Although the educational programs for the LPN/LVN and the ADN student may appear to be similar, close examination reveals major differences between the two. The LPN/LVN practitioner has a directed, prescriptive role, providing safe and high-quality care as outlined and directed by medical and nursing professionals. The expanded role of the professional nurse includes the acquisition and application of increased theory, analysis of data, examination of legal issues and ethical dilemmas, reflection and critical thinking, clinical reasoning and judgment, the ability to make nursing diagnoses, informatics, resource management, quality management, and economics, to name a few. The registered nursing student develops into a professional nurse, designing customized plans of care for individual and family clients, and working collaboratively with other healthcare team professionals to provide holistic, high-quality care.

You may at first think the only difference between the two programs is some additional science background and technical skill development with more complex procedures. However, you will find that developing professional competence involves learning and thinking in a whole new way. Qualities of professional competence include initiative, sensitivity to one's own sensitivity, evidence-based decision-making, and self-evaluation. Clinical judgment is the foundation of professional competence for registered nurses. Noticing a situation exists and having the ability to interpret that situation requires a high level of reasoning to respond and to take action. Nursing students develop clinical judgment during clinical experiences and simulations by making evidence-based decisions to solve problems. The process of reflecting on patient care situations and determining needed changes builds strong professional competence for practice (Hambach et al., 2023).

PHILOSOPHIES AND CONCEPTUAL MODELS

Each nursing program is built on a philosophy developed and shared by that program's nursing faculty. Although both levels of nursing programs (LPN/LVN and ADN) set forth beliefs about the practice of nursing in their philosophy statements, the ADN program's philosophy generally provides greater depth in its view of nursing, defining such central concepts as human (patient/client or person), health, environment, nursing, caring, teaching, and learning.

The **conceptual model** is the template of theoretical concepts and principles that is a basis for developing the curricular content for the nursing program. The conceptual model is derived from the program's philosophy and guides the development of course objectives and competencies. LPN/LVN programs may be built on either a medical or nursing model. The LPN/LVN operates as a member of the nursing profession and the healthcare team, providing care to clients as prescribed by physicians, nurses, and other healthcare professionals. In this directed role, the LPN/LVN carries out physicians' orders and contributes to the planning, implementation, and evaluation of care to individual clients based on nursing diagnoses established by the RN.

The LPN/LVN programs that use a nursing model (i.e., based on nursing theory and nursing diagnoses rather than medical diagnoses) often choose a human needs approach because this model fits well with the directed scope of practice of the LPN/LVN. ADN programs often use an integrated nursing model for their conceptual framework, drawing on the research of nurse theorists and incorporating nursing diagnoses to guide the developing autonomous practice of the RN student. These models allow for the nurse with an associate degree to practice both independently and collaboratively with other healthcare providers, within their scope of practice.

CURRICULAR FRAMEWORKS

The curricular frameworks for each of these levels of nursing programs are consistent with their state nurse practice acts, National Council of State Boards of Nursing (NCSBN) test plans (NCSBN, 2023a, 2023b), and competencies identified by such professional organizations as the National League for Nursing (NLN, 2012). Each state's nurse practice act outlines the educational preparation needed for licensure in that state as an LPN (LVN in Texas and California), an RN, or an advanced practice RN.

Each nursing school's curricula must be approved by its state board of nursing for it to be accredited so that program graduates will be eligible for licensure through the NCLEX after completion. In addition, most ADN programs have adopted student learning outcomes (SLOs) for each course, for the program, and for the associate degree consistent with the college's institution-level SLOs as required by the institution's regional accrediting body.

The NLN (2012) has identified the outcomes and competencies of all programs in nursing from the practical/vocational level to the doctoral level. Four broad outcomes are applicable to all nursing programs. Graduates should be prepared (a) to promote and enhance *human flourishing* for patients, families, communities, and themselves; (b) to show sound *nursing judgment*; (c) to continually develop their *professional identity*; and (d) to maintain a *spirit of* inquiry as they move into the world of nursing practice, and beyond (NLN, 2012).

CURRICULAR CONTENT AND LEARNING DOMAINS

In the mid-1900s, Benjamin S. Bloom (1956) identified three **learning domains** into which curricular content falls and from which educational objectives are written. The **cognitive** domain is the area of learning in which you acquire knowledge. The **affective** domain is the area of learning involving values and attitudes. The **psychomotor** domain is the area of learning in which you develop manipulative skills in the discipline.

THINKING CRITICALLY

To gain a better understanding of the three learning domains, think about the last time you attended a nursing in-service at work. What cognitive learning took place? What words, procedures, and rules did you need to learn and apply to participate in the in-service? What affective learning took place? What attitudes did you need to change or develop? How did your beliefs or views about nursing and the type of people involved change? What psychomotor learning took place? What hands-on skills did you need to learn?

Both LPN/LVN and ADN education programs contain curricular content in all three learning domains. For example, both programs require knowledge of body structure and function (cognitive domain), an appreciation for the self-image changes confronting the aging individual (affective domain), and the ability to take accurate vital signs (psychomotor domain). However, more in-depth content in each domain is included in the ADN program curriculum. A review of the curriculum content in each of the two program levels reveals that additional content or course work is required for the ADN program in such areas as the biologic and behavioral sciences; computational, communication, and language skills; advanced medical-surgical nursing; psychiatric nursing; and management and leadership skills.

LEARNING ACHIEVEMENT LEVELS

Within the cognitive domain, Bloom (1956) identified six **learning achievement levels**: **knowledge**, **comprehension**, **application**, **analysis**, **synthesis**, and **evaluation**. Bloom developed the Taxonomy of Educational Objectives to differentiate the various types of thinking. Objectives were developed for the cognitive, affective, and psychomotor domains, and educators have used these for curriculum planning over the decades. During the 1990s, Lorin Anderson (a former student of Bloom) led a team of cognitive psychologists to review and revise the taxonomy for the 21st century, including the terminology, structure, and emphasis within the cognitive domain. Box 5.2 shows a comparison of Bloom's original and Anderson's revised Taxonomy of Educational Objectives (Anderson & Krathwohl, 2001; Bloom, 1956). These two taxonomies continue to provide the foundation for NCLEX-PN and NCLEX-RN Test Plans today.

Competencies at the LPN/LVN level include the knowledge, comprehension, and application of content within the scope of practice of the LPN/LVN. Competencies at the ADN level include all six cognitive learning achievement levels. Whether your ADN program uses the original or the revised taxonomy, the ability to analyze, synthesize, evaluate, and create is essential to the RN in evidence-based research, clinical reflection, critical thinking, and clinical reasoning necessary for making appropriate nursing diagnoses, designing nursing care plans, and managing client care. Curriculum content and learning activities in the ADN program support learning achievement at these higher-order learning levels.

BOX 5.2 Comparison of Bloom's Original (1956) and Anderson's Revised (2001) Taxonomy of Educational Objectives in the Cognitive Domain

Bloom's Original Taxonomy	Anderson's Revised Taxonomy
Knowledge	Remembering
Comprehension	Understanding
Application	Applying
Analysis	Analyzing
Synthesis	Evaluating
Evaluation	Creating

Source: Bloom, B. S. (Ed.). (1974). *The taxonomy of educational objectives: Affective and cognitive domains.* David McKay; Anderson, L. W., & Krathwohl, D. R. (Eds.). (2001). *A taxonomy for learning, teaching, and assessing: A revision of Bloom's taxonomy of educational objects.* Longman.

NURSING PROCESS AND NURSING DIAGNOSIS

Taylor et al. (2023) describe the **nursing process** as a systematic method that progresses through five phases: assessment, analysis and **nursing diagnosis**, planning, implementation, and evaluation. Nurses implement their roles through the nursing process, which integrates both the art and science of nursing. The nursing process is used by the nurse to identify the patient's healthcare needs and strengths, to establish and carry out a plan of care to meet those needs, and to evaluate the effectiveness of the plan to meet established outcomes.

Both the LPN/LVN and the RN participate in the nursing process within their respective scopes of practice. However, the roles played by each differ. Table 5.1 provides a comparison of the roles of LPN/LVNs and RNs with regard to nursing process and nursing diagnosis. The LPN/LVN collects data, assists with patient assessment, contributes to the planning phase, implements basic therapeutic and preventive measures outlined in the plan, and evaluates the effectiveness of such measures. The RN collects data and performs patient assessment, analyzes and groups data, draws conclusions and uses judgment in establishing nursing diagnoses, designs a plan of care collaborating with other healthcare providers, develops an implementation plan with short- and long-term goals, and provides outcomes of the plan, redesigning as needed.

The test plan for the NCLEX-PN outlines the role of the LPN/LVN and this practitioner's role in relation to the nursing process. The practical/vocational nurse provides care to individuals in various settings under the direction of qualified health professionals. Using the nursing process, the practical/vocational nurse contributes to the interdisciplinary team by collecting and organizing relevant healthcare data and assisting in identifying client health needs and problems. The practical/vocational nurse at the entry

TABLE 5.1 Comparison of the Role Played by LPN/LVNs and RNs in Nursing Process and Nursing Diagnosis

Nursing Process Phase	Role of LPN/LVN	Role of RN Beyond LPN/LVN Scope of Practice
Assessment	Gathers data Performs patient assessment Identifies patient strengths	Gathers more extensive biopsychosocial data Groups and analyzes data Researches additional data needed Identifies client resources
Nursing Diagnosis	Not applicable	Draws conclusions Uses judgment Makes diagnoses
Planning	Contributes to development of care plans	Sets short- and long-term client goals Establishes priorities Collaborates and refers
Implementation	Provides basic therapeutic and preventive nursing measures Provides client teaching Records client information	Manages client care (performs and delegates) Provides client and family teaching Provides referrals Records and exchanges client information with health team
Evaluation	Evaluates effects of care given	Evaluates effectiveness of overall plan Analyzes new data Modifies and redesigns plan Collaborates with other professionals and members of the healthcare team

level exhibits the fundamental skills required to care for patients with common health problems with predictable outcomes (NCSBN, 2023b). The entry-level practical nurse acts in a more dependent role when participating in the planning and evaluation phases of the nursing process and acts in a more independent role when participating in the data collecting and implementing phases of the nursing process.

In contrast, the test plan for the National Council Licensure Examination for Registered Nurses (NCSBN, 2023a) recognizes the role of the RN in all five phases of the nursing process, including the analysis (nursing diagnosis) phase. Nursing process is integrated across the client needs areas, as are these four processes: caring, communication and documentation, teaching/learning, and culture and spirituality. The client needs areas include safe and effective care environment, health promotion and maintenance, psychosocial integrity, and physiological integrity. Test questions are based on the job analysis study of practicing RNs (NCSBN, 2022). More in-depth information on nursing process is covered in Chapter 10.

DIFFERENCES IN THE LEARNING PROCESS AND CHANGES IN THE EDUCATIONAL ENVIRONMENT

As you enter the ADN program, you may discover differences in the learning process from that encountered in the LPN/LVN program you attended. These differences may be attributed partly to the length of time between the programs, especially if it has been many years since your participation in the LPN/LVN program. However, even if you just recently completed the LPN/LVN program, you will encounter differences attributable to the areas discussed in this chapter: program philosophies; conceptual models; curricular frameworks; curricular content within learning domains; addition of the analysis, synthesis, and evaluation learning achievement levels; and role in nursing process and nursing diagnosis.

As has been mentioned several times throughout this text, learning at the ADN level is much different than that at the LPN/LVN level. As a returning student, you may not be familiar with nursing theory. Because theory is abstract in nature, you may be anxious because you previously learned in educational environments that were concrete and structured, and you previously functioned professionally using technical expertise (Kearney-Nunnery, 2020).

Additionally, the science of nursing is ever evolving. Even if you just recently completed your LPN/LVN training, you will discover new problem-solving theory as you progress through the RN program. For example, in the most recent NCLEX-RN Test Plan, the five-step problem-solving method of the nursing process is evolving into the four-step clinical judgment model of noticing, interpreting, responding, and reflecting (Ignatavicius, 2021).

Another area that is relatively new in higher education is the move away from "learning objectives," toward "student learning outcomes." As a student, you will be evaluated on higher-level thinking skills and practice-based competencies. As Cherry and Jacob (2022) note, this approach results in a movement away from the traditional lecture format of students trying to memorize readings and class notes and requires instead a wide array of classroom learning activities and different evaluation methods to promote and assess the student's problem-solving, critical thinking, and clinical reasoning skills.

Because the goal of the ADN program is to enable you to function in the independent and interdependent (collaborative) modes, use higher-level thinking skills, and make nursing diagnoses using analysis and judgment, you will experience two key differences in the educational process: (a) an active learning process will mostly likely be the mode of operation and (b) learning activities will include a focus on developing your ability to analyze, synthesize, and apply curricular content to achieve identified learning outcomes.

Active learning is the act or process of acquiring knowledge or skills by being engaged in action or activity. Participating actively provides learners with several advantages. By interacting with others, learners have the opportunity to clarify thoughts and observations, to process course material, and to gain insight into content (Kearney-Nunnery, 2020). The active learning environment of the ADN program, when compared perhaps to your LPN/LVN training, will require you to be resourceful, disciplined, self-directed, and proactive in seeking those learning opportunities that will build both your confidence and your competence to function as a professional nurse. In today's workplace, the ability to effectively self-direct one's work is becoming more and more important. However, educators occasionally meet individuals who lack self-confidence or are reluctant to take ownership of their education, which is most commonly caused by one of the below factors:

- The adult has not been socialized to see themselves as in control of their own learning.
- The adult's experiences in school or in the specific field of learning have generally been negative or unsuccessful.
- The adult does not think they have a choice as to whether or not they participate in the learning or training experience.

Adult learners frequently need training not so much because they want the training but rather because they need the job, promotion, and money for which these learning experiences are essential. For many adults, they might feel powerless to change the situation they are in and may often respond with, "Just tell me what to do" (Bergin et al., 2023). At times, you may feel this way within the active learning environment of the ADN program.

In addition to traditional lecture, laboratory, and clinical experiences, learning activities in the ADN program include classroom activities and out-of-class assignments that require active participation and reflection on one's own values, beliefs, and practices. Such exercises are designed to build self-confidence, develop communication skills, develop analytical skills, and foster critical thinking to prepare you for the autonomous professional role you will be expected to assume after graduation. No longer will the correct response be to report findings to the RN or physician. You will now need to analyze information, think critically, use judgment, establish nursing diagnoses, confront ethical issues, take action, manage client care, and delegate interventions while maintaining responsibility for clients under your care. The active learning process in the ADN program and learning activities that focus on developing your ability to analyze and synthesize curricular content will prepare you for these new challenges.

Your nursing instructors and other faculty on campus teaching at the associate degree level are preparing you for today's world of work where problem-solving, critical thinking, and lifelong learning are vital to your success as an RN. Contemporary instructors focus less on teaching and more on facilitating learning so that both you and the instructor are focused on your learning. Instructors who are learner-centered link students to resources. They provide tasks and activities that keep students interested and support learning in both individual and group settings (Dashew & Gayeski, 2023).

> **BOX 5.3**
>
> ### The Faculty Role in Adult Learner–Centered Teaching
>
> 1. Create a supportive and inclusive learning environment in which adult learners feel empowered to explore new ideas, question established norms, and embrace change.
> 2. Provide resources such as reading materials, online tools, templates, and videos.
> 3. Facilitate self-directed learning by guiding learners in setting goals, designing study plans, and accessing support services.
> 4. Facilitate collaborative learning environments by guiding group discussions, peer activities, and projects.
> 5. Facilitate experiential learning by emphasizing the connection of real-life experiences to theoretical concepts.
> 6. Provide opportunities for reflection on learning activities and application of new knowledge and skills to practical scenarios.
> 7. Assess progress and provide feedback that enables the learner to identify areas for improvement and take ownership of their learning.
> 8. Promote a culture of lifelong learning, intellectual growth, and professional development.

Source: Dashew, B., & Gayeski, D. (2023). Instructional design: Applying principles of adult education. In A. Belzer & B. Dashew (Eds.). *Understanding the adult learner: Perspectives and practices* (pp. 255–274). Taylor Francis Group.

An outline of the faculty role in learner-centered teaching is presented in Box 5.3. Longworth (2003) added that the old method of imposing large quantities of information onto students and hoping they remember it is obsolete. The world is changing at a rapid pace, and the need for lifelong learning means that "what to think" is superseded by "how to think."

Lastly, especially if you have been out of the educational environment for a while, you may find the campus and classroom learning environments and library very different than when you were enrolled in the LPN/LVN program. Huston (2023) describes the evolution of the educational environment and the challenges you may face as a returning adult student. Today's nursing students must be literate in not only computers but also virtual learning spaces and online research.

Today's classroom involves both face-to-face and virtual/online courses and learning management systems (e.g., Blackboard and Canvas). The on-campus laboratory may have high-tech simulation systems for you to access for assignments. Threaded discussions, chat rooms, online-guided discussions, and other **virtual learning spaces** may be part of the curriculum's required learning activities. Some coursework may be incorporated from **Massive Open Online Courses (MOOCs)**, and/or **Open Education Resources (OERs)** may be used.

Your library research for written assignments, research on patients/clients, and nursing care plans will likely be conducted in an online environment, using qualified websites, online journals, and other research sources. You will need to know how to discern between quality research sources and social media. These educational environments and approaches may be uncomfortable for you. Developing ease in their use as you begin your ADN program will strengthen not only your comfort but also your success in the program. Additionally, this may be an excellent opportunity for you to engage with your study group. They may seek your experiential knowledge as a practicing LPN/LVN while you seek their assistance with challenges you may have with technology or navigating this new educational environment.

LEARNING STRATEGIES FOR SUCCESS

As an adult learner, you can adopt learning strategies that will maximize your success in the ADN program by increasing your self-awareness, establishing self-directed goals, becoming an active learner, and adopting techniques to stimulate your thinking.

SELF-AWARENESS

As you return to school to pursue registered nursing, your success will be enhanced with increased self-awareness. Each individual, and each nursing student, is unique. The more one is familiar with oneself, the more the uniqueness can be accessed as a support.

Addressing Your Learning Style

In Chapter 1, you learned about learning styles and how individuals have different ways in which they best learn in an educational setting. You reflected on this material to determine your own learning style(s) or ways you learn best. You may have taken advantage of the Learning Styles Inventory by Ellis (2022a) to discover how you, as an individual, learn. Are you an auditory, visual, or kinesthetic learner? Do you rely primarily on thinking, feeling, doing, or watching? Do you need to role-play or in other ways "experience" the content you are trying to learn?

Learners must know how they learn best and be aware of their strengths and weaknesses in the learning process. This self-awareness then leads to being a more confident and self-directed learner. Exploring new forms of study habits or redesigning group study sessions to address your learning style(s) may enhance your success. In addition, make sure your instructor knows how you learn best. When teachers are aware of your particular learning style, they can incorporate into their teaching methods and strategies that will be particularly helpful to you. Oermann et al. (2023), however, note that it also is good for you to diversify your learning style and try new methods as a strategy to achieve success in both current and future learning activities.

Accommodating for Disabilities

Many individuals with physical, mental, or learning disabilities have experienced success in pursuing a career at the ADN level. The law requires all educational institutions to provide reasonable accommodation to individuals with disabilities, but it is up to the individual to request such accommodation.

Some students may have experienced difficulty in school without knowing they had a learning disability. Several indicators of possible learning disabilities are shown in Box 5.4.

The key to overcoming a learning disability and achieving success in the ADN program is to identify and understand the learning disability and then to seek accommodation for the disability. If requested by the student, the college will provide testing to identify learning disabilities as well as support services and referrals for students with disabilities. The college learning disability specialist can work with you and your instructors to identify effective accommodation strategies for you, but this service must be requested by you. Hunt (2015) notes, "Being your own advocate is extremely important because unfortunately some nurses and faculty may unknowingly or knowingly discriminate against students with disabilities, which is often related to lack of knowledge and/or well-developed policies" (p. 25).

BOX 5.4 Indicators of Possible Learning Problems or Learning Disabilities

Visual Perceptual Problems
- Reverses letters and order of letters
- Omits endings of words
- Cannot edit own work
- Mismarks computerized scoring sheets
- Loses place while reading (marks place with finger or piece of paper)
- Has difficulty lining up numbers correctly (uses graph paper to do math)
- Is confused by complex visual fields (when doing a worksheet, blocks out all but essential item)

Auditory Perceptual Problems
- Cannot differentiate sounds (e and i, m and n)
- Has difficulty sounding out unknown words
- Is poor at spelling
- Is highly distracted by background noise
- Cannot locate emphasis in words or sentences

Spatial Perceptual Problems
- Has trouble differentiating left from right
- Has trouble following directions (gets lost easily)
- Is slow to learn dance routines

Visual–Motor Problems
- Miscopies information
- Has poor handwriting

Integration Problems
- Understands concepts but forgets facts, dates, and names
- Frequently has difficulty recalling commonly known words
- Is poor at spelling (cannot remember order of letters)
- Understands mathematical concepts but cannot remember the order of steps to solve math problems
- Has poor organizational skills

Attention Deficit
- Has trouble sitting still for an extended time
- Is highly distractible
- Is unable to concentrate for an extended time
- Jumps from task to task

Addressing Age, Gender, Sexual Orientation, and Cultural Differences

As described in Chapter 1, LPN/LVNs enrolling in ADN programs may experience barriers to achievement of course objectives and competencies because of age, gender, sexual orientation, or cultural differences in relation to other students or social roles. The re-entry nurse may feel uncomfortable if classmates or peers in study or clinical groups are much younger. The male student who acquired his LPN/LVN through military service may be participating for the first time in an educational setting in which peers and instructors are predominantly female. He or his peers may be uncomfortable in group learning activities, or he may be called on in the clinical area to help move patients or do other physical activities, thus impeding his ability to work on clinical objectives and competencies in his student role.

Cultural mores may also hamper success in the program. The submissive role of women in some cultures may prevent female students from those cultures from teaching male clients, developing autonomy, collaborating with physicians, and developing leadership and management skills. Cultural views of time, acceptable verbal and nonverbal communication skills, and **proxemics** (comfort in spatial relations) may prevent the student from meeting clinical competencies involving these areas of interpersonal skills and responsibilities.

The increased diversity among nursing students today, however, may actually provide you with opportunities to interact with individuals that are more accepting of your uniqueness than in the past. The increased diversity among nursing students contributes to each student's opportunity to develop **transcultural literacy** via group work and team activities in class. The American Nurses Association (2021) encourages development of transcultural literacy as a framework in providing holistic nursing care to culturally diverse individuals, groups, and communities. Strategies for success for students experiencing difficulties because of age, gender, sexual orientation, or cultural differences are shown in Box 5.5.

Many resources are now available to assist students from underrepresented groups on how to succeed. Books, periodicals, and online resources discuss the following:

- Success strategies for students from underrepresented groups—including those who are lesbian, gay, bisexual, transgender, queer and/or questioning, intersex, asexual, and more (LGBTQIA+)—and those with disabilities
- How to deal with racism
- Effective ways to approach moral and ethical decisions students may face based on their ethnic, cultural, or religious values.

SELF-DIRECTED GOALS

A second strategy for maximizing success is to establish self-directed goals. Chapter 1 describes breaking up reading and other learning activities into smaller time blocks and scheduling time in advance for study as important in the goal-setting process. Doing research online or preparing questions for discussion before a study group

---

BOX 5.5 Strategies for Success for Students Experiencing Difficulties Because of Age, Gender, Sexual Orientation, or Cultural Differences

1. Identify situations that generate discomfort.
2. Discuss these areas with the instructor.
3. Share and confront such issues openly in class discussions and clinical conferences.
4. Explore successful coping and accommodation strategies that have been used by other students and nurses.

session will enhance your learning at the session. Proactively seeking clinical skills during each clinical session will ensure completion of clinical skill checklists by the end of the term.

ACTIVE LEARNING

The ADN program will include learning activities for students to work with peers and other healthcare professionals in a variety of ways. There are many benefits of active participation by adult learners who are often distracted by personal problems yet have a wealth of firsthand experience to contribute. Active participation in class enables you to put any worries and issues from your personal life aside while you engage in course content. This focus will strengthen what you learn and improve retention of content for later use on exams and in the clinical area. Through the active learning process, students develop the ability to apply curricular content, analyze and problem solve, think critically, and perform independently, as they advance from the LPN/LVN to the RN level of practice.

A variety of active learning activities will likely be included in the design of your ADN educational program. Commonly found are such activities as brainstorming, small group discussion, role-playing, threaded discussions and other virtual learning activities, group projects, and formal debates. The student who takes a proactive approach in creating their own active learning strategies will enhance success. Forming study groups, posing problems to solve, writing study questions to exchange with peers, and designing care plans in a collaborative process are examples of ways you can strengthen the learning process for both you and your peers.

THINKING CRITICALLY

If you have started courses in the registered nursing program, examine the learning activities and assignments in the course syllabus. Are these different than those you experienced in your LVN/LPN training? Do some of these involve active learning? How is the instructor guiding you into an active learning model?

TECHNIQUES TO STIMULATE THINKING

A similar learning strategy for success is to develop techniques to stimulate thinking about curricular content in each of the three learning domains. One of the best strategies for stimulating thinking is to continually ask yourself questions about the learning being acquired (the what, where, why, who, how, and what if questions). Sample questions are included in the subsections below.

Another learning strategy for success is to take into account your individual uniqueness. In Chapter 6, you will have an opportunity to design your own personal education plan. Other strategies for developing your critical thinking skills are addressed in Chapter 9.

Stimulating Questions in the Cognitive Domain

- What is the meaning of this content?
- How does it relate to last week's learning?

- How does it relate to prior content or courses?
- How would I explain this to someone else?
- How would I apply this in practice?
- How would this apply to clients of different ages, the different genders, different cultures, or those who are disabled?
- What are opposing viewpoints to this content?

Stimulating Questions in the Affective Domain

- How would I feel if I or a family member was experiencing this disorder, dysfunction, or difficulty?
- How would I react if this were happening to someone close to me?
- How do I value this type of response or behavior?
- How might someone experience this whose age, gender, cultural background, or sexual orientation was different than mine?
- What values or beliefs underlie this patient's or nurse's comments?
- What ethical dilemmas might arise in this situation, and how would I confront them?
- Do I need to develop my emotional intelligence?

For this last question, to stretch your thinking in the affective domain, you should develop an awareness of your emotional intelligence and strive to enhance it. da Silva (2022) offers a definition of emotional intelligence to help build a better understanding of the concept and gives tips for developing one's emotional intelligence.

Stimulating Questions in the Psychomotor Domain

- What are the principles underlying this procedure (aseptic techniques, ethical considerations, protection of privacy, body mechanics, energy conservation, resource conservation, and therapeutic effect)?
- How else could this be performed while maintaining these principles?
- How would I teach this to a client?
- How could this procedure be performed on a patient in traction or with mobility limitations?
- How could this be done in a home environment?
- What verbal and nonverbal communication is occurring?
- What shortcuts can I take to save time or supplies while still maintaining the principles involved?

The NCLEX-RN *Might Ask* 5.1

The nursing student is teaching a client with a colostomy about irrigation of the stoma. The type of learning domain the student would use to teach the client is:
a. cognitive.
b. psychomotor.
c. affective.
d. communicative.

- See Appendix A for correct answer and rationale.

TRANSITION NEEDS UNIQUE TO THE LPN/LVN-TO-ADN STUDENT

In this chapter, you have been learning about the process of transitioning from the LPN/LVN role to the ADN student role. As an LPN/LVN, you are entering the ADN program in one of three entry patterns. Transition needs of LPN/LVNs vary somewhat among the three patterns.

LPN/LVNs ENTERING A GENERIC ADN POPULATION

The generic ADN student starts at the beginning of the ADN program and progresses through the curriculum to completion of the program. Generic ADN students are provided with an orientation at the start of the program and learn about the history and development of ADN nursing and registered nursing in general. An overview of the program philosophy, conceptual model, and curriculum framework is usually presented, and the student is socialized into the role and expectations of the RN scope of practice.

The LPN/LVN who enters a generic ADN class is usually advance-placed 25% to 50% of the way through the program. They may be a lone enrollee or may be accompanied by others advance-placed at this point of entry. The orientation and socialization (transition) process varies according to nursing program policies and practices, but most programs provide only a minimal orientation/socialization process. Material and student exercises presented in this text are designed to enhance the success of students who have been provided with a formal transition course or process as well as those who have not.

The unique needs of LPN/LVNs entering a generic ADN population center on socialization not only into the program culture but also into the class culture. These cultures include the unwritten and written rules and acceptable behaviors of student participants. The LPN/LVN who takes a proactive approach in seeking assistance from faculty and classmates in getting to know the ropes and trying to fit in with study groups increases their chance of success. This is especially important if you are the lone LPN/LVN entrant, or one of only a few, with few peers experiencing similar challenges.

STRAIGHT-THROUGH LPN/LVN-TO-ADN STUDENTS

The straight-through LPN/LVN-to-ADN student is one who has participated in the school's LPN/LVN program and has continued directly into the ADN program (usually at the second-year level). When large groups of students are involved in this entry pattern, or if the college offers only a career ladder (LPN/LVN-to-RN) "bridge" program and no generic program, the transition is usually smoother. The culture of the school will be familiar, including instructional support areas (e.g., library, computer lab, and skills center), and the student may already know faculty in the program. The ADN program generally provides a formalized orientation or transition course for these students.

The unique needs of LPN/LVN-to-ADN students in this entry pattern center on the role transition required to move to the registered nursing scope of practice. The learning environment may shift from a more passive learning process to a more active learning process. Performance that was considered acceptable and competent in the LPN/LVN program can now be considered inadequate, as faculty foster independent thinking, problem-solving, and self-directed learning in these students.

TIME-OUT LPN/LVN-TO-ADN STUDENTS

The time-out LPN/LVN-to-ADN student completes an LPN/LVN program and then steps away from education before later embarking on the ADN program. The time out may be as short as 1 year or as long as a decade or more. Individuals might work during this period, or they might not. Thus, the needs of these students are individualized according to the length of time out, whether the individual worked as an LPN/LVN and in what job role, and whether the individual is attending the same or a different school.

DIFFERENTIATING ADN STUDENT AND LPN/LVN PRACTICE ROLES

A difficulty encountered by most LPN/LVNs returning to school to pursue registered nursing is the role confusion that emerges in the clinical setting. What was once a comfortable setting may now seem awkward, restrictive, and cumbersome. Additionally, your course requirements will include the application of theory to your patient assignments, more in-depth analysis and evaluation, and the use of the nursing process to establish nursing diagnoses and to design comprehensive nursing care plans.

Oermann et al. (2023) provides an overview of rights and responsibilities of students in the clinical setting. They note that the student must abide by laws in that state, policies of the clinical agency, and of the nursing school. Often this means that procedures you are familiar with performing in your LPN/LVN practice are "off limits" in your new role. Practice concerns, issues of liability, legal parameters, and the level of autonomy can be confusing and problematic for the ADN student who is an LPN/LVN.

PRACTICE CONCERNS

As you first encounter the clinical setting in your new ADN student role, you may find yourself asking the following questions to yourself, to other LPN/LVNs who also just entered the program, or to your instructor:

- Don't they know I already know how to take care of this kind of patient?
- Don't they trust me? Why are they checking every little thing I do?
- Why do I need to look up all these meds? I've been administering them for years now!
- Why do I need to "wait for my instructor" to perform this procedure? I've done it lots of times!
- Why am I not allowed to do things I'm already licensed to do as an LPN/LVN?
- Why do I need to do all this paperwork? I'd rather be taking care of patients!
- Why do I need to write out a whole long care plan when I already know how to care for patients with diabetes and heart problems…we learned all that in LPN/LVN training!

These are all questions asked by LPN/LVN-to-RN students in their first weeks of clinical. The practice concerns you may encounter, and questions such as the above, are common but do have rational answers. After several weeks, you will become more comfortable in your role and will begin to see the expanded level of thinking you are doing in preparation for professional nursing practice.

As previously discussed, the registered nursing practice for which you are now preparing is a different practice level than that of your current license. The autonomous, independent practice of the RN differs from the more dependent, directed, and prescriptive practice of the LPN/LVN. One area where this is especially important is in the use of the nursing process to develop nursing diagnoses. The care plans you develop as a student will be somewhat different than those used in practice upon graduation. Your clinical assignments provide you with opportunities to use data, apply theory, and collaborate with other professional practitioners in new ways for a comprehensive, holistic approach to care planning, individualized for your specific patient/client. As you develop experience at the RN level, much of the thinking behind nursing diagnoses and care planning will become "second nature" to you, just as much of your LPN/LVN practice is to you currently.

ISSUES OF LIABILITY

There are also issues of liability related to your new role as a student nurse. As a student in the ADN program, the LPN/LVN is bound by contract language in the agreement between the school and the clinical agency, policies of the clinical agency, policies of the ADN program, and course-by-course objectives and competencies in the curriculum. For example, the LPN/LVN may work at an agency other than that of the clinical assignment as an ADN student. Differences in policies, standardized procedures, and protocol between the two agencies may cause frustration for the student, particularly if they are still employed as an LPN/LVN on days alternating with the student experience and thus is operating out of two different agencies.

As a second example, procedures the LPN/LVN performs regularly in their licensed practice because they have had additional training (e.g., complex procedures, intravenous therapy, etc.) may be beyond the curriculum level or contract language for the course in which they are enrolled in the ADN program and not allowed. This has nothing to do with your abilities and skill sets you have as an LPN/LVN and should not be taken as such. Keeping in close contact with the instructor at the clinical site and verifying interventions planned are essential when dealing with liability issues; it also helps minimize frustration.

OTHER LEGAL ASPECTS

In addition to these liability issues, several legal aspects must be considered by the LPN/LVN in the ADN student role. While in the student role, the LPN/LVN is not functioning as a licensed person but rather as a student in the ADN program. As such, they practice as all other program students do, within the legal parameters of that role. As an example, handling controlled substances and signing for insulin, blood, and narcotics should be performed by the LPN/LVN in the student role under the same guidelines as such procedures would be performed by other unlicensed ADN students.

AUTONOMY AND PARAMETERS FOR INSTRUCTOR SUPERVISION

LPN/LVNs in the ADN student role may also experience a feeling of loss of autonomy at the very time faculty are advocating increased autonomy in the RN role. This may cause some role confusion for the LPN/LVN-to-RN student. In particular, the time-out LPN/LVN-to-ADN student who has gained clinical expertise and has been given increasing responsibilities in the practice setting may experience this loss the greatest. Patient assessment and nursing interventions that the LPN/LVN has been performing independently may now have to be done under the supervision of the instructor, such as procedures and medication administration. The instructor may also notice poor practices that need to be corrected, which can cause even further frustration. The LPN/LVN-to-ADN student must have a clear understanding of the level of independence allowed in relation to nursing care activities according to program policies and each course's clinical guidelines and must discuss areas of role conflict with the instructor.

The NCLEX-RN *Might Ask* 5.2

The LPN/LVN-to-RN student nurse is assigned to a client in an ambulatory surgical setting. The LPN in this setting is held to the legal accountability of a(an):
a. layman.
b. student.
c. LPN/LVN.
d. RN.

• See Appendix A for correct answer and rationale.

CONCLUSION

This chapter is built on information presented in previous chapters about ADN education programs. Adult learning theory can inform how you as an adult learner can enhance your success in the ADN program. LPN/LVN and ADN education programs have different philosophies and conceptual models, curricular frameworks, curricular content and learning domains, learning achievement levels, nursing process and nursing diagnosis, and learning processes.

You will need to keep in mind the learning strategies covered in this chapter, including knowing your learning style; accommodating for disabilities; addressing differences in age, gender, sexual orientation, and cultural background; establishing self-directed goals; engaging in active learning activities; and adopting techniques to stimulate thinking. You will also need to consider what transition needs you have depending on your unique situation as you enter an ADN program.

STUDENT *Exercises*

Exercise 5.1

Obtain a school catalog or access an online catalog with course descriptions of the curricula for the ADN program you are planning to enter (or have entered). Review nursing and non-nursing course titles, course descriptions, and breakdown of lecture and laboratory time spent in each course. In the following space, write key concepts or phrases from the course descriptions that indicate learning you will gain in each of the three learning domains as you complete course work for the program.

Learning Domain	Course Number	Key Concepts/Phrases
1. Cognitive domain (knowledge)		
2. Affective domain (values, attitudes)		
3. Psychomotor domain (skills)		

REFERENCES

American Nurses Association. (2021). *Nursing: Scope and standards of practice* (4th ed.).

Anderson, L. W., & Krathwohl, D. R. (Eds.). (2001). *A taxonomy for learning, teaching, and assessing: A revision of Bloom's taxonomy of educational objects.* Longmans.

Bergin, D. A., Bergin, C. A., & Prewitt, S. L. (2023). Motivating adult learners. In A. Belzer & B. Dashew (Eds.). *Understanding the adult learner: Perspectives and practices* (pp. 59–78). Taylor Francis Group.

Bloom, B. S. (Ed.). (1956). *Taxonomy of educational objectives: The classification of educational goals.* Longmans, Green.

Bradshaw, M. J., Hultquist, B. L., & Hagler, D. (2021). *Innovative teaching strategies in nursing and related health professions* (8th ed.). Jones and Bartlett.

Cherry, B., & Jacob, S. R. (2022). *Contemporary nursing: Issues, trends, & management* (9th ed.). Elsevier.

Covey, S. R. (2004). *The 8th habit: From effectiveness to greatness*. Free Press.
Dashew, B., & Gayeski, D. (2023). Instructional design: Applying principles of adult education. In A. Belzer & B. Dashew (Eds.). *Understanding the adult learner: Perspectives and practices* (pp. 255–274). Taylor Francis Group.
da Silva, T. H. R. (2022). Emotional awareness and emotional intelligence. *British Journal of Community Nursing*, 27(12), 573–574. https://doi.org/10.12968/bjcn.2022.27.12.573
Ellis, D. (2022a). *Becoming a master student: Making the career connection* (17th ed.). Cengage Learning.
Ellis, D. (2022b). *The essential guide to becoming a master student: Making the career connection* (6th ed.). Cengage Learning.
Hambach, C., Cantrell, M. A., & Mariani, B. (2023). A program of simulated learning experiences to develop clinical judgment and clinical competence among sophomore baccalaureate nursing students. *Clinical Simulation in Nursing*, 80, 55–63. https://doi.org/10.1016/j.ecns.2023.04.005
Hunt, D. D. (2015). *The nurse professional: Leveraging your education for transition to practice*. Springer Publishing.
Huston, C. J. (2023). *Professional issues in nursing: Challenges and opportunities* (6th ed.). Wolters Kluwer.
Ignatavicius, D. (2021). Preparing for the new nursing licensure exam: The next-generation NCLEX. *Nursing*, 51(5), 35–41. https://doi.org/10.1097/01.NURSE.0000743100.95536.9b
Kearney-Nunnery, R. (Ed.). (2020). *Advancing your career: Concepts of professional nursing* (7th ed.). F.A. Davis.
Knowles, M. S., Holton III, E. F., Swanson, R. A., & Robinson, P. A. (2020). *The adult learner: The definitive classic in adult education and human resource development* (9th ed.). Routledge.
Longworth, N. (2003). *Lifelong learning in action: Transforming education in the 21st century*. Routledge/Falmer.
National Council of State Boards of Nursing. (2022). *2021 RN practice analysis: Linking the NCLEX-RN examination to practice*. https://www.ncsbn.org/public-files/21_NCLEX_RN_PA.pdf
National Council of State Boards of Nursing. (2023a). *Next generation NCLEX: NCLEX-RN test plan effective April 2023*. https://www.ncsbn.org/public-files/2023_RN_Test%20Plan_English_FINAL.pdf
National Council of State Boards of Nursing. (2023b). *Next generation NCLEX: NCLEX-PN test plan effective April 2023*. https://www.ncsbn.org/public-files/2023_PN_Test%20Plan_FINAL.pdf
National League for Nursing. (2012). *Outcomes and competencies for graduates of Practical/Vocational, Diploma, Associate Degree, Baccalaureate, Master's, Practice Doctorate, and Research Doctorate Programs in nursing*.
Oermann, M. H., Shellenbarger, T., & Gaberson, K. B. (2023). *Clinical teaching strategies in nursing*. Springer Publishing.
Poore, J. A., & Cooper, D. D. (2020). Interprofessional simulation: From the classroom to clinical practice. *Annual Review of Nursing Research*, 39(1), 105–125.
Taylor, C., Lynn, P., & Bartlett, J. L. (2023). *Fundamentals of nursing: The art and science of person-centered nursing care* (10th ed.). Wolters Kluwer.

On the WEB

National Council of State Boards of Nursing: http://www.ncsbn.org

National Council of State Boards of Nursing NGN Sample Packs: https://nurseachieve.com/ncsbn-ngn-sample-pack

Accrediting Commission for Education in Nursing: http://www.acenursing.org

National Student Nurses Association: http://www.nsna.org

CHAPTER 6

Individualizing a Plan for Role Transition

LEARNING OUTCOMES

By the end of this chapter, the student will be able to:
1. Assess preparedness for the student role.
2. Describe your learning style(s).
3. Assess your own uniqueness as an adult learner.
4. Identify prior cognitive, affective, and psychomotor learning achieved through formal education and experience.
5. Design a personal education plan (PEP) to enhance success in the ADN program.
6. Apply concepts learned to establish an effective instructor–student partnership.

KEY TERMS

experiential learning
feedback mechanism
instructor–student partnership
mentor
mutual goal setting
nonstandardized test
personal education plan (PEP)
proactive learner
standardized test
strategic learner
time management

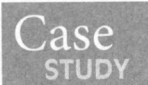

Case STUDY

Sherry Williams is an LPN in her first semester of ADN school and is meeting with her nursing advisor. Sherry has opted to take an advanced placement course via the internet and is not sure where to start with a needs assessment that she has been assigned to perform.

ADVISOR: Hi, Sherry. Thanks for scheduling an appointment with me. I enjoy seeing my students, but sometimes they don't come in until after the first exam. I'm happy that you're proactive and contacting me early in the course. How can I help you?

SHERRY: I see you've sent me a needs assessment. I'm not sure why we're doing this, and I'm a little intimidated with the length of the form. Can you help me understand the purpose for this and how to complete it?

ADVISOR: Because you've opted to take the advanced placement course for LVNs via the Web, faculty want to tailor your course so that it concentrates on your needs. For example, if you're a whiz at math, we want to spend less time on that and more on, say, nursing planning—especially if your exposure to that has been minimal in your current position.

SHERRY: So, this is similar to how we deal with teaching a patient with diabetes. If the client and family know about insulins and can return demonstrate an injection, we might concentrate more on their diet, especially if blood sugars aren't under control.

ADVISOR: Exactly. We realize that our students in this course come from a wide variety of backgrounds. Some haven't been in school for years, some have been away for only a few years, and some are fresh out of LPN school.

SHERRY: I didn't realize that. I guess it's sort of like a new employee working at our nursing home. Everyone comes with different experiences, and being new, you have to get adjusted. We have learned a lot from people just out of school as well as from other workplaces.

ADVISOR: The same will be true with this course. I'll send everyone a list of course participants' e-mail addresses so that even though you won't meet each other face to face, you can "talk" to each other online. I hope this will help you share experiences.

SHERRY: Okay, now on to the assessment…

ADVISOR: The reason this is so in-depth is that it makes you think about what you are good at. Perhaps you are an expert at administering tube feedings or inserting urinary catheters but need more help with fluid and electrolytes or medication theory. If so, we can concentrate more on those topics, and you may want to attend the parallel course that meets here on campus for more hands-on work in the lab or more classroom work as needed.

SHERRY: I see now. It's all falling into place… I think I can take it from here.

ADVISOR: Great. Let me know if you would like me to help you complete the first page.

SHERRY: I have to pick my kids up now. I'll have to work on it tonight.

ADVISOR: Later, if you'd like more help we can meet via Zoom to go over more details. When you're finished in a day or two, you can hand it in here, you can mail it, or you can scan it and e-mail it to me.

SHERRY: I'll e-mail it to you by tomorrow. Thanks for your help!

In this chapter, you are given the opportunity to apply knowledge gained from the preceding chapters to yourself, assess prior knowledge and experience, and design a **personal education plan (PEP)** specific to your individual needs. You will assess your preparedness for the student role, examine your learning style, and reflect on the unique characteristics and needs you bring to the ADN program. As described in Chapter 1, the PEP you develop in this chapter can become part of your portfolio as you meet with your nursing adviser to plan for your return to school and success in pursuit of your RN.

Several methods for assessing your theoretical and experiential knowledge and abilities are discussed in this chapter, and you will also use these in developing your PEP at the end of this chapter (see Box 6.2 later in this chapter). A reflection of who you are, your strengths, how you best learn, and those areas where you will want to focus your efforts over the next year or so in the ADN program will be reflected in your PEP. The PEP will be helpful to both you and your instructors to support your success in the ADN program and also on the NCLEX-RN, which you will take after you complete the ADN program.

This chapter also discusses the instructor–student partnership. Strategies for fostering a successful partnership are explored, as are techniques for individualizing your learning activities and strengthening your clinical practicum in the ADN program. This chapter presents such concepts as **mutual goal setting** and **feedback mechanisms**, and as part of your PEP development, you will outline areas for discussion with your faculty advisor at your individual conference.

ASSESSING PREPAREDNESS FOR THE STUDENT ROLE

The first step in individualizing a plan for role transition is to examine your preparedness for returning to school and moving back into a student role, as discussed in Chapter 1. If you recently completed the LPN/LVN nursing program or have been recently completing course work and receiving academic advising in preparing for the ADN program, you may already feel comfortable with or settled into the student role. In assessing your preparedness for the student role, four areas of preparedness, which have been explored in previous chapters, will be reviewed:

- The reentry process
- The school setting
- Student success strategies
- Time management

REENTRY PROCESS

For those who have been away from the educational setting for some time or who have acquired their LPN/LVN license in a pathway other than formal education (eg, military or other service experience), moving into the college student role may feel awkward and uncomfortable. It is important to find out the demographics of the ADN program you plan to enter to know how your characteristics and biases will fit with the class you will enter. What have been the age, gender, and ethnic distributions of classes during the last few years at this nursing school? How many other LPN/LVNs will be entering this class, and what percentage of the class as a whole will be represented by the LPN/LVN constituency? Are the LPN/LVNs in this group advanced placement, straight-through, or time-out students (as described in Chapter 5)?

THINKING CRITICALLY
Write down how you are similar to and different from the typical student in the ADN program you will enter. Consider age, gender, ethnicity, and nursing experience. In areas in which you are different, cite strengths you will bring to the class to enhance others' learning, and identify actions you can take to develop comfort with the reentry process. (Save this information for use in designing your PEP.)

THE SCHOOL SETTING

Feeling prepared to enter (or reenter) the school setting develops self-confidence and comfort in the student role. "Knowing the ropes" or knowing where to find things on campus and how to function within the processes and systems of the school can assist you in this process. Chapters 1 and 5 described today's educational environment and examined strategies for success in the student role in this setting. Ask yourself these questions:

- Do you have a campus map?
- Do you know the location of such areas as counseling, registration, student services, health center, child care services (if needed), nursing office, library, computer lab, and bookstore?
- Do you know how to register for classes, apply for financial aid or scholarships, and seek assistance for learning disabilities or for tutoring?
- Do you know how to use the library/learning resource center, research a topic, and use online systems and the Cumulative Index for Nursing and Allied Health Literature (CINAHL) to locate periodical (journal) articles?
- If you do not have a computer, do you know where on campus you can access one to complete an assignment or how to obtain one through the school's loan program or student discounts?
- Do you know how to navigate the school's virtual learning spaces (eg, Blackboard or Canvas) and engage in web-conferencing, chat rooms, and threaded discussions with your instructor and peer students?
- Do you know where and how to access copying services?
- Are there any orientation sessions, printed materials, or student success courses you can take to prepare yourself better for the school setting?
- How much of the above can you access online to develop familiarity with such resources prior to arriving on campus?

STUDENT SUCCESS STRATEGIES

As described in previous chapters, many strategies can be used to support your success in the ADN program. Preparing for the student role involves identifying student success strategies that meet your individual needs and with which you feel comfortable. Review your notes from previous chapters, and summarize student success strategies applicable to you. Several learning techniques are highlighted below, along with discussion of learning techniques, networking, mentors, and study groups.

THINKING CRITICALLY

Take a moment to reflect on the previous questions, your school setting and its educational environment, and the list of student success strategies you made that seem applicable to your situation. What strategies do you need to research further or take action on to further develop? Write down several actions you can take to better prepare yourself for the school setting and its educational environment. (Save this information for use in designing your PEP.)

Learning Techniques

Have you developed effective learning techniques and study skills to be successful in this more complex ADN course work? To achieve learning outcomes and competencies identified for the ADN program, you need to not only gain knowledge, comprehension, and the ability to apply content learned but also must analyze data, draw conclusions, use clinical judgment, synthesize information, and make decisions by thinking critically about course content, case studies, simulations, and patient assignments during classroom and clinical learning activities. Critical thinking and clinical judgment for decision-making are discussed in Chapter 9. What learning techniques do you possess, and what resources have you developed to support you in this process?

Becoming a Proactive, Strategic Learner

Previous chapters discussed the value of and need for active learning for higher-level thinking in the ADN program. The advantage of your being proactive in the learning environment was also mentioned. Reflect on your learning style. Have you learned how to be a proactive learner? What does this mean to you?

The **proactive learner** seeks experiences to add knowledge, skills, and abilities to their expertise, as opposed to just waiting to see what is assigned. Professional nurses are lifelong learners, which means developing the skill to be proactive in the process is critical for professional nursing practice. This book and the PEP you will complete later in this chapter are geared toward developing your ability to be a proactive learner, seeking the learning necessary for you as an individual to be more successful in the ADN program, on NCLEX-RN, and in your professional practice.

It is an expectation that professional nurses will readily embrace learning throughout their careers by placing themselves into new learning situations to achieve identified learning goals. The science of nursing knowledge is rapidly increasing and will continue to grow (Coyne & Chatham, 2020). Most authors revise their textbooks every 3 to 5 years to keep information current for learners, with the process to research changes in the field of nursing and in education sometimes taking up to 18 months.

The ANA (2021) revises its definition of nursing, *Social Policy Statement*, *Code of Ethics*, and *Scope and Standards of Practice*, every 5 to 7 years, based on extensive research and input from practicing nurses across the country. The NCSBN (2023a, 2023b) revises its test plans for registered nursing and licensed practical/vocational nursing every 3 years, based on in-depth studies and analyses of the current practice of RNs and LPN/LVNs, respectively. Likewise, the dozens of professional nursing organizations revise their mission statements, produce position papers, and update practices frequently based on research in the field of nursing.

Your nursing practice requires this "updating" and "refresh" as well, which is why relicensure requirements include Cistus. In the NLN's Education Competencies Model (NLN, 2012), personal/professional development is described as "a lifelong process of learning, refining, and integrating values and behaviors" (p. 68). The model emphasizes that acquiring knowledge and enhancing skills that align with the core values and ethical principles of the nursing profession are important concepts that differentiate nurses from other healthcare professionals. Continuing education and professional development foster a commitment to continuously enhance patient care and empower nurses to adapt to the evolving healthcare environment.

As you move through the ADN program, you will likely be surprised at how much has changed even since you completed your LPN/LVN training. New fields are rapidly developing for nursing in such areas as geriatrics, palliative care, holistic nursing, global health, spiritual nursing, transcultural nursing, and nursing informatics, to name a few. New fields continue to emerge through nursing research and evidence-based practice, and many new developments can be seen also in clinical care in the traditional areas of medical, surgical, obstetrical, pediatric, and psychiatric/mental health nursing.

Another area that has received increased attention in recent years is the need for more interprofessional collaboration to provide more comprehensive care between the professions of medicine and nursing, with some nursing diagnoses (eg, "At risk for…") sharing the foreground with medical diagnoses. Nursing associations, such as the ANA and NLN, and the Institute of Medicine (2011) stress the need for more collaboration between the two professions, including the need to initiate this collaboration during educational programs prior to graduation (Benner et al., 2010).

Lifelong learning is essential. One must become self-directed, resourceful, a critical and creative thinker, and a **strategic learner**. Scheckel (2020) identifies tools to assist the student in developing current workplace skills, including the use of social media and strategies for applying what is learned to workplace situations, using analytical, creative, and practical skills. Are you taking advantage of college resources, Web resources, college orientation and success courses, textbooks, and online resources to access these learning opportunities in alignment with your goals? Are you assessing those clinical skills you will want to seek once you are in the clinical setting to brush up on your techniques? These are all aspects of becoming a proactive learner.

THINKING CRITICALLY

Assess your study skills and resources. Identify those you possess and those you need to develop to support yourself in the ADN program. Are you a strategic learner? What can you do to develop yourself in this area? (Save this information for use in designing your PEP.)

Networking and Developing Mentors

Another strategy for success as you enter the ADN program is building networks and developing mentors. You probably have a network of nurses and other healthcare professionals that you consult in your current practice as an LPN/LVN. In your new role as an ADN student, you will find it extremely helpful to develop a new network of individuals on whom you can rely to assist you with learning activities and student success strategies. This network will include other classmates and nurses or assistants working in the nursing skills and simulations labs and may also include other campus resource personnel in the library, learning resource center, tutoring, and learning disabilities center if you have a learning disability. These individuals can help you with technology concerns, study skills, research services, use of online services, etc. They can also help you find group study areas and refer you to community resources if you are not from the area.

In addition to building your new network, it is important to develop mentors to support you in your progress through the ADN program. Mentors are especially important during times of transition, such as in your LPN/LVN-to-RN role transition (Twedell, 2023). A **mentor** is someone with whom you can consult, who will give you advice, and who will counsel, guide, and help you in the learning process. Mentors open doors, create opportunities, provide wisdom, and inspire their mentees (Hood, 2021). More advanced students, program graduates, practicing RNs, and your nursing advisor are examples of people who may be appropriate mentors for you. A good mentor will be honest with you, assist you in times when you are "stuck," and offer you moral support when you are discouraged, are frustrated, or have lost confidence.

At times, nursing students become overwhelmed with all the studying, intensity, and work in the nursing program. If they get behind or lose confidence in their ability to perform well, they may find themselves taking shortcuts, plagiarizing material, or cheating. A good mentor can help you avoid falling into these traps by assisting you with time management, study habits, and strategies for success. Mentorship is crucial to both personal and professional growth. Mentors foster career success by proving guidance and direction, and they have a significant impact on self and career development (Ellis, 2020).

Buckway and Sowerby (2023) describe a mentor as someone who actively supports the growth and professional development of another person. A mentor is usually an experienced professional in a given field who develops a supportive relationship with a less experienced individual and provides advice and emotional support. Important aspects of the mentor–mentee relationship, as described by Buckway and Sowerby (2023), are shown in Box 6.1.

BOX 6.1 Important Aspects of the Mentor–Mentee Relationship

The mentor:
- Develops a supportive relationship with the mentee
- Provides advice and emotional support for the mentee
- Assists the mentee with career and personal development
- Provides personal support, acceptance, and counseling
- Facilitates the mentee's advancement within the organization by helping to establish networks and organizational know-how
- Provides help in learning how to work effectively within the system
- Is an effective and experienced practitioner who serves as a role model of effective practice
- Maintains a positive attitude, a caring approach toward others, and effective communication

Adapted from Buckway, A. J., & Sowerby, H. (2023). *Nursing in today's world: Trends, issues, and management* (12th ed.). Wolters Kluwer.

Much has been written about the value of mentoring, especially in today's world, where information changes rapidly and job turnover often occurs every 2 to 3 years. Mentoring is a one-to-one professional connection that empowers and improves practice by not only leading, supervising, and training but also assisting in navigating challenging situations by providing guidance and support. The relationship should be a positive one and should enhance one's sense of worth (Claire & Reising, 2023).

When choosing a mentor, you must decide on qualities in prospective mentors that will enhance your success based on your individual learning style and personality. An individual who is a good mentor for one student may be a poor one for another. For example, do you want a mentor who will challenge you with prodding questions about program content or one who will act as a sounding board for your ideas? Do you want a mentor who will be nurturing and offer words of encouragement or one who will challenge you and assist you in disciplining yourself to study? What role(s) do you want your mentor to play?

Choosing a mentor is an area in which you need to be proactive. Duff (1999) emphasized the importance of:

- Women mentoring women as career professionals with job and personal lives
- Not "waiting" for a mentor to appear, but rather taking the initiative to seek a mentor
- Overcoming the fear of appearing demanding, needy, or weak or the fear of being rejected
- Choosing a mentor you admire, respect, and can confide in and whose values are those with which you feel comfortable

You should not be hesitant to ask a new program graduate or experienced RN to be your mentor. In fact, the nurse you ask will most likely be honored and will gain as much from the mentor–mentee relationship as you will.

Study Groups

Forming or joining a study group can greatly enhance thinking, problem-solving, and decision-making skills. However, selecting or forming a study group must take into account your preference(s) for learning. The ground rules for the study group must be clear. For example, does each member read all material and then discuss it with the group, or does each member take a portion of the assignment and then present or teach it to the others? Will the purpose of the study group be to meet frequently and discuss the content or to infrequently meet, bringing up only unanswered questions or problems? What will be the format of the sessions? How small or large will it be? These questions must be addressed early in the process to avoid conflict between group members and to ensure the time spent is productive and enhances your learning.

In addition to enhancing thinking skills, study groups allow members to discuss and complete assignments. Study groups have two other benefits:

- Experiential knowledge will differ among study group members. Differences in age, life experiences, and nursing practice experiences can provide a rich conversation among study group members. Multiple approaches to nursing care can be explored, and information is likely to "stick" better because of the discussion and its meaning to members' personal lives.
- As nursing class demographics have become more diverse, members of your study group may be of a different background than your own. This can provide for a

rich discussion of diverse opinions about nursing care. As Bradshaw et al. (2021) describe, questioning, discussion, and expressing different viewpoints and perspectives within a diverse student group contributes to learning. Disagreement or disharmony should be explored in an objective fashion to expand the thinking of all.

THINKING CRITICALLY

Think about the type of learning required in an ADN program and the strengths and growth needed to achieve this learning level. On a piece of paper, make a large box with four quadrants. Label the four quadrants as follows: mentor characteristics, mentor role, study group characteristics, and study group role. Fill in each box, and examine your results. Do you know anyone who will meet your needs to be your mentor? Do you know classmates with whom you might work well in a study group? (Save this information for use in designing your PEP.)

TIME MANAGEMENT

A last important area to examine in assessing your preparedness for the student role is the area of **time management**. Often, the LPN/LVN entering an ADN program must balance a number of roles, such as spouse, caregiver, student, worker, and community citizen. The nursing program can be very demanding at times. As discussed in Chapter 1, preparing for the student role involves such time management success strategies as balancing personal, career, and student roles; reassessing commitments to committees, boards, and service groups; and enlisting the support of significant others through the use of win–win agreements.

Covey et al. (1994) advocated the identification of your key roles in life—that is, caregiver, spouse/partner, friend, community service worker, LPN/LVN, etc.—and establishing weekly goals in each role. Then, by completing a weekly time map that includes these goals for the week, and scheduling time for each, your time management will be focused on your highest priorities, and all roles will receive the attention they deserve. Other activities can then be scheduled around these high-priority items so that the most important, rather than just the daily urgent tasks, are accomplished. It also avoids the sense nursing students sometimes feel that they are working in a "crisis mode" all the time.

By focusing on your "roles and goals" each week, you will be more productive and feel more satisfied with a sense of completion by the end of the week. This also helps with (1) breaking up large projects into "bite sizes" to make progress and not be stressed near the due date, (2) developing confidence in yourself as you see progress each week, and (3) minimizing any guilt you may be experiencing by not devoting specific time to a particular role (e.g., caregiver or spouse/partner role).

In Chapter 1, you were also encouraged to develop a win–win agreement with the significant others in your life. This is an important support structure for you but also assists with time management. Review the win–win agreement you developed. In light of your new "roles and goals" approach to time management, are there adjustments that need to be made in either the roles or the goals for them to work effectively together?

The aforementioned techniques can assist you in your time management in the clinical area and in your nursing practice as well, which will be discussed later in Chapter 14.

THINKING CRITICALLY

On a sheet of paper, identify your roles, group commitments, and significant others. Write an action plan for time management that takes into account these three items, the win–win agreement(s) you developed in Chapter 1, and any revisions you have made for these to work in concert with one another. (Save this action plan for use in designing your PEP.)

ASSESSING LEARNING STYLE

The second step in individualizing a plan for transition from the LPN/LVN to the ADN level is to assess your learning style. In previous chapters, you learned about the characteristics of adult learners and that we each learn best in different ways. Some people are visual learners, whereas others are auditory learners. Some learn best through teaching strategies in which the learner uses manipulative skills or body kinetic (motion) or kinesthetic (sensory) approaches to learn course content. Take a moment and review the four styles of learners presented in Chapter 1, your Learning Styles Inventory (if you completed it), and the characteristics of adult learners discussed throughout Unit 1. For a more in-depth discussion of learning styles, and/or to take the Learning Styles Inventory, refer to Ellis (2022a, 2022b).

THINKING CRITICALLY

Based on material presented throughout Unit 1, the exercises you have completed thus far, and reflecting on learning activities that have been the most helpful to you in the past, assess and write in your own words a description of your learning style. Give examples of study techniques and approaches to learning activities that fit your learning style. (Save this information for use in designing your PEP.)

THE REFLECTIVE PROCESS: ASSESSING ADULT LEARNER UNIQUENESS

The third step in individualizing a plan for role transition is to identify your unique characteristics as an adult learner. In Chapter 5, you learned about the characteristics of adult learners and the driving forces that motivate such learners in the educational setting. Adult learners bring with them to the educational setting a variety of personal and professional life experiences. Assessing learning needs, including knowledge gaps, and being aware of learning styles are important in developing a learning plan. Exposure to different learning methods ensures that students are able to utilize the learning style that best meets their needs and that creates a less stressful environment (Scheckel, 2020). Chapter 5 also emphasized the need to be proactive in seeking support for any learning disabilities you may have or think you might have. This should be included in your PEP as well.

Each adult learner has developed values, biases, and fears; each is motivated by their own unique driving forces. Each has identified personal and career goals that guide them in the learning process. As you transition to the RN role, you will assume more of a leadership role, in which others will be taking directions from you and following your lead. To assume a lead role, you must be able to envision yourself in that role. As you begin your transition from the LPN/LVN to the RN role, how do you view yourself? Can you see yourself in the lead role?

THINKING CRITICALLY

Reflect on yourself as an adult learner. Write down specific areas of nursing expertise you believe that you have developed in the practice of nursing, things that motivate you to learn in classroom and clinical settings, and personal goals you hope to achieve by participating in the ADN program. (Save this information for use in designing your PEP.)

ASSESSING PRIOR LEARNING: STANDARDIZED AND NONSTANDARDIZED TESTS

The fourth step in individualizing a plan for role transition from the LPN/LVN to the ADN level is to assess your prior learning. You acquire knowledge, skills, and abilities in the cognitive, affective, and psychomotor domains through formal education and **experiential learning** processes. (For a discussion of the three learning domains, refer to Chapter 5.)

In addition to a review of transcripts for course work completed, assessment tests are available to assist you in assessing your knowledge base and to guide you as you pursue a career as an RN. Many standardized tests are available for individual use, and many nursing schools use standardized or nonstandardized tests for assessment and selection purposes. A **standardized test** has undergone numerous validity and reliability research studies to ensure that content is valid and unbiased and that test takers would provide the same answers if the same test was administered again or by a different test administrator. It has also been administered to several populations, resulting in available normative data (information on the norms from various populations of test takers). Standardized tests are often published by formal organizations and are usually copyrighted. In contrast, **nonstandardized tests** are locally prepared (often by a teacher or a school) and may contain regional questions.

ASSESSMENT TESTS FOR GENERAL EDUCATION

Many standardized tests are available to assess reading, writing, and mathematical computation skills. Most 2-year colleges require some form of general education assessment in their college admissions process. You will need to find out if any tests are required by the college or by the nursing program you are about to enter. Some commonly used tests are shown below.

- ACT: American College Test
- SAT: Scholastic Achievement Test

- TABE: Test of Adult Basic Education
- Accuplacer: Assessment test used by many community and technical colleges for English and Mathematics for placement purposes
- TEAS: Test of Essential Academic Skills for students applying to nursing and allied health programs
- NET: Nurse Entrance Test
- DET: Diagnostic Entrance Test
- RNEE: Registered Nurse Entrance Exam
- COMPASS: Computer Adaptive Placement Assessment and Support System
- TOEFL: Test of English as a Foreign Language

Some of these tests can be taken more than once, and many have workbooks, textbooks, workshops, and online resources for preparing for the exam that are available on the internet and may be available on campus or in the college bookstore. Students must be academically prepared to be successful in college, and often reentry students do not do as well in general education classes as those straight out of high school because they learned the content a long time prior and have not used many of the concepts recently. Most students improve their test scores by taking a refresher workshop or a self-paced refresher module prior to assessment testing. These are readily available online and can be completed in a relatively short time. Often, a refresher is all that is needed for you to recall some concepts you may have forgotten while you have been away from the academic setting.

SUBJECT AREA ASSESSMENT TESTS FOR NURSING AND SUPPORT CURRICULA

Assessment tests are available to assist LPN/LVNs in assessing knowledge in specific nursing curricular areas. Test areas include nursing fundamentals, medical surgical nursing, obstetric nursing, pediatric nursing, nutrition, pharmacology, anatomy and physiology, microbiology, and the behavioral sciences. Your nursing school may require some of these, but you also may want to take some of these on your own. Professional organizations (e.g., NLN and ANA) and the private sector (e.g., American College Testing and College-Level Examination Program) have assessment tests for specific subject areas in the discipline of nursing.

INTEGRATED NURSING ASSESSMENT TESTS

Because many tests you will take during your ADN education (and ultimately the NCLEX-RN) include primarily multiple-choice, multiple-option, and scenario-based questions, you might want to examine your test-taking skills. Many books on test-taking strategies that offer excellent suggestions for how to take tests made up of multiple-choice and alternative format questions can be found in your school's library and/or learning resources center. These resources include suggestions for how to select the correct answer by reading questions well, understanding the intent of the question, and eliminating answer choices as a result. Other test-taking strategies—for example, time management and completing short essays—can also be found in your college library or learning resource center, as well as online. In addition, student success courses provide suggestions on test-taking strategies. Specific examples of types of test questions are covered in Chapter 7.

NURSING REVIEW TEXTS

An additional self-evaluation technique LPN/LVNs have found useful in assessing their prior learning in preparation for role transition to the ADN level is published review texts. Subject-specific and integrated nursing review texts are available, providing the opportunity not only to assess strong and weak areas in your knowledge base but also to practice answering multiple-choice, multiple-option, and scenario-based test questions in preparation for your nursing courses and the NCLEX-RN, which you will take after you complete the ADN program (Ignatavicious, 2021).

THINKING CRITICALLY

Examine the course work in the ADN program for which you will receive challenge credit or equivalency credit (or beyond which you will be advance placed). Reflecting on your own learning needs, identify in writing the methods or tests you would like to use, and those required by your nursing program, to assess your prior learning in nursing. Contact your school's nursing department, counseling office, bookstore, or testing center to determine the process for accessing the assessment tests you have identified. (Save this information for use in designing your PEP.)

INSTRUCTOR–STUDENT PARTNERSHIP

Throughout this chapter, you have worked through several Thinking Critically exercises for self-assessment. In preparing to develop your PEP, you have assessed your preparedness for the student role, learning style, adult learner uniqueness, prior learning, and student success strategies that are a good "fit" for you. As you use this information to design your PEP, another area to consider is the **instructor–student partnership**. The instructor–student partnership has one goal: your success.

For the majority of adult learners, a somewhat vague feeling of inclusion or exclusion serves as an initial indicator of the strength of the instructor–student relationship. Adult learners lose their enthusiasm and motivation if they feel excluded (Bergin et al., 2023). The culturally responsive teacher will build motivation in adult learners by establishing inclusion, enhancing meaning, and engendering competence (Bergin et al., 2023). Your relationship with your faculty advisor will be critical for these motivational goals and will serve as a positive resource to you if you are struggling during the program. For this reason, it is important to establish a positive rapport with your faculty advisor early in the program.

The goal of the instructor–student partnership is the success of the student. The more the instructor understands your learning style, strengths, areas for growth, and individual uniqueness, the more the partnership will be able to meet your learning needs. Positive instructor–student partnerships foster independence and responsibility for patient care, giving students the opportunity to practice various skills and to make connections between theory and practice (Mathisen et al., 2023).

Do you share some of these same perceptions?

Scheele (2005) noted that returning students often make one of two errors: either overplaying their role by reminding instructors that they too have experience or underplaying it (acting dumb). Even though a student may believe they have equal or more experience than the teacher, returning learners need advice and direction. Students should not assume a position of leadership based on their perceived experience or maturity because, as learners, they are similar to traditional students. Likewise, if you are a returning student, you should not make the error of reverting to a submissive role out of fear of failing. Recognize that you are a student, yet maintain your adult maturity.

Meeting with your instructor/advisor early and sharing your PEP—including information about how you learn best, your fears, your goals, barriers to overcome, accommodations needed, clinical experiences needed, and methods of feedback that are most helpful to you—will maximize the ability of your partnership with the instructor to reach its goal: your success. This is also an opportunity to share with the instructor your strengths, your clinical and life experiences, and the contributions you can make to the class and learning experience. Lastly, you can ask questions, get tips, and advice from your instructor as to what strategies lead to success for students in this program, and determine how to contact each other (phone, e-mail, text, etc.) in case the need arises.

INITIATING YOUR STUDENT PORTFOLIO

Completing your PEP is a good first step in developing your student portfolio. A portfolio is a snapshot of your accomplishments. As a nursing student, your development of a portfolio provides you, your instructor, and others with a snapshot of your accomplishments in preparation for and during the ADN program. Many students maintain an e-portfolio in today's virtual environment, and some schools even provide a repository for student portfolios. Calacci and Hagler (2023) advocate the maintenance of a portfolio throughout your nursing program as a means for demonstrating achievement of course and program outcomes and also as a tool for your own reflection on your development as a nurse professional.

As you progress through the program, snapshots of your accomplishments can be added to your portfolio and, as you graduate, this portfolio may be helpful to you in securing positions as an RN. Clinical competency achievements, sample nursing care plans, reflective papers, a self-evaluation, and a well-developed professional resume are also recommended additions to your portfolio. Your nursing instructor/advisor can also recommend additions to your portfolio as you progress through the program.

CONCLUSION

This chapter presented you with the opportunity to synthesize and apply to yourself knowledge gained from the preceding chapters. You now have the necessary information to design a PEP specific to your individual needs. Assessing your preparedness for the student role, examining your learning style, and reflecting on the unique characteristics and needs you bring to the ADN program are critical for your success. The PEP you develop can become part of your portfolio as you meet with your nursing adviser to plan for the successful pursuit of your RN.

You can use several methods to assess your theoretical and experiential knowledge and abilities, and you can use these in developing your PEP (see Box 6.2). In addition, these should enhance your success in the ADN program and on the NCLEX-RN, which you will take after you complete the ADN program.

The instructor–student partnership is important, and effective strategies are needed to foster a successful partnership. In addition, you should utilize techniques for individualizing your learning activities and strengthening your clinical practicum in the ADN program. Your success will depend on your focus on the concepts of mutual goal setting and feedback mechanisms as part of your PEP development. With these tools in hand you should have everything you need for building a mutually satisfying instructor–student partnership, initiating your student portfolio, and experiencing success in your LPN/LVN-to-RN role transition.

BOX 6.2 Personal Education Plan for Successful LPN/LVN-to-RN Role Transition

Name _____ Date _____

School I will be attending _____

Review the Thinking Critically sections of the chapter, and use your written responses to complete the following plan.

I. **Action Plan: Preparedness for the Student Role**
   A. Overcoming reentry barriers
      Examine the demographics of the ADN program you will enter (e.g., ages, genders, culture diversity, and generic vs. advance placed members).
      1. Identify strengths you will bring to the class based on your personal uniqueness and how these can be used.

      _____
      _____
      _____
      _____
      _____
      _____
      _____
      _____

      2. Identify potential barriers you anticipate, based on your personal uniqueness (e.g., cultural background, fears, and self-confidence) and your plan to overcome these potential barriers.

      _____
      _____
      _____
      _____
      _____
      _____
      _____
      _____
      _____

   B. Preparing for the school setting and educational environment
      1. List the areas you need to locate and familiarize yourself with on campus. Obtain a campus map, and plot a self-guided tour.

      _____
      _____
      _____
      _____
      _____

BOX 6.2 (Continued)

2. List the campus processes or systems with which you need to familiarize yourself and who you need to see or where you need to go to obtain information.

   Process/System   Who or Where
   _____
   _____
   _____
   _____
   _____
   _____
   _____

3. List the library and research skills you need to acquire to become oriented to the library and to use it effectively. Be sure to include online services.

   _____
   _____
   _____
   _____
   _____
   _____
   _____
   _____

C. Developing student success strategies

1. List the print and online texts and other resources you will need to buy or borrow to prepare for the nursing program.

   _____
   _____
   _____
   _____
   _____
   _____
   _____

(Continued)

Unit I • The Transition Process

BOX 6.2 (Continued)

2. List the traits (characteristics) and roles of mentors and study groups that will enhance your success at the ADN level.

Mentor Traits   **Mentor Roles**

_____   _____
_____   _____
_____   _____
_____   _____
_____   _____
_____   _____
_____   _____

Study Group Traits   **Study Group Roles**

_____   _____
_____   _____
_____   _____
_____   _____
_____   _____
_____   _____
_____   _____

D. **Time management**

Write down your action plan for effective time management as you transition to the student role. Include elements of the win–win agreements you established with significant others and your "roles and goals" weekly time map.

_____
_____
_____
_____
_____
_____
_____
_____

II. **Action Plan for Needed Course Work**

List all course work needed to complete ADN requirements and college graduation requirements. Note course work completed or in progress. If course work was completed at another school or if you received equivalency or advance standing credit, indicate course(s) or experience for which you were granted that status. For course work needed, indicate the term and year you plan to take each course.

BOX 6.2 (Continued)

Nursing and Graduation Requirements At This School (Term/Year) *(IP = In Progress)*	Course Completed Name of School Another School Equivalency *(Course, School)*	Course Planned Term/Year *(IP = In Progress)*

III. Information for the Instructor–Student Partnership Meeting

Complete the four areas (A–D) below in preparation for the first meeting you will have with your nursing instructor/advisor.

A. Information I need to share, or of which my instructor/advisor needs to be aware, about myself and/or the program (e.g., issues, fears, concerns, etc.).

B. Questions I want to ask about the program and my transition process.

(Continued)

BOX 6.2 (Continued)

C. Resources/referrals that I may need, and information on obtaining them.

D. Advice and counsel from my nursing instructor/advisor; special tips, advice, etc., for success in the program. (Leave this section blank and complete it during the first appointment with your nursing instructor/advisor.)

STUDENT Exercises

Exercise 6.1
Now that you have completed the Thinking Critically sections of this chapter, you are ready to develop your PEP (see Box 6.2). Gather all the exercises you have completed throughout the text for entry into your PEP and complete all sections.

Exercise 6.2
Schedule an appointment with your instructor/advisor to review the PEP, and you have already made some great first steps toward success in your new role as you embark on the transition to professional registered nursing practice!

REFERENCES

American Nurses Association. (2021). *Nursing: Scope and standards of practice* (4th ed.).

Benner, P., Sutphen, M., Leonard, V., Day, L., & Schulman, L. S. (2010). *Educating nurses: A call for radical transformation*. Jossey-Bass.

Bergin, D. A., Bergin, C. A., & Prewitt, S. L. (2023). Motivating adult learners. In A. Belzer & B. Dashew (Eds.). *Understanding the adult learner: Perspectives and practices* (pp. 59–78). Taylor Francis Group.

Bradshaw, M. J., Hultquist, B. L., & Hagler, D. (2021). *Innovative teaching strategies in nursing and related health professions* (8th ed.). Jones and Bartlett.

Buckway, A. J., & Sowerby, H. (2023). *Nursing in today's world: Trends, issues, and management* (12th ed.). Wolters Kluwer.

Calacci, M. M., & Hagler, D. (2023). Managing your career. In P. S. Yoder-Wise & S. Sportsman (Eds.). *Leading and managing in nursing* (8th ed., pp. 470–488). Elsevier.

Claire, B. D., & Reising, D. L. (2023). Mentoring-as-partnership: The meaning of mentoring among novice nurse faculty. *Journal of Nursing Education*, 62(2), 83–88. https://doi.org/10.3928/01484834-20221213-03

Covey, S. R., Merrill, A. R., & Merrill, R. R. (1994). *First things first: To live, to love, to leave a legacy*. Simon & Schuster.

Coyne, M. L., & Chatham, C. (2020). Advancing and managing your professional nursing career. In K. Masters (Ed.), *Role development in professional nursing practice* (6th ed., pp. 161–180). Jones & Bartlett.

Duff, C. S. (1999). *Learning from other women: How to benefit from the knowledge, wisdom, and experience of female mentors*. American Management Association.

Ellis, D. (2022a). *Becoming a master student: Making the career connection* (17th ed.). Cengage Learning.

Ellis, D. (2022b). *The essential guide to becoming a master student: Making the career connection* (6th ed.). Cengage Learning.

Ellis, P. (2020). Systematic program evaluation. In D. M. Billings & J. A. Halstead (Eds.). *Teaching in nursing: A guide for faculty* (6th ed., pp. 514–559). Elsevier.

Hood, L. (2021). *Leddy & Pepper's professional nursing* (10th ed.). Kluwer.

Ignatavicius, D. (2021). Preparing for the new nursing licensure exam: The next-generation NCLEX. *Nursing*, 51(5), 35–41. https://doi.org/10.1097/01.NURSE.0000743100.95536.9b

Institute of Medicine. (2011). *The future of nursing: Leading change, advancing health*. The Academies Press.

Mathisen, C., Bjørk, I. T., Heyn, L. G., Jacobsen, T. I., & Hansen, E. H. (2023). Practice education facilitators perceptions and experiences of their role in the clinical learning environment for nursing students: A qualitative study. *BMC Nursing*, 22(1), 165. https://doi.org/10.1186/s12912-023-01328-3

National Council of State Boards of Nursing. (2023a). *2023 NCLEX-RN test plan*. https://www.ncsbn.org/public-files/2023_RN_Test%20Plan_English_FINAL.pdf

National Council of State Boards of Nursing. (2023b). *2023 NCLEX-PN test plan*. https://www.ncsbn.org/public-files/2023_PN_Test%20Plan_FINAL.pdf

National League for Nursing. (2012). *Outcomes and competencies for graduates of practical/vocational. Diploma, Associate Degree, Baccalaureate, Master's, Practice Doctorate, and Research Doctorate Programs in Nursing*.

Scheckel, M. (2020). Designing courses and learning experiences. In D. M. Billings & J. A. Halstead (Eds.). *Teaching in nursing: A guide for faculty* (6th ed., pp. 181–201). Elsevier.

Scheele, A. M. (2005). *Launch your career in college: Strategies for students, educators, and parents*. Praeger.

Twedell, D. M. (2023). Role transition. In P. S. Yoder-Wise & S. Sportsman (Eds.). *Leading and managing in nursing* (8th ed., pp. 470–488). Elsevier.

On the WEB

Back to College: A website with answers to frequently asked questions for individuals returning to school: http://www.back2college.com:

National Council of State Boards of Nursing: http://www.ncsbn.org

CHAPTER 7

Test Success and the Challenge of NCLEX-RN Questions

LEARNING OUTCOMES

By the end of this chapter, the student will be able to:
1. Describe the benefits of computerized adaptive testing (CAT).
2. List the four main categories of client needs according to the NCLEX-RN test plan.
3. Describe the components of a test question.
4. Analyze the complexity of questions used, from knowledge through evaluation.
5. Explain the range of item types used on the NCLEX-RN exam.
6. Describe the process of clinical judgment.
7. Develop a plan for student success on exams using before-, during-, and after-test strategies.

KEY TERMS

acronym
acrostic
analysis questions
application questions
Bloom's Taxonomy of Educational Objectives
comprehension questions
computerized adaptive testing (CAT)
correct option
creating questions
knowledge questions
mnemonic
NCLEX-RN
NCLEX-RN test plan
paraphrasing
reciprocal teaching
synthesis questions
test distractors
test item
test options
test stem

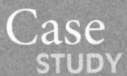

Case STUDY

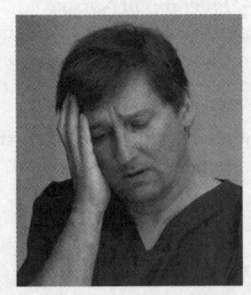

Randy Caruthers has been an LVN for 15 years and is a serious, hardworking student. He has sacrificed financially, going part time to complete his schooling. His wife is now supporting him and his 5-year-old son. It worries him that he is giving up time with his son and is stressing his wife to complete his course requirements. He has just received the results of his first nursing test and is stunned to see that he is barely passing. He is confused about what to do and where to start. He approaches his course professor looking bewildered and frustrated.

> **RANDY:** What is it with these nursing tests? I have an A average in all my other courses, and even with all the time I put into this, I barely passed with a C!
>
> **PROFESSOR:** You seem angry and upset! And I know you need to work through these feelings, but I'm not the enemy. I'm here to help.
>
> **RANDY:** You bet I'm angry and confused. And now, I don't know whether I can do this! I've got too much at stake to fail!
>
> **PROFESSOR:** What we need to do, Randy, is to sit down and look at your test together. I know that you attended the test review, and I know you take your studies seriously. We need to channel that confusion and frustration into an action plan. Together we can assess your content strengths and needs, look at your current study habits, and develop a plan that might help you be more successful. The first step is to assess your needs.
>
> **RANDY:** Now that I think about it ... I didn't do very well on my PN tests either. I was young and didn't realize how serious studies are for safe patient care. I sure would appreciate the extra help.

The situation in which Randy and his professor are engaged is the beginning of a collaborative dialogue that will help him to be successful. Taking a test is an anxiety-producing and high-stakes situation for both student and professor. In today's society, where students like Randy carry such heavy personal and professional loads, failure to live up to expectations on an exam can take a heavy toll on the student's psychosocial state and financial future. Acceptance into nursing school is competitive. Nursing schools have a vested interest in not only the recruitment but also the retention of students. Students often need help to be successful, and there are an almost overwhelming number of resources. Increasing the odds of your success is the objective of this chapter. To better understand the nursing examination process, this chapter will describe how test questions are written; identify components of Bloom's Taxonomy of Educational Objectives; summarize the National Council of State Boards of Nursing (NCSBN) Clinical Judgment Measurement Model (NCJMM); walk you through what to do before, during, and after an exam; and describe helpful hints to reduce anxiety when preparing for nursing exams.

DEVELOPMENT OF THE NCLEX-RN

As an LVN/LPN, you are familiar with the testing processes used in nursing. However, if you did not graduate recently, you may not be aware of the changes that were implemented in the NCLEX beginning in 2023. This section briefly describes the historical development of the NCLEX-RN, the incorporation of **computerized adaptive testing (CAT)**, and the implementation of next generation style questions in 2023, as well as how the NCLEX adapts to an ever-changing healthcare environment.

HISTORICAL DEVELOPMENT OF THE NCLEX

Testing is designed for one main purpose: To ensure that nurses are safe and effective (NCSBN, 2023). The **NCLEX-RN** is administered to graduates of nursing schools to test the knowledge, abilities, and skills necessary for safe entry-level nursing practice.

Designed with safety in mind, the NCLEX exam evaluates the nurse's minimum competency level in meeting basic patient needs.

In the 1960s to 1990s, NCLEX-PN and NCLEX-RN used a paper-and-pencil examination. In the 1990s, NCLEX exams became computerized. Like Randy, as a PN you have already established a minimum competency level by successfully passing the computerized NCLEX-PN. To be a candidate for the NCLEX-PN, you had to take proficiency tests in school and graduate. After graduation, you decided the date and time you would take the NCLEX-PN exam.

Computerized Adaptive Testing

In 1994, CAT was implemented for testing on the NCLEX-RN. This was the first time that the state boards of nursing used computerized testing. CAT afforded many advantages (see Box 7.1), including allowing nursing graduates to be tested at multiple sites with greater frequency, therefore decreasing the time between graduation and taking or retaking the examination. CAT technology individualizes the question sequence for each test taker. On a CAT exam, each test question presented to the student is based on the student's ability to successfully meet the passing standard set for the previous question; if a candidate exhibits proficiency, the next question's passing standard increases in difficulty. If a candidate does not successfully meet the passing standard set for that question, the next question's passing standard decreases in difficulty. During CAT, students are given questions until it is determined whether the student exhibits the proficiency to meet passing standards or the student lacks proficiency and fails. Students cannot return to questions to change answers. Being aware that this is a feature of the exam will help you to prepare, and you will probably have exams in school that will be administered in the same way. The minimum number of test items a test taker will receive is 85. Once the computer determines that the minimum safe competency level and the passing standard for the exam has been met or not met, the test ends.

How Questions Are Formed and Changed

The NCLEX-RN test plan is revised every 3 years using results from a job practice analysis completed by working RNs, educators, and managers. Skills, interventions, and critical incidents of nursing practice are reviewed by the NCSBN through the National Council Examination Committee. This process supports the clinical relevance and validity of the examination. The job practice analysis focus of the committee is the knowledge needed by new graduate nurses who are at an entry level of practice. Questions are written by experienced nurse educators and screened through a rigorous examination by the committee (NCSBN, n.d.-a). New questions are then included in NCLEX exams on a trial basis (i.e., they are not included in the test taker's score). Through this method, the questions are evaluated and, if determined to be suitable for inclusion in the test, are

---

BOX 7.1

Advantages of CAT

- Quick
- Individualized
- Multiple sites of administration
- Multiple times of administration
- Less wait time than paper-and-pencil tests if a re-examination is needed
- Less wait time between graduation and testing than paper-and-pencil tests

then added to the question pool for future NCLEX exams. The NCSBN revised its test plan for 2023. You can review the test plan by visiting the NCSBN website at https://www.ncsbn.org/public-files/2023_RN_Test%20Plan_English_FINAL.pdf

MAIN CATEGORIES OF THE NCLEX-RN TEST PLAN

Much like an architectural blueprint provides the direction or the step-by-step plan for a building, the **NCLEX-RN test plan** is a roadmap that faculty and students can follow to determine priorities of content on a nursing exam. The NCLEX-RN test plan incorporates the nursing process in four main categories of client needs. It is important for students to become familiar with test plans and blueprints to anticipate the content, scope, and areas covered in exams (Ignatavicius, 2021). Before administering exams, nursing instructors should share their test plans and blueprints with students to ensure that students are aware of the significance of the nursing concepts being tested (McDonald, 2018). When faculty share their test plans, it helps to calm test anxiety.

FOUR MAIN CATEGORIES OF CLIENT NEEDS

The NCLEX-RN test plan focuses on four categories of client needs (Table 7.1). Students taking a nursing school exam and the NCLEX-RN should anticipate demonstrating their competence in these areas on nursing examinations. In addition, nursing tests are based on processes that are fundamental to the practice of nursing that are listed in Box 7.2. These frameworks are also the foundation for the tests in your nursing courses.

The NCLEX-RN *Might Ask* 7.1

A nursing student is studying the NCLEX-RN test plan. Which of the following main content categories does it include? (Select all that apply.)

a. Caring
b. Nursing process
c. Teaching/learning
d. Safe, effective care environment
e. Health promotion and maintenance
f. Psychosocial integrity
g. Physiological integrity

TABLE 7.1 Four Main Categories of Client Needs

Client Needs	Subcategories
Safe and effective care environment	• Management of care • Safety and infection control
Health promotion and maintenance	
Psychosocial integrity	
Physiological integrity	• Basic care and comfort • Pharmacologic and parenteral therapies • Reduction of risk potential • Physiological adaptation

Source: NCSBN. (2023). *Next Generation NCLEX: NCLEX-RN Test Plan, Effective April 2023.* https://www.nclex.com/files/2023_RN_Test%20Plan_English_FINAL.pdf

BOX 7.2 Processes That Are Fundamental to the Process of Nursing

- Caring
- Clinical judgment
- Communication and documentation
- Culture and spirituality
- Nursing process
- Teaching/learning

Source: NCSBN. (2023). *Next Generation NCLEX: NCLEX-RN Test Plan, Effective April 2023.* https://www.nclex.com/files/2023_RN_Test%20Plan_English_FINAL.pdf

TEST LANGUAGE: KEY COMPONENTS TO A TEST

To correctly interpret test questions, the test taker must understand the question's construction and language. If the test questions are poor quality, the test will not evaluate the intended criteria. In preparation for nursing school exams and the NCLEX-RN exam, students need to know the structure of the types of questions that will be presented. In the Next Generation NCLEX (NGN) exam, there are numerous item types including case studies, matrix/grid, bow-tie, drop-down menus, drag and drop, highlight items, extended multiple response, multiple response select all that apply, and multiple response. Items may include charts, tables, and graphic images. Let's start with the basics.

Test questions should be directly related to course learning outcomes (McDonald, 2018). Randy's nursing professor will likely advise him to be attentive to the course outcomes in his reading list. Each test question is called a **test item**. The part of the test item that states the problem is called the **test stem**. In a multiple-response question, all potential choices to the question are called **test options**. The options that the student must eliminate, or the incorrect answers, are called the **test distractors**. In a multiple-choice exam, there are three distractors and one **correct option** (Box 7.3). Students need to carefully read each question on the exam, eliminate the distractors, and choose the correct option.

NCLEX style test questions are written so that they involve a simulated nurse/patient situation (see Box 7.4). Because of this scenario style, questions can become quite long and involved. For the test taker, **paraphrasing** what the test item is specifically asking becomes key to answering the question. Paraphrasing is rewording the question without

BOX 7.3 Structure of a Multiple-Choice Question (Test Item)

The nurse is performing a physical assessment on a client with a pneumothorax. The nurse palpates a crackling, popping sound under her hands near a chest tube site. This finding indicates		The Test Stem
A. tactile fremitus	DISTRACTOR	The Test Options
B. subcutaneous emphysema	CORRECT OPTION	
C. egophony	DISTRACTOR	
D. whispered pectoriloquy	DISTRACTOR	

BOX 7.4 Comparison of an NCLEX Style and a Non-NCLEX Style Test Question

Non–NCLEX Style Question	NCLEX Style Question
A risk factor for coronary artery disease includes A. Height B. Cancer C. Weight D. **High cholesterol**	The nurse is assessing the client's risk factors for coronary artery disease. Which of the following indicates a high risk for this potential health problem? A. Height B. Cancer C. Weight D. **High cholesterol**

Bold indicates the correct option.

stating it word for word. Although paraphrasing can be challenging, the technique helps to identify the heart of the meaning of the question.

Because patient care is complex, nursing instructors write exams so that questions simulate the critical thinking, decision-making, and problem-solving needed by the nurse in the clinical setting. As you progress through your courses, test questions will increase in level of difficulty from simple to complex. Understanding how the level of difficulty is determined will help you to correctly answer increasingly complex test questions.

THINKING CRITICALLY

Read the NCLEX style question in Box 7.4. Identify the test stem, test options, and distractors.

BLOOM'S TAXONOMY AND LEVEL OF DIFFICULTY

The most widely used theory by educators to help categorize the level of difficulty for test items, which is also used by the NCSBN, is **Bloom's Taxonomy of Educational Objectives** (Bloom et al., 1956) (see Table 7.2).

TABLE 7.2 Comparison of Bloom's Taxonomy and NCLEX-RN Style Questions

Bloom's Taxonomy	NCLEX-RN Taxonomy
Knowledge/Remembering	Knowledge
Comprehension/Understanding	Comprehension
Application/Applying	Application
Analysis/Analyzing	Analysis
Synthesis/Evaluating	Evaluation
Evaluation/Creating	Creation

TABLE 7.3 Levels of Complexity and Types of NCLEX-RN Questions

Taxonomy	Definition	Types of Questions
Knowledge/Remembering	Recallable Learned by memorization/repetition	Definitions Steps in a procedure Common terms/facts Medication doses, side effects
Comprehension/Understanding	Understanding Paraphrasing Meaning/intent Translate Interpret	The how and why of information use
Application/Applying	Using information that is understood	Using information in a new setting by demonstrating, solving, changing, and modifying. Making judgments
Analysis/Analyzing	Looking at information and examining the essential features in relationship to each other Priority setting Recognizing effects	Comparing and contrasting information Best or better answer Highest priority or initial response
Synthesis/Evaluating	Make a decision or provide a solution based on specified criteria, standards, or supporting data	Client response to treatment Delegating tasks
Evaluation/Creating	Apply knowledge to develop something new	Develop a plan of care Create a quality improvement project

The structure that Bloom created goes from simple questions that are knowledge based to questions that are quite complex and involve evaluation and analysis of information. The NCLEX-RN exam design includes nursing questions from knowledge through evaluation levels (Table 7.3).

KNOWLEDGE/REMEMBERING QUESTIONS

Information that a student has recalled and that is easily recallable is called knowledge (Billings & Hensel, 2024). Knowledge is concrete and easily identified in the textbook or other sources from where the topic was presented. Knowledge-based questions require the fewest steps by the student to determine the answer. A student either knows or does not know the answer. Types of **knowledge questions** that may be used are as follows:

- Definitions
- Steps in a procedure
- Common terms or facts
- Identifying a medication, a normal dose, or its side effects

Students usually think that these are the easiest questions to answer, because the success of answering correctly depends on memorizing and recalling material. Knowledge questions can be made more difficult if the concept being tested is one that is difficult to understand. An example of a knowledge-level question is shown on the next page.

To demonstrate how a question can be changed to reflect a higher level of difficulty in the same content area, hematocrit lab tests are used in the following sections.

EXAMPLE 7.1 Knowledge Question
The nurse knows an adult patient's hematocrit value normally is:
A. 10% to 20%.
B. 21% to 45%.
C. 35% to 65%.
D. 35% to 52%.
(D is the correct answer.)

COMPREHENSION/UNDERSTANDING QUESTIONS
The second type of question a student will possibly answer is focused on the comprehension of presented material. Comprehension questions are one level higher in difficulty than knowledge questions and require the student to understand the material and to interpret the importance of the information. Types of **comprehension questions** that may be used are as follows:

- Understanding a definition or term
- Knowing why a lab result is important
- Recognizing what and why a step in a procedure is important
- Identifying why or how a medication will work

Students usually find these questions are a bit more difficult to answer, because answering them correctly depends not only on memorizing material but also on truly understanding the material and its relationship to nursing practice. An example of a comprehension-level question is shown below.

EXAMPLE 7.2 Comprehension Question
The nurse is assessing a patient's complete blood cell count. The hematocrit value is a reflection of:
A. the number of red cells circulating in the body.
B. the type of anemia a patient has.
C. the percentage of red cells to serum.
D. the infection-fighting ability of the body.
(C is the correct answer.)

In this question, the student must understand not only the meaning of the concept but also how it relates to the patient's body function.

APPLICATION/APPLYING QUESTIONS
A third type of question a student will possibly answer is an application question. Application questions are a step higher and more difficult than comprehension questions and require a student to know the material and to use it in a concrete or new situation. An application question may ask the student to solve a problem, change a nursing action, or manipulate variables in a given situation. Types of **application questions** that may be used are as follows:

- Apply a definition or term to a new/unique situation.
- Assess the importance of a lab result in relationship to a disease.
- Prioritize what steps in a procedure are important or when they occur.
- Evaluate a response to a medication.

Students usually report that application questions are among the most difficult to answer. Successful elimination of distractors and identification of the correct answer depends on memorizing and understanding the material and then applying the material to a new nursing situation. An example of an application question is shown below.

EXAMPLE 7.3 Application Question
The nurse is evaluating a patient's complete blood cell count after administration of a unit of packed red blood cells. The hematocrit value is 75%. This value indicates which of the following regarding fluid balance?
A. Too much circulating volume
B. A decrease in circulating fluid levels
C. A higher level of circulating oxygen
D. Not enough red blood cells
(The correct answer is B.)

In this question, the student needs to know the range of normal values of hematocrit levels (knowledge) and hematocrit's role as a vascular component of blood (application). The student also has to apply the concepts to the presented distractors. The three-step process requires students to think critically and to integrate applied knowledge.

ANALYSIS/ANALYZING QUESTIONS
As the difficulty of questions increases, analysis questions challenge the student to analyze data and to draw logical conclusions. Analysis questions include information that must be broken down into components for understanding and require students to understand the complex relationships of concepts and topics. Analysis questions require knowledge, understanding, and the ability to apply, dissect, and scrutinize elements. In analysis-type questions, all answer choices may be correct for the presented scenario; however, students are required to determine the correct answer by identifying the best or highest priority option. Types of **analysis questions** that may be used are

- Choosing the best definition or term to a new situation
- Anticipating lab test results with a client's history/diagnosis
- Prioritizing the first step of action to perform when a given set of symptoms occurs
- Identifying the best medication to give a client according to their symptoms and variables given in the stem

Analysis questions require a high degree of critical thinking. The correct answer depends on all of the previous types of cognitive-level reasoning. The test-taker must successfully eliminate distractors by identifying the data presented in the stem and eliminating many variables. An example of an analysis question is shown below.

EXAMPLE 7.4 Analysis Question
The nurse is evaluating the complete blood cell counts of four patients. One of the patients has a hematocrit value of 75%. This value is most reflective of which of the following patients?
A. A 45-year-old man with chronic sickle cell disease
B. A 55-year-old man with a history of chronic lung disease admitted with shortness of breath
C. A 65-year-old woman with ovarian cancer
D. A 75-year-old woman with chronic right-sided heart failure
(The correct answer is B.)

To answer the question successfully, the student must know the normal hematocrit value range, *anticipate* the hematocrit value for each client, and *predict* which client is most likely to have a hematocrit value of 75%. The example question simulates the complex clinical judgment commonly required for the day-to-day screening and safety of clients.

SYNTHESIS/EVALUATING QUESTIONS

To demonstrate a higher level of reasoning, synthesis questions require the student to make a judgment or to provide a solution based on presented criteria, standards, or evidence. When answering synthesis questions, students assess supplied information to provide their perspective on such concepts as delegation, confirming client teachings, interventions, or client status. Types of synthesis questions that may be used are as follows:

- Assessing the effectiveness of nursing interventions to make judgments about the best course of action for client care
- Application of professional standards, guidelines, and evidence-based practices to evaluate the quality and effectiveness of nursing care
- Examining ethical dilemmas or moral principles that require nurses to consider the ethical implications of their actions and decisions in client care

Synthesis questions require students to synthesize client care by critiquing the significance of data, understanding the underlying structure of a concept, identifying patterns or trends, and recognizing cause-and-effect relationships to choose the best course of action based on given criteria. Synthesis questions may include the keywords assess, compare, contrast, determine, recommend, justify, or select. Synthesis questions are a high level of cognitive complexity in Bloom's taxonomy and represent advanced critical thinking skills. An example of a synthesis question is shown below.

EXAMPLE 7.5 Synthesis Question

A 72-year-old client with a history of heart failure (HF) is admitted to the cardiac care unit (CCU) with worsening dyspnea, orthopnea, and bilateral lower extremity edema. The nurse reviews the client's laboratory results, which reveal elevated levels of B-type natriuretic peptide (BNP) and serum creatinine. The client's vital signs include a blood pressure of 90/60 mm Hg, heart rate of 110 beats per minute, respiratory rate of 24 breaths per minute, and oxygen saturation of 88% on room air. Based on these data, what is the most appropriate nursing intervention?
A. Administer intravenous diuretics to reduce fluid overload.
B. Initiate continuous positive airway pressure (CPAP) therapy.
C. Prepare for emergent intubation and mechanical ventilation.
D. Administer intravenous vasopressors to increase blood pressure.
(The correct answer is A.)

To answer the question successfully, the student must critically *evaluate* the significance of data, understand underlying concepts related to heart failure pathophysiology, and recognize cause-and-effect relationships to choose the best course of action based on the client's problems.

EVALUATION/CREATING QUESTIONS

The highest level of question complexity is **creating questions**. The focus of creating questions is on encouraging students to generate new ideas or ways of thinking by combining existing knowledge and concepts in innovative ways. Create questions challenge students to use their creativity and problem-solving skills to produce new ideas, structures, or patterns, such as quality improvement projects or plans of care. Types of create questions that may be used are as follows:

- Developing innovative approaches to address healthcare challenges or to improve patient outcomes
- Identifying problems or areas for improvement in patient care and developing creative solutions
- Integrating knowledge from various sources, including evidence-based practices, clinical expertise, and patient preferences, to develop comprehensive and effective interventions
- Demonstrating collaboration with interdisciplinary teams, clients, and caregivers to cocreate solutions that meet the diverse needs of clients and improve healthcare delivery

To respond to create questions, students must demonstrate their ability to evaluate and synthesize information from several sources, to apply critical thinking skills, and to develop solutions. Keywords in create level questions may include create, develop, manage, modify, plan, or prepare. Create questions provide valuable insight into student clinical reasoning and clinical judgment. An example of a create question is shown below.

EXAMPLE 7.6 Create Question
The nurse is working in a pediatric oncology unit. Despite the nurse's best efforts, a 10-year-old client undergoing chemotherapy for leukemia is experiencing significant anxiety and distress during their treatments. What interventions should the nurse plan to help alleviate the child's anxiety and to enhance coping mechanisms during chemotherapy sessions? (Select all that apply.)
A. Provide virtual reality goggles or handheld video games during chemotherapy sessions.
B. Incorporate play therapy activities tailored to the child's interests.
C. Administer sedative medications to the child before chemotherapy sessions.
D. Restrain the child physically to prevent movement or resistance during treatment.
E. Provide a reward system where the child earns stickers, small toys, or privileges for completing each chemotherapy session.
(The correct answers are A, B, and E.)

To answer the question successfully, the student must think creatively and develop an original intervention plan tailored to address the unique needs of the pediatric oncology patient. *Creating* requires the student to integrate knowledge of child development, therapeutic communication, psychosocial support, and creative interventions to promote the child's well-being during chemotherapy sessions.

CLINICAL JUDGMENT

As nursing care continues to become increasingly complex, to enter practice students are required to develop clinical judgment using critical thinking, clinical reasoning, nursing knowledge, and nursing skills. To identify if students are ready to enter practice,

TABLE 7.4 Dimensions of Tanner's Clinical Judgment Model

Dimension	Nurse's Function
Noticing	Examines the situation and the patient's condition; identifies important information
Interpreting	Exhibits understanding, analyzes facts, comes to conclusions; determines meanings, recognizes patterns and trends
Responding	Identifies priorities, determines goals, plans and implements care
Reflecting	Evaluates the patient's response, determines effectiveness of care; identifies errors in judgment to apply to future patient care

Source: Tanner, C. A. (2006). Thinking like a nurse: A research-based model of clinical judgment in nursing. *Journal of Nursing Education, 45*(6), 204–211.

nursing exams need to test more than clinical knowledge; they also need to evaluate each student's judgment, decision-making, and critical thinking skills. Increasing the difficulty of test items using the various taxonomy levels (as discussed in the previous section) evaluates the test taker's nursing knowledge and critical thinking skills, but it falls short of effectively evaluating clinical reasoning skills and clinical judgment.

Although the nurse uses characteristics such as experience, knowledge, and level of expertise to make decisions, numerous other factors such as observations, task complexity, and cultural competence influence clinical judgment. Tanner's (2006) model of clinical judgment describes the process through which nurses progress in making clinical decisions. The model consists of the dimensions of noticing, interpreting, responding, and reflecting. See Table 7.4 for detailed descriptions of each dimension.

After reviewing the results from the 2013–2014 NCSBN Strategic Practice Analysis, the NCSBN recognized that a better method was needed to evaluate the test taker's understanding of nursing skills and clinical judgment. To revise and improve the NCLEX-RN exam, the NCSBN then completed an in-depth analysis of testing, decision theory, and nursing literature to identify a valid and reliable method of measuring clinical judgment. The result was the NCJMM evaluation framework. Although the framework includes concepts from nursing theories and nursing models, the NCJMM is specific to testing and provides a systematic, evidence-based framework for measuring nurse licensure candidate minimal competence of clinical judgment and decision-making (NCSBN, n.d.-b).

The NCJMM reflects concepts similar to Tanner's (2006) clinical judgment model incorporated with the nursing process (see Table 7.5). With the framework in place as

TABLE 7.5 Comparison of Concepts of the Nursing Process, Tanner's Clinical Judgment Model, and the NCSBN Clinical Judgment Measurement Model (NCJMM)

The Nursing Process	Tanner's Clinical Judgment Model	The NCSBN Clinical Judgment Measurement Model (NCJMM)
Assessment	Noticing	Recognize cues
Diagnosis	Interpreting	Analyze cues
Diagnosis	Interpreting	Prioritize hypotheses
Planning	Responding	Generate solutions
Implementation	Responding	Take action
Evaluation	Reflecting	Evaluate outcomes

the foundation, the NCSBN developed the NGN exam. Developed to improve patient outcomes and improve readiness for practice, test items are constructed to reflect working environments. During your nursing program, you will probably be introduced to NGN style test items that evaluate your ability to recognize cues, interpret situations, respond appropriately, and reflect on care that would be given.

TEST ITEM FORMATS

The evolution to NGN allows for a wide variety of test item types in the NCLEX-RN (see Table 7.6). There are no established norms for the number of items using the new formats to be included on the NCLEX-RN; however, a hallmark of NGN exams are case studies. The case studies are designed to evaluate your clinical judgment in complex, real-world scenarios. Patient case studies include a series of questions that require you to identify clinical issues, prioritize nursing actions, and evaluate outcomes.

PREPARATION FOR AN NCLEX-RN STYLE EXAM

Preparation for class and exams is an important activity for students and professors in your program. Acceptance into nursing school is highly competitive, and you are

TABLE 7.6 NGN Test Item Formats

Type of Questions	Examples
Single best response	Select one correct answer
Multiple response: Students must identify multiple correct answers	Performing steps in a procedure Selecting correct nursing interventions for a particular diagnosis
Fill in the blanks	Calculating medication Prioritizing nursing actions
Mathematical calculations	Determining a score on assessment tool scales
Use of graphic images, pictures, charts, or tables • Hot spot • Exhibit	Determining physical locations on a patient model
Case study	A patient scenario consisting of vital signs, admission notes, nurse's notes, and other chart information
Matrix/grid	Choose multiple options in a column and/or row of a table of answer options
Drop-down menu	Select answers from provided choices in tables, charts, or paragraphs
Drag and drop	Use the computer mouse to drag and drop the options in order of priority. May not use all answer choices
Highlight	Use computer mouse to highlight text in patient charts or paragraphs
Bowtie	Analyze electronic health record or patient scenario. Determine the patient medical condition, nursing actions, and data to monitor
Ordered response	Use the computer mouse to drag and drop the options in order of priority

Source: National Council of State Boards of Nursing. (2022). *Next generation NCLEX®: NCLEX-RN® exam preview.* https://ncsbn.az1.qualtrics.com/WRQualtricsControlPanel/File.php?F=F_bpBwY7Is4EoRiWa; National Council of State Boards of Nursing. (2021). *Next generation NCLEX®: Sample pack.* https://ncsbn.az1.qualtrics.com/WRQualtricsControlPanel/File.php?F=F_eR8xOxTNt8iyUiG

invested in being successful. Preparing for the work ahead will clear your path to positive achievement in your nursing courses.

BEFORE THE EXAM
Planning
Planning is a good study habit that provides a foundation for the discipline you will need to succeed in robust, rigorous programs. For each of your nursing courses, once you receive the syllabus and course outline, you should immediately use a planning calendar to write down due dates for assignments, projects, and exams. At a minimum, for every hour you spend in class, 2 hours should be devoted to study and preparation. Thus, if you have a weekly 3-hour nursing lab, a minimum of 6 hours a week should be devoted to studying for that lab. So, in your planning calendar, block out times during the week to devote to this prep time. Planning regular study time prevents "cramming" before examinations. Although cramming may help with retaining information for knowledge-type questions, it does not increase learning and is rarely beneficial for questions at the application and analysis levels.

The ideal study time is 1- to 2-hour blocks of concentrated time, with short breaks. You will also want to use any downtime in your busy schedule to your advantage. When Randy and his professor looked at his class schedule, they blocked out weekly study time so that Randy could be consistent in his study habits. Together they also found some extra study time for Randy by using his commute time. His professor suggested that he use his phone to record himself talking about important concepts missed in his first exam and listen to those recordings during his bus ride. Randy also found that he could download podcasts and listen to some of his instructor's lectures while working out at the gym. Together, they also found extra study time while he waited at his son's karate lessons.

Using Class/Professor Time Wisely
During your study time, you should read for comprehension. Some students read important review concepts out loud. You should ask yourself, "Do I understand this material?" Using either a notepad and pencil or a laptop or tablet, write down what you do not understand. Most professors will start a lecture, class, or lab by asking if there are any questions; use this time as an opportunity to ask questions. Do not feel alone. Chances are, if you do not understand the material, there are other students also in the same situation. Be assertive in your learning needs. If you do not want to ask your questions in class, set up a regular appointment to meet with the professor outside class. Use the appointment time to get your questions answered and your needs met. Having a regular appointment allows the instructor to get to know you as an individual and helps the instructor become familiar with your needs.

Memorization
Building a knowledge foundation will require that you memorize some material. There are many memory aids to help with what seems to be an overwhelming amount of information. A **mnemonic** is any device that provides an easy way to increase memory by improving retention of foundational knowledge (see https://en.wikipedia.org/wiki/List_of_medical_mnemonics for more information).

Acrostics and acronyms, described below, are two types of mnemonics that involve words. If these words are coupled with a picture or diagram, they enhance learning for both auditory and visual nursing students.

An **acrostic** is an arrangement of words into a phrase that helps you to recall information. Below is an example of an acrostic that is helpful for students.

EXAMPLE 7.7 Acrostic

The letters APE, T, and M in "Ape To Man" can help a student remember the heart values for auscultation of heart sounds:

We evolve **Ape To M**an **A**ortic
          Pulmonic
         Erb's point
         Tricuspid
         Mitral

Another type of memory enhancer is an **acronym**. Acronyms are words that are formed using the first letter of other words. See the below example.

EXAMPLE 7.8 Acronym

A common nursing acronym that helps students remember the order of steps for treating heart failure is:

UNLOADME
This acronym stands for:
Upright positioning
Nitrates
Lasix
Oxygen
Albuterol
Dobutamine
Morphine
Extremities

Mnemonics are not beneficial for every student; in fact, learning the mnemonic can sometimes be more difficult for students than learning the material. Try to stick with what works for you. Randy's professor noted that he was creative and could develop mnemonics that worked well for him. Randy started writing mnemonics on index cards and taking them with him to study while his son went to healthcare appointments. He also used his cards to study during breaks between his classes. At home, his wife used his cards to quiz him while they prepared supper. His wife was happy to be involved in his learning, and she began adding pictures to the cards to illustrate facts. With instructor encouragement, Randy decided to share his learning techniques with the class, giving his classmates valuable ideas for developing their own learning materials.

Making Reading Come Alive

Reading a textbook is usually a passive process, with no interaction on the part of the reader. One of the keys to successful learning is to interact with textbooks. Some ways to interact are highlighting in the textbook, writing down questions about your reading to have answered by the instructor during lecture, forming study groups, and using the publisher's interactive tools that come with the textbook. You might write notes about the more difficult concepts or topics. Writing down information forces you to think about the content and helps you to retain more of what you have read.

Using a Highlighter

Using a highlighter to mark key concepts makes you think critically about the material by identifying important information and facilitates the process of reviewing that key content later much easier. However, highlighting can become a problem when important information is misinterpreted or students become so overwhelmed with the volume of presented information that they overuse highlighting. Here are some guidelines for highlighting effectively.

- Completely read a paragraph or a section, then determine and highlight the main concepts. Why is the point you are highlighting critical? How would a nurse put this information to use?
- Limit highlighting to only one sentence or phrase per paragraph.
- Highlight key words and phrases instead of full sentences.
- Consider color-coding by using one color of highlighter for definitions, another color for key points, and another color for examples.

Writing Down Questions About Your Reading

Another way to make reading active is to have a conversation with the author while reading. If the author was in the same room while you were reading, what would you want to ask them? What concepts are not clear? What doesn't make sense to you? Write your questions out. Use the list to ask questions at the beginning of your professor's lecture. Most instructors like to answer questions that clarify important nursing concepts at the beginning of lecture. If you are in a study group with other students, use the questions as study topics to get others' viewpoints. If the textbook has a list of important concepts/questions in the chapters, make sure you understand concept meanings and answer the practice questions. Be assertive in seeking clarification of meanings to make sure your needs are met.

Forming Study Groups

Study groups promote active learning through reciprocal teaching, in which students help each other learn material. **Reciprocal teaching** uses four strategies: summarizing, question generating, clarifying, and predicting. Reciprocal learning is typical of postconference activities, in which instructors encourage students to share information about actual clinical situations (Billings & Hensel, 2024).

Student study groups should be structured so each participant is responsible for a block of the material to summarize, to teach to other students, and then to develop and present multiple-choice questions that stress the importance of the information. Designing mnemonics and drawing pictures may help the learning process. This approach forces each group participant to hear oneself think when talking out loud, to clarify important concepts, and to rationalize answers.

Using Interactive Tools

Most textbooks come with interactive learning tools that may include workbooks, online resources, case studies, and interactive graphics (such as choosing items needed to place on a patient body for a particular assessment or moving items appropriately in a nursing care room). Although interactive tools add to the student workload, they are designed to enhance the learning process. The use of interactive tools encourages students to engage with the nursing curriculum by moving the student from being a passive to an active participant. Interaction is important because what you hear, you may forget; what you see, you sometimes remember; but what you do, you learn for a lifetime. Interactive tools are not only helpful for studying course material, but they are also helpful in preparing for clinical.

EXAM DAY

There are some key things you can do before you take an exam that will improve your chances of success (see Box 7.5). Prepping your body to take an exam should be similar to an athlete preparing for a contest. The day before an exam, it is important to get a good night's sleep. If you have been studying all night, you won't perform at your best. Stop studying early on the evening before the test and plan something enjoyable for the rest of the evening.

Before going to bed, lay out what you will wear the next dad. The temperature of the testing room is out of your control, so it's best to be ready to add or remove clothing as necessary to stay comfortable. Always choose comfort over fashion on exam days. Prepare everything you will need for the exam, organizing items in a convenient place where you can locate them easily before you leave. These items may include your laptop computer or tablet, power cord or charging cables, sharpened pencils, a calculator, extra paper, watch, earplugs, and/or examination book. Ensure that your laptop or tablet are fully charged. If your school utilizes computer exams, be sure you know your password. If you will use your own laptop or tablet, be sure that you have the latest exam and browser software uploaded on your device. And don't forget to set your alarm.

The morning of exam day, eat a well-balanced, high-protein breakfast, which consists of complex carbohydrates and proteins that will sustain you throughout the day. Eggs, peanut butter, milk, and oats or nuts are high in protein. Breakfasts that will help maintain your blood glucose level and prevent blood sugar spikes and dips might include a glass of milk and a bagel with peanut butter (or other protein source), or cereal with milk and fruit. Take a water bottle with you to the exam so you will stay hydrated.

Leave home early and arrive to the testing room early; an unexpected bus delay or traffic jam can cause stress. Don't engage in negative conversations or negative thoughts; you have organized your study time and you have prepared for the exam, so believe in your abilities. If you are anxious or nervous, try stress-relieving techniques such as breathing exercises or brief meditation. A brisk 10-minute walk will stimulate your sympathetic nervous system, making you more alert and expending any nervous energy that may block your critical thinking ability. Turn your cell phone off.

BOX 7.5 Tips for Success Before an Examination

1. Prepare items needed for the exam the night before. (You can even pack your car that night.)
2. Get a good night's sleep.
3. Eat a well-balanced, high-protein breakfast.
4. Arrive at the testing site early.
5. Consider a brisk walk before the exam.
6. Ask whether you can use earplugs during the exam.
7. Synchronize your watch to the classroom clock.

DURING THE EXAM

Depending on your class and your school's examination policy, you may complete exams using paper and pencil, on a computer, by demonstrating skills, or by some other method of evaluation. There are several strategies you can use during exams to decrease your stress, help you focus, and improve your performance. Most exams have a time limit for completion. Before beginning an exam, you will want to estimate the amount of time you can spend to answer each question by dividing the total number of questions by the allotted time. You will want to allow enough time for every question and a few minutes for review at the end. Having an estimate for timing will help prevent a last-minute rush to answer remaining questions.

Types of Exams
Paper and Pencil Exams

Once your instructor has distributed the exams and has indicated that you can begin, you will want to skim through the exam. The professor will often write on the exam how the questions are weighted or how the points will be distributed. If there are short answer, ordered response, or case study questions that are weighted more, answer those first. Because multiple-choice questions are usually quicker to answer and may be weighted less, try to leave the multiple-choice section for last.

After you have skimmed the exam, go back to the beginning and read each question carefully. Respond first to questions for which you are certain of the answer. If determining the answer to a question takes you longer than 1 minute or you do not initially understand the question stem, do not choose an answer and proceed to the next question; this is especially important during timed tests, so that you don't waste valuable time on one question. If you spend too much time on one question, you may experience anxiety that will possibly affect your ability to answer the next question. Occasionally, content in the next few questions may jog your memory and help you to determine the correct response to the skipped question. Be sure to flag your answer sheet or the exam copy so that you will not forget to go back to skipped questions.

When completing the especially difficult questions, underline or circle key words and the question stem. Cross out the distractors one by one. If allowed, physically cross off the answer on the copy of the exam to give you a visual cue of choice elimination. If time permits, write a brief note about why you chose a particular answer. When you meet with your professor after the exam, your notes will help identify your thought process and any faulty thinking.

Computer Exams

If your school utilizes computer exams, questions will be presented in one of two ways: one question at a time or all questions at once. When exam questions are presented all at once, similar to paper and pencil exams, you have the option of skipping questions. Many computer exam programs allow students to "flag" skipped questions. Then, students can go back and answer the flagged questions after answering the questions for which they are sure of their responses.

When questions are presented one at a time, students usually do not have the option to skip questions and return to them later. If this is the case, you will want to limit the amount of time you spend to answer each question. If you know how many total questions are on the exam, allot an equal amount of time to answer each question. Depending on the course or how far along students are in a program, computer exams may initially present questions all at once. However, to prepare students for the NCLEX-RN, exams in later courses, close to graduation, may present questions one at a time.

Similar to paper and pencil exams, many computerized exams may allow students to use a "highlighter" to emphasize information in test items. Your professor might also allow you to write down notes on scratch paper. Do not use the scratch paper to write down test items; copying test items will take up much of your time and a violation of academic integrity at most schools. In most circumstances, you will have to place your name on your scratch paper and return the paper, even if it is blank, to your professor at the end of the exam.

Demonstration Exams

During your previous LPN/LVN classes, your nursing skills and abilities were evaluated through skills demonstrations. Depending on school and program requirements, when studying to be an RN you may again be required to demonstrate nursing skills. Skills demonstrations are anxiety producing even when the skill is a task that you have performed daily for a great length of time. The idea of being watched closely can erode concentration and destroy confidence. Whether the skills being tested are ones you learned previously or are new, you should prepare for skills demonstration tests to build your confidence and to prevent errors in technique. Always review and practice a skill using the skill checklist for that skill. As you practice a skill, write down notes for technique, especially for any areas where you have difficulty. Keep a list of questions to present to your instructor and, to gain clarity, ask the instructor to demonstrate the skill.

Many skills demonstrations also include written documentation of the skill performed. Although you may have developed your own personal documentation style, be sure to review the course requirements for information that should be included in the documentation. Documentation by a registered nurse may include more information than you have written in the past.

Common Issues During Exams

Completing an exam can be an anxiety-producing endeavor. Even after studying and preparing, you may confront a question that confusions you or stops your momentum. What should you do if you don't know what the question is asking? First and most important, do not panic. Take a deep breath. Read the question again. Paraphrase the question. What is it asking? What important nursing concepts apply?

Remember, for multiple-choice questions you have a 25% chance of choosing the correct answer. Carefully examine the answer choices. Eliminate any "all or every" answers, because absolutes are rarely correct answers. If all choices seem correct, look for similarities in the options; if two choices are the same but worded differently, cross them off. Also, remember that if a choice is only partially incorrect, the entire choice is incorrect. If the question refers to the best choice, choose the one that is all encompassing or has a broader focus.

For test-taking tips, see Box 7.6.

Sometimes students may not identify important aspects that indicate the focus of the question. If you find yourself saying "what if" when answering exam questions, you may be considering issues beyond the information presented or reading things into the question that are not there. To prevent this, carefully read the question and look for key words and key phrases, identify the subject of the question, and identify the parts of the question. Visualize the scenario, and do not imagine anything beyond what is included in the question.

> **BOX 7.6**
>
> **Tips for Success During an Examination**
> 1. Skim through the test, answering what you know is absolutely correct.
> 2. Read each question carefully.
> 3. Skip questions that are confusing.
> 4. Ask the proctor if you do not understand a question.
> 5. For harder questions, use a highlighter (if allowed) to highlight important aspects of the question.
> 6. Paraphrase the question: What is it asking?
> 7. Cross out the distractors.
> 8. If two distractors seem equally correct, what nursing concepts make one better than the other?
> 9. Always consider patient safety.
> 10. Watch out for and disregard absolutes.
> 11. After answering questions, do not change your answers.
> 12. Look for the best answer.

Sometimes students struggle with nursing prioritization questions—that is, questions with phrases such as "what is the nurse's best action," "what will the nurse do first" and with keywords such as "best," "primary," "immediate," "highest priority," "most appropriate," or "initial response." Priority questions are often connected to patient safety. Nurses prioritize using ABC—airway, breathing, and circulation—to order nursing actions and keep patients safe. The nursing process, ADPIE (assessment, diagnosis, plan, intervention/implementation, and evaluation), is the strategy for methodically providing patient care. Maslow hierarchy of needs identifies requirements that must be met to effectively care for patients. After recalling these ordering acronyms, if you still cannot make a decision, the bottom line in prioritization is determining the aspect of the patient condition that is most serious (i.e., "what will kill the patient first?") and doing an intervention to address it.

Determining how to assign tasks or when to call a provider can also be problematic for students. Delegation questions require you to understand and apply the scope of practice for registered nurses versus other members of the care team. Knowing the scope of practice and roles of the care team will help you determine which tasks can be assigned and which ones cannot. You may also need to determine the appropriate time to call a provider. If an answer choice includes calling the provider, you must first determine if there is enough assessment information for the nurse to intervene—a strategy termed "assess versus implement." If the nurse cannot perform the task independently and within the scope of practice, the best choice may be to contact the provider.

Once you choose an answer, do not change it unless you are 100% sure that your original choice is incorrect. The first choice, or your "gut reaction," is usually the best.

AS YOU FINISH THE EXAM
Paper and Pencil Exams
Before you turn in your paper exam, look everything over to see if you've missed anything or left something out. Make sure your name is on the paper exam and the answer sheet. If you had to complete a scannable bubble sheet, be sure you have completely

filled in the bubbles and have not left any blank. Review all questions, and make sure you have answered them to your best ability. Do not forget the back sides of the pages. Because tests are often double sided, always check the backs of pages before you turn in an exam.

Computer Exams

Before you click "save and submit" in a computer exam, check that you have answered all the questions. Did you go back and review any flagged questions? Do not open other browsers or click out of the exam before it is submitted. Depending on how your professor has set up the exam, you may or may not see items you missed.

AFTER THE EXAM: DECOMPRESSING, REVIEWING, AND GETTING HELP

Once you have turned in the exam, take time to do something enjoyable. You cannot change the outcome now, but you can reward yourself for doing your best. Take a long-awaited hike, read a passage in your favorite book, enjoy an ice cream cone, go for a jog in the park, or buy something special. Forget about the exam until it is graded.

After you receive the test results, schedule an exam review with your professor to examine missed questions for trends and patterns. If you did not perform as well as you had hoped, examine your study plan. Did you complete all the assigned reading and any homework? Did you review chapter vocabulary and concepts, lecture outlines and notes, and any interactive tools? A test review with the professor will help you identify the types of questions you had trouble answering, identify your strengths in answering questions, and identify how you can improve your study and exam skills. The professor can also explain the rationale for each question. You may want to ask if you can meet on a regular basis if you continue to have difficulty. If an NCLEX-RN review text is not required, ask if there is one that the faculty member recommends. Also, many schools use outside learning companies that offer NCLEX-RN style tests with personalized reviews.

You may benefit from other services available at your college to help you master course content and NCLEX-RN style questions. Many schools have a variety of support systems designed for nursing students; these may include student tutors (especially for math and English). Student tutors are less likely to elicit anxiety than instructors and are available at a variety of time intervals. Other services available might include learning specialists for time management, to teach anxiety-reducing techniques, to ascertain your learning style, and to provide general tips for test taking. Many of these services are free to you because they are covered in your tuition.

Your instructors are there to help you. Instructors schedule office hours so they are available to students who need one-on-one guidance. Many instructors also schedule mid-semester appointments to check in with students. Attending a mid-semester evaluation is beneficial to both you and your instructor. By then, you will have had time to become acquainted with the course expectations and course content, and your instructor will have had a chance to get to know you better. The mid-semester evaluation also gives the instructor the opportunity to better evaluate your progress over several weeks. But remember, if you are having difficulty in the course, it is your responsibility to seek out help. Your faculty want you to be successful.

> **THINKING CRITICALLY**
> For additional study tips for the NCLEX exam, visit the NCSBN Prepare for Success webpage at https://nclex.com/prepare.page. Explore this website and the exam preview. What types of questions are available to students at this website? What resources are available there to help students prepare for the NCLEX exam? Does this website include links to visit for other information?

CONCLUSION

Test-taking skills are not easily attained for all nursing students. Because the higher level of critical thinking in the clinical judgment model of the NCLEX-RN may not be familiar to you, you may need help in achieving success. It is important to review the NCLEX-RN test model, what is included in the exam, and the overall test plan developed by the NCSBN. Test questions are based on the NCJMM, and students can study in several ways to improve their scores and to decrease their test anxiety. Applying improvement strategies before, during, and after the examination will benefit the student in increasing test success.

STUDENT *Exercises*

Exercise 7.1
Arrange to meet with one of your professors to review your first test. Make a list of the questions you missed. According to the NCJMM, what dimension of clinical judgment are those questions in? What subject matter are they testing? Are there any trends you can identify that will be helpful for the next exam?

Exercise 7.2
Keep a diary of how you feel before tests. How do you prepare? What makes you nervous? What calms you? Keep track of these aspects over the semester. What did you discover about your test-taking preparation that is successful? What needs to be changed? Discuss in a group setting.

Exercise 7.3
Meet with a group of students in the class. Discuss the following: What was your worst testing experience? What made it that way? What was your best testing experience, and what made it that way? What are the strategies you are using that help you master material before an exam? Create a document with your findings. Share this information with your course instructor, and see if they have any additional recommendations.

Exercise 7.4
Visit the NCSBN NCLEX Candidate Prepare for Success page at https://nclex.com/prepare.page. What resources have you accessed? Has your group accessed any of the resources? If you could add a content area to the site, what would you add?

REFERENCES

Billings, D., & Hensel, D. (2024). *Lippincott Q&A review for NCLEX-RN* (14th ed.). Wolters Kluwer.

Bloom, B. S., Englehart, M. B., Furst, E. J., Hill, W. H., & Krathwohl, D. R. (1956). *Taxonomy of educational objectives. The classification of educational goals. Handbook I: Cognitive domain*. Longmans Green.

Ignatavicius, D. (2021). Preparing for the new nursing licensure exam: The next-generation NCLEX. *Nursing2021, 51*(5), 35–41. https://doi.org/10.1097/01.NURSE.0000743100.95536.9b

McDonald, M. (2018). *The nurse educator's guide to assessing learning outcomes* (4th ed.). Jones and Bartlett.

National Council of State Boards of Nursing. (2021). *Next generation NCLEX®: Sample pack*. https://ncsbn.az1.qualtrics.com/WRQualtricsControlPanel/File.php?F=F_eR8xOxTNt8iyUiG

National Council of State Boards of Nursing. (2022). *Next generation NCLEX®: NCLEX-RN® exam preview*. https://ncsbn.az1.qualtrics.com/WRQualtricsControlPanel/File.php?F=F_bpBwY7Is4EoRiWa

National Council of State Boards of Nursing. (2023). *Next generation NCLEX: NCLEX-RN® test plan effective April 2023*. https://www.ncsbn.org/public-files/2023_RN_Test%20Plan_English_FINAL.pdf

National Council of State Boards of Nursing. (n.d.-a). *About the NCLEX: A behind-the-scenes look at the exam*. https://www.nclex.com/About.page

National Council of State Boards of Nursing. (n.d.-b). *Clinical judgment measurement model: A framework to measure clinical judgment & decision making*. https://www.nclex.com/clinical-judgment-measurement-model.page

Tanner, C. A. (2006). Thinking like a nurse: A research-based model of clinical judgment in nursing. *Journal of Nursing Education, 45*(6), 204–211.

SUGGESTED READING

De Lima, M., Macey-Stewart, K., Salas, R., Smetana, R., & Woodroof, M. (2023). Faculty collaboration in transitioning to NGN test item writing. *Teaching and Learning in Nursing, 18*(1), 188–192. https://doi.org/10.1016/j.teln.2022.11.001

Irwin, B., & Burckhardt, J. A. (2023). *Next generation NCLEX-RN prep 2023–2024: Practice test + proven strategies (Kaplan test prep)*. Kaplan Publishing.

Nugent, P. M., & Vitale, B. A. (2023). *Test success: Test-taking techniques for beginning nursing students* (10th ed.). F.A. Davis.

Pence, P. (2023). Nursing students' perceptions of learning with NGN-style case studies. *Nurse Educator, 48*(2), 103–107. https://doi.org/10.1097/NNE.0000000000001292

Silvestri, L. A., & Silvestri, A. E. (2023). *Saunders comprehensive review for the NCLEX-RN® examination* (9th ed.). Elsevier Saunders.

On the WEB

HowToStudy.org: Provides practical resources for students about the best ways to study: http://www.howtostudy.org

Medical mnemonics: https://en.wikipedia.org/wiki/List_of_medical_mnemonics

NCLEX Test Plans: https://www.nclex.com/test-plans.page

NCSBN Prepare for Success: https://nclex.com/prepare.page

Unit II

Core Competencies for Professional Nursing Practice

Practicing Within Regulatory Frameworks

CHAPTER 8

LEARNING OUTCOMES

By the end of this chapter, the student will be able to:
1. Compare differences among regulations, policies, and standards of practice in nursing.
2. Identify boundaries and restrictions of practice of the LPN/LVN.
3. Describe the differences between LPN/LVN and RN scopes of practice.
4. Discuss the need for regulation language in nurse practice acts.
5. Examine nurse practice acts, and write a statement that reflects the scope of practice of the RN in the United States.
6. Differentiate among directed, autonomous, and collaborative nursing practices.
7. Analyze sample situations to determine directed, autonomous, and collaborative nursing practices in action.
8. Describe mechanisms for identifying differences in the knowledge and roles of LPN/LVNs and RNs.
9. Differentiate between the NCSBN test plans for LPN/LVNs and RNs.
10. Differentiate between the roles of the LPN/LVNs and RNs in the nursing process.
11. Explain the differences between core competencies for the LPN/LVN and those for the RN.

KEY TERMS

affective	competency	policy
American Nurses Association (ANA)	directed nursing practice	psychomotor
	learning domains	regulation
autonomous nursing practice	mutual recognition	restrictive language
	National League for Nursing (NLN)	scope of practice
cognitive		standards of practice
collaborative nursing practice	nurse practice acts	state board of nursing
	permissive language	

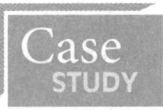

Case STUDY LoriAnn, LPN, is talking with another LPN-to-RN student, Randall, LPN, about entering an ADN program. They have been discussing the difference in clinical practice for the LPN and RN.

LORIANN: I have been an LPN for 20 years. In that time, I have done multiple catheterizations, charted on hundreds of clients, monitored rhythm disturbances by telemetry, and passed medications effectively and safely. Why do I have to do this all over again? Why do I have to demonstrate performance in skills I have already mastered as an LPN?

RANDALL: I haven't been an LPN as long as you have, but I've performed a lot of skills too. I heard some of the other students say that we have to learn skills that we haven't performed before. Along with administering medications and performing tasks, we have to learn to coordinate patient care, perform diagnostic procedures and analyze the results, provide patients with education about how to manage their illnesses, and oversee other healthcare staff like CNAs and LPNs.

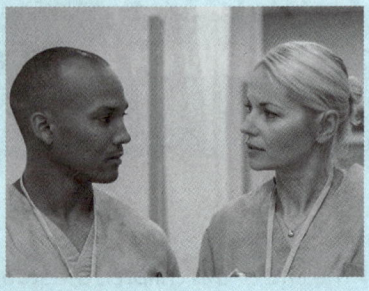

LORIANN: It's going to feel strange to be in charge of so many things, and a little scary too.

RANDALL: That's why we're learning the role of being an RN.

As you enter the RN program, you are embarking on a new scope of practice level. Perhaps you have felt like the LPNs in the case study. As an LPN/LVN, you have practiced under the direction of the RN or the provider to whom you have reported. Your role has been an important yet directed role, partly restricted. State law has dictated that you are restricted to performing certain nursing procedures, administering medications, and performing some intravenous therapy procedures.

In answer to the question of the nursing student in the case study: Your **scope of practice** as an RN not only will be broader in the types and complexity of procedures/assessments you perform but also will require additional knowledge, independent thinking, problem-solving, and teaching skills. As an RN, you will be expected to utilize evidence-based practice, which is the collection and application of evidence from research to maintain and upgrade your nursing practice. Evidence-based practice is described by the Institute of Medicine (2003) as the best "research with clinical expertise and patient values for optimal care" (p. 4). (For more information about EBP, see Chapter 9.) You will acquire the ability to collaborate with other members of the healthcare team to design plans of comprehensive care for patients and clients and to teach prevention and self-care among these healthcare consumers.

REGULATIONS, POLICIES, AND STANDARDS

Regulations, policies, and standards all play a role in defining the practice of the RN. A thorough understanding of each is essential as you embark on an RN educational program.

REGULATIONS

Regulations are those guidelines for nursing practice established through the state boards of nursing in the United States and territories in Canada. Legislatures grant power through statutory laws by regulations. State legislatures set nursing regulations and give state administrative agencies many of the enforcement responsibilities through **nurse practice acts**. Regulation of nursing practice matters because of risk of harm to the public if practiced by someone who is unprepared and incompetent. Because the public may not have sufficient information and experience to identify an unqualified healthcare provider, they are vulnerable to unsafe and incompetent practitioners. State and federal regulations exist to govern various aspects of the healthcare industry and healthcare professionals.

Regulations at the state/province level define the scope of practice, requirements for licensure and relicensing, certification and continuing education requirements, and disciplinary consequences for healthcare practitioners. Regulations that define the practice of individuals licensed in a particular area are called practice acts. Nurse practice acts are laws established in a state or province to regulate the practice of nursing (Potter et al., 2023). Although practice acts may differ from state to province, similarity and support of **mutual recognition** are increasingly evident as states attempt to meet the needs of consumers, healthcare workers, and the healthcare industry. At the present time, 41 states have granted mutual recognition that enables a nurse with an unencumbered license to practice in another state; this is called the nursing licensure compact. You can find more information about which states participate in multistate licensure at the NCSBN website https://www.nursecompact.com/index.page#map. Extensive use of the NCLEX-RN throughout the United States is an example of this effort. Practice acts define the practice of RNs and LPN/LVNs and are publicly available online.

Regulations, especially those with the purpose of defining the scope of practice of various healthcare professionals, can be written with either restrictive or permissive language. **Restrictive language** restricts the practitioner to performing only the functions and procedures outlined in the regulation. LPN/LVN practice acts are often written in this manner.

Permissive language in regulations allows practitioners to use judgment and make decisions to serve their purpose in performing their roles. Box 8.1 contrasts restrictive and permissive language in LPN/LVN and RN practice acts in the state of Kansas. Permissive language is used for the more autonomous practice of the RN. Similar restrictive and permissive language for LPN/LVN and RN practice acts, respectively, exists in many other states.

POLICIES

To implement and enforce regulations, governing bodies (often in the form of appointed boards) are established to develop policies. A **policy** is a rule, plan, or course of action for specific situations. Policies are usually established by a group of people, such as committees, organizations, the government, or political parties. In nursing, each state establishes one or more state boards of nursing to institute policies, to develop guidelines for interpreting regulations, and to ensure implementation of policies consistent with that state's regulations. The boards include members of the public to ensure consumer protection as regulations are implemented. Some states have separate boards of nursing for governing the practice of the LPN/LVN and the RN, whereas others have a single **state board of nursing** to oversee both.

An example of a regulation by the Pennsylvania State Board of Nursing is shown in Box 8.2. The policy is an encouragement to get nursing school graduates to complete their NCLEX-RN/PN within a year.

STANDARDS

Regulations and policies denote only minimal requirements for licensed nurses. When nurses became more independent and accountable for their actions, they began to develop standards of practice. The practice of nursing is controlled through the standards of practice, licensure, and nurse practice acts. A standard is established by an authority as a level of quality or a rule for the measure of value or quality. **Standards of practice** define

> **BOX 8.1** **Restrictive and Permissive Language in Practical/Vocational and Registered Nurse Practice Acts in the State of Kansas**
>
> **Restrictive Language for the Practical Nurse**
>
> 60-16-102 Scope of Practice for Licensed Practical Nurse Performing Intravenous Fluid Therapy
>
> A licensed practical nurse under the supervision of a registered professional nurse may engage in a limited scope of intravenous fluid treatment, including the following:
> 1. Monitoring
> 2. Maintaining basic fluids
> 3. Discontinuing intravenous flow and an intravenous access device not exceeding three inches in length in peripheral sites only
> 4. Changing dressings for intravenous access devices not exceeding three inches in length in peripheral sites only
>
> **Permissive Language for the Registered Nurse**
>
> 65-1113 Definitions
>
> The practice of professional nursing as performed by a registered professional nurse for compensation or gratuitously, except as permitted by K.S.A. 65-1124, and amendments thereto, means the process in which substantial specialized knowledge derived from the biological, physical, and behavioral sciences is applied to the care, diagnosis, treatment, counsel, and health teaching of persons who are experiencing changes in the normal health processes or who require assistance in the maintenance of health or the prevention or management of illness, injury, or infirmity; administration, supervision, or teaching of the process as defined in this section; and the execution of the medical regimen as prescribed by a person licensed to practice medicine and surgery or a person licensed to practice dentistry.

Reprinted from Kansas State Board of Nursing. (2023, July). *Nurse practice act statutes & administrative regulations.* https://ksbn.kansas.gov/wp-content/uploads/NPA/npa.pdf

actions that constitute safe, prudent care for which the nurse is accountable. Therefore, they become legal guidelines to evaluate the quality of care given (Roux & Halstead, 2018).

Professional organizations play a key role in further defining the discipline of nursing, identifying entry-level competencies, and establishing standards of practice. The **American Nurses Association (ANA)** and the **National League for Nursing (NLN)** are two professional organizations that establish general standards of practice for the discipline of nursing. Other specialty organizations, such as the American Association of Critical-Care Nurses (AACN), have standards that are based on those general standards but are more specific for nurses who work in a specialty area, for example, in the critical care units. Many states have a state chapter of each organization (e.g., Pennsylvania

> **BOX 8.2** **Example of a Regulation**
>
> A candidate for licensure shall take the examination for the first time within 1 year of completing the professional nursing education program unless prevented by emergency, illness, military service or other good cause shown, or the candidate holds a license to practice nursing in another state or country.

Reprinted from Licenses, Chapter 21 State Board of Nursing, § 21.23. (2022). *Qualifications of applicant for examination.* https://www.pacodeandbulletin.gov/secure/pacode/data/049/chapter21/049_0021.pdf

Nursing Association [PNA], Pennsylvania League for Nursing). One of the most notable publications by the ANA (2021) is the *Nursing: Scope and Standards of Practice*. The first social policy statement (ANA, 2010 was groundbreaking and provided clarity on the definition of nursing as a discipline, identifying it as an entity discrete from medicine, with its own unique purpose and autonomous practice. This social policy statement was updated and expanded in 1995 and 2003.

> **The NCLEX-RN** *Might Ask* **8.1**
>
> An RN is explaining to a student nurse that the scope of an RN's practice is governed by the state nurse practice acts. These acts are considered:
> a. regulations.
> b. policies.
> c. permissive language.
> d. standards of care.
>
> • See Appendix A for correct answer and rationale.

Both the ANA and the NLN, each of which is composed of nurses who pay dues as members of the discipline, continue to set standards and to publish documents that identify nursing's role in the healthcare industry, entry-level competencies of practitioners in the discipline of nursing, and professional accrediting standards for nursing education programs.

NURSE PRACTICE ACTS

Nurse practice acts exist in each state as part of the state's regulations/laws (Potter et al., 2023). States provide additional clarity and interpretation of the practice of nursing through policies established by the state boards of nursing. State nurse practice acts are available online and can be reached through the NCSB of nursing as well.

Changing regulations and laws requires a lengthy political process. The choice of the extent to which specifics of nursing practice are incorporated into law is at the discretion of the state and may or may not be desirable, depending on the state's desire for flexibility and ease of change of such language. However, policies can be changed by the state board of nursing as needed. Because the role of nurse practice acts and subsequent policies by the state board of nursing for implementing and enforcing such laws is to protect the consumer, public hearings are often held when major regulation or policy changes are proposed.

Nursing organizations like the ANA, NLN, and AACN play key roles in shaping nurse practice acts and in providing guidance to states in restructuring nurse practice act language. Nurses need to keep in contact with their nursing organizations to continue to have a voice and an impact on the continually evolving nurse practice acts.

LoriAnn and her LPN friend are aware of these rules and regulations in their own state, but LoriAnn is considering working for a telehealth company and always wondered how her license could be accepted by another state. She is happy she got the chance to review what her state board regulations and policies are and how to find information about other states easily online. But she is still confused about how the roles of an RN and LPN differ.

DIRECTED, AUTONOMOUS, AND COLLABORATIVE NURSING PRACTICE

A key factor differentiating the scopes of practice of LPN/LVNs and RNs is the extent of independence legislated by nurse practice act language.

DIRECTED NURSING PRACTICE

The restrictive language used in outlining the scope of practice of the LPN/LVN limits this nurse's practice to a directed role. Directed roles are supervised or regulated by an individual. Although many LPN/LVNs have achieved a great deal of independence in their practice, particularly as it relates to caring for clients with common disorders or dysfunctions, their practice remains by law a **directed nursing practice**. Most states define a practical nurse as someone who performs certain nursing practices, including the administration of medications, treatments, health maintenance, and wellness promotion of others under the direction of a registered nurse, an advanced practice registered nurse, a licensed provider, a licensed dentist, or other appropriate healthcare provider. The ANA (n.d.) defines the role of the practical/vocational nurse as someone who provides basic client care and assists registered nurses (RNs) or providers by monitoring client health, updating health records, and administering treatments.

The educational preparation of the LPN/LVN provides this practitioner with the basic knowledge for practice in a directed role. It also allows the LPN/LVN to use standardized procedures within that directed role.

Consistent with the ANA's definition of practical/vocational nursing is the NCSBN's (2021a, 2021b) Model Act, which defines the role of the practical/vocational nursing program graduate as one who practices

> under the direction of a registered professional nurse, an advanced practice registered nurse, a licensed physician, a licensed dentist, or other appropriate healthcare provider which acts do not require the substantial specialized skill, judgment and knowledge required in professional nursing. (p. 2)

Nursing standards established or recognized by Boards of Nursing specify the practice of the licensed practical/vocational nurse. The standards for LPN/LVN practice can be viewed on page 3 of The National Council of Boards of Nursing website at https://www.ncsbn.org/public-files/21_Model_Act.pdf.

AUTONOMOUS NURSING PRACTICE

Autonomous nursing practice is engaging in the practice of nursing independently, without supervision. The NCSBN (2021a, 2021b) Model Act contrasts the practice of nursing (i.e., registered nursing) with the practice of practical nursing. The standards for RN practice can be viewed on pages 4 and 5 of The National Council of Boards of Nursing website at https://www.ncsbn.org/public-files/21_Model_Act.pdf.

Substantial specialized knowledge enables the RN to exercise judgment, design and implement plans of care and engage in various independent functions. Both LPN/LVNs and RNs collect assessment data, collaborate with other health professionals, and advocate for clients; however, the major difference between LPN/LVNs and RNs lies in their level of autonomy and decision-making authority. Whereas LVN/LPNs work under the supervision of RNs or providers, RNs have greater autonomy and are tasked with making more independent clinical judgments and decisions regarding client care. RNs have a broader scope of practice and are responsible for more complex nursing tasks, including assessing client conditions, identifying nursing diagnoses, developing care plans, determining appropriate interventions to achieve optimal outcomes, administering medications, performing treatments and procedures, and providing client education. Although LPNs use their judgment in carrying out routine tasks, they generally have less independence in decision-making compared to RNs. LoriAnn's reaction to this new information is a bit more positive and less perplexed. She has never had the time in those 20 years to follow an RN to see the differences in responsibilities. LoriAnn has been too focused on her own responsibilities to see the differences in assessment, teaching, and coordination of care. She is awed and a bit uneasy about these new responsibilities.

> **The NCLEX-RN** *Might Ask* **8.2**
>
> In working with clients, the nurse uses the resources of many other healthcare workers to achieve acceptable outcomes in client care. In this role, the nurse is working:
> a. independently.
> b. as an advocate.
> c. autonomously.
> d. collaboratively.
>
> • See Appendix A for correct answer and rationale.

> **THINKING CRITICALLY**
> Compare and contrast the areas in your personal life in which you perform in a directed role versus an autonomous role. What additional specialized knowledge enables you to exercise judgment and to perform independently when in the autonomous role?

COLLABORATION IN NURSING PRACTICE

Collaboration and working together with other healthcare providers is essential for meeting an array of client needs and fostering health in a holistic manner. **Collaborative nursing practice**, also called interdependent nursing practice, is working jointly with others (providers, physical therapists, etc.) in performing nursing roles within the legislated scope of practice.

The registered nurse and the provider practice autonomously in making nursing diagnoses and medical diagnoses, respectively. However, collaboration improves comprehensiveness, efficiency, and consistency in fostering health in clients. Many states have created practice act language to allow for the development of standardized procedures, developed jointly by providers and nurses. Standardized procedures developed for use in organized healthcare systems (e.g., hospitals, clinics, home health agencies, community health services, providers' offices) enhance the nurse's ability to function independently.

MECHANISMS FOR IDENTIFYING DIFFERENCES IN KNOWLEDGE AND ROLES

Although there is a common core of knowledge and competencies in the practice of LPN/LVNs and RNs, the knowledge base and practice roles differ between these two licensed healthcare providers. How does an individual, organization, council, or licensing board determine the knowledge and roles of a specific practitioner? How do the knowledge and roles of the LPN/LVN differ from those of the RN? What expectations should an employer have of these two levels of practitioners? What additional knowledge and role abilities should the LPN/LVN expect to gain by participating in and completing an ADN educational program? What knowledge, skills, and abilities should be tested under the governance of the state boards of nursing to assure the public that individuals are competent to be licensed to practice within the scope of practice outlined by state law? These questions are addressed in this chapter as the knowledge and roles of the LPN/LVN and the RN are explored, explained, compared, and contrasted. Several mechanisms are used to identify such differences in knowledge and roles. These include periodic job analysis studies, licensure examination test plans, licensure requirements and nurse practice acts, and professional organization standards.

JOB ANALYSIS STUDIES

An important mechanism for determining the knowledge needed and the roles played by a particular licensed healthcare provider is to survey those already in the work setting who are licensed to practice at that level. The National Council of State Boards of Nursing regularly conducts a job analysis of both levels of practitioners—RNs and LPN/LVNs. The most recent analyses for each were conducted in 2021 and published in 2022 (NCSBN, 2022a, 2022b). These updated job analyses are then used to design the new test plans for the NCLEX-RN and NCLEX-PN exams (NCSBN, 2022a, 2022b). The cycle is repeated approximately every 3 years.

THINKING CRITICALLY

Visit the NCSBN 2021 RN Practice Analysis document at https://www.ncsbn.org/public-files/21_NCLEX_RN_PA.pdf. Scan through the document, especially the "Applicability of Activities to Practice Setting" section and the corresponding tables. The NCSBN lists, in priority order, many procedures that newly graduated RNs need to know and do. Write down five of them and discuss them in a group. Did any of them surprise you? Did the priority of any of the procedures surprise you?

LICENSURE EXAMINATION TEST PLANS

Job analysis studies play a key role in the design of licensure examination test plans. It is critical that such test plans identify the knowledge and roles of practitioners at the designated licensure level. In addition to job analysis studies, the NCSBN examines the scope of practice for that licensure level by its member jurisdictions and uses item writers (nurses and nurse educators) to operationalize the test plan for actual test construction. The NCLEX-PN differs from the NCLEX-RN in relation to the results of the respective job analyses, the scopes of practice as defined by member jurisdictions, and the levels of knowledge, skills, and abilities tested.

LICENSURE REQUIREMENTS AND NURSE PRACTICE ACTS

The nurse practice act in each state outlines eligibility and requirements for licensure within that state. Most states use the same NCLEX-PN and NCLEX-RN examination to determine eligibility for licensure. Minimum examination scores needed for licensure eligibility are determined according to the nurse practice act language in each state.

The nurse practice act in each state also clearly describes the nursing education program content and clinical experience needed for the program to be accredited by the state board of nursing and for the program graduate to be eligible for licensure. In addition to behavioral sciences, biological sciences, and core nursing content, some states specify a certain number of hours of education in such areas as communication skills, communicable diseases, pharmacology, abuse of children and older adults, and substance use. Nurse practice acts may also designate specific roles for LPN/LVNs and RNs related to such areas as medication administration, intravenous therapy, blood administration or withdrawal, and chemotherapy.

PROFESSIONAL ORGANIZATION STANDARDS

Although job analysis studies identify activities being performed by newly licensed LPN/LVNs and RNs, and state boards of nursing establish licensure eligibility, these represent only minimal competencies for licensed practice. An additional mechanism for identifying differences in the knowledge and roles of LPN/LVNs and RNs is the standards set by professional organizations.

The NLN's (2012) *Outcomes and competencies for graduates of Practical/Vocational, Diploma, Associate Degree, Baccalaureate, Master's, Practice Doctorate, and Research Doctorate Programs in nursing* describes the role and competencies that should be expected from graduates of nursing programs. Knowledge critical to each role and the expected competencies of graduates are outlined in the document. Prelicensure nursing education must prepare students for generalist practice. Focusing on practice across the life span and diverse populations, the AACN identifies four spheres of care: promotion of health and well-being/disease prevention; chronic disease care; regenerative or restorative care; and hospice/palliative/supportive care. The AACN (2021) identifies domains and core competencies essential to nursing education at https://www.aacnnursing.org/Portals/0/PDFs/Publications/Essentials-2021.pdf.

NATIONAL COUNCIL LICENSURE EXAMINATIONS
PRACTICAL/VOCATIONAL NURSING TEST PLAN

The *Test Plan for the NCLEX Examination for Practical Nurses* (NCSBN, 2023a) provides a concise summary of the content and scope of the NCLEX-PN examination and serves as a guide for candidates preparing to take the examination and for those individuals involved in creating it. The test plan provides the foundation for the development of each licensure examination, so that each NCLEX-PN examination reflects the knowledge, skills, and abilities essential for the application of the phases of the nursing process to meet the needs of clients with commonly occurring health problems having predictable outcomes. As indicated, the test plan designed by the NCSBN is based on job analysis studies. The exam includes test items at the knowledge, comprehension, application, and analysis levels.

The test plan notes that the LPN/LVN functions in a directed role, contributing to care planning and participating in the nursing process. The NCSBN/NLN states that at the entry level, the LPN/LVN, under supervision, ensures competent care for clients with common healthcare needs that have stable, predictable outcomes. Both the LPN/LVN and the RN use the nursing process to collect and to summarize important healthcare data that assists in identifying needs/problems of clients in a variety of settings throughout the span of a client's life.

The *Test Plan for the NCLEX Examination for Practical Nurses* (NCSBN, 2023a) details client needs that can be addressed by the LPN/LVN and emphasizes that this level practitioner requires "basic" knowledge of nursing in four major categories: safe, effective care; health promotion and maintenance; psychosocial integrity; and physiological integrity. The following elements are integrated throughout the NCLEX-PN exam: clinical problem-solving process (nursing process), caring, communication and documentation, and teaching/learning.

REGISTERED NURSING TEST PLAN

The *Test Plan for the NCLEX Examination for Registered Nurses* (NCSBN, 2023b), similar to that for practical nursing, serves as a guide for those preparing to take the NCLEX-RN examination and for item writers in their development of the exam. The test plan continues to be developed based on job analysis. In contrast with the test plan for the NCLEX-PN, test items for the NCLEX-RN includes some test items at the knowledge level but mostly at the comprehension, application, analysis, synthesis, and creating levels.

The NCLEX-RN *Might Ask* 8.3

An LPN/LVN is asking an RN about the NCLEX-RN test. The LPN/LVN is correct when they say that passing NCLEX-RN demonstrates:

a. specialty competency.
b. excellence in practice.
c. average competency.
d. minimal competency.

- See Appendix A for correct answer and rationale.

The test plan for registered nursing describes the RN practitioner's role in nursing process, noting (in contrast with that of practical nursing) autonomous functions, such as assessment, nursing diagnosis, plan development, and evaluation; and collaborative functions, such as planning with other health team members, delegating, and providing referrals. Similar to the test plan for practical nursing, the test plan for registered nursing outlines the knowledge, skills, and abilities needed to address client needs. However, unlike the practical nursing test plan, the test plan for registered nursing calls for a more in-depth knowledge base and skills in teaching, communication, and management.

PRACTICAL/VOCATIONAL NURSING ROLES AND COMPETENCIES

As you begin your new nursing role as an RN, it is important to define and to compare the roles and competencies of the LPN/LVN and the RN. The following role and **competency** review for LPNs/LVNs and RNs will decrease the chance of role confusion in practice.

PRACTICAL/VOCATIONAL NURSING ROLES

The NCSBN (n.d.) defines an LPN/LVN and their role as follows:

> An individual who has completed a state-approved practical or vocational nursing program, passed the NCLEX-PN Examination, and is licensed by a state board of nursing to provide patient care. Normally works under the supervision of a registered nurse, advanced practice registered nurse, or physician. (para 2)

This definition designates two roles for the LPN/LVN: care provider and member of the discipline of nursing.

COMPETENCIES IN THE CARE PROVIDER ROLE
Within the care provider role, the LPN/LVN is actively involved in four of the five phases of the nursing process: assessment, planning, implementation, and evaluation.

Assessment
In the assessment phase, the LPN/LVN assesses basic needs of clients by collecting data and by identifying deviations from normal. They document these data and communicate findings.

Planning
In the planning phase, the LPN/LVN contributes to the development of nursing care plans, determines client care need priorities, and assists in revising such care plans. They use established nursing diagnoses in this planning process for clients with common, well-defined health problems.

Implementation
In the implementation phase, the LPN/LVN provides care using effective communication, collaborating with other health team members, and instructing clients regarding health maintenance. They use accepted standards of practice, and they record and report implementation activities. The LPN/LVN also maintains the privacy and dignity of clients.

Evaluation
In the evaluation phase, the LPN/LVN seeks guidance and continues collaboration with others in modifying nursing approaches and in revising nursing care plans.

COMPETENCIES IN THE MEMBER OF THE DISCIPLINE ROLE
As a member of the discipline of nursing, the LPN/LVN's primary role is in the delivery of healthcare; this complies with each state's nurse practice act. As part of ongoing competency, the LPN/LVN identifies personal strengths, weaknesses, and potential, using educational opportunities; they not only adhere to nursing's code of ethics but also function as a healthcare consumer advocate.

ASSOCIATE DEGREE NURSING ROLES AND COMPETENCIES
In 1990, the NLN identified three interrelated roles of the associate degree nurse: provider of care, manager of care, and member within the discipline of nursing. In a 2000 revision of that document, the NLN Council of Associate Degree Competencies Task Force believed that the role expectancies would be simpler and duplication would be avoided by organizing expected competencies into eight core components that crossed the traditional boundaries of the three roles of provider of care, manager of care, and member within the discipline of nursing. In 2010, the NLN further refined these delineated competencies into four broad outcomes that range from the practical/vocational level to the doctoral. As mentioned in Chapter 5, these outcomes are human flourishing, nursing judgment, professional identity, and spirit of inquiry.

COMPETENCIES IN THE CARE PROVIDER ROLE
The associate degree nurse uses the nursing process when engaging in the care provider role.

Assessment
In addition to competencies specified at the practical nursing level, the associate degree nurse conducts a more extensive data collection process, using various resources. They contribute this information to a database and are able to identify changes in the client's health status.

Diagnosis
Unlike the practical nurse, the associate degree nurse has the educational preparation to analyze and interpret data, identifying actual or potential healthcare needs and selecting nursing diagnoses.

Planning
In addition to competencies at the practical nursing level, the associate degree nurse establishes client-centered goals, develops client-specific care plans, and develops individualized teaching plans in collaboration with other healthcare workers.

Implementation
In addition to competencies at the practical nursing level, the associate degree nurse initiates nursing interventions, implementing care plans according to priorities of goals and making adjustments as client situations change. The associate degree nurse also fosters a health-supportive environment, promoting rehabilitation potential, providing for physical and psychological safety, and using communication techniques that assist clients with coping and problem solving. Individualized, client-centered care management and teaching plans are implemented, providing continuity of care, and referrals are provided as needed.

Evaluation
The associate degree nurse evaluates the client's progress toward goals and the effects of interventions, revising care plans as needed.

LICENSED PRACTICAL/VOCATIONAL VERSUS REGISTERED NURSE KNOWLEDGE, SKILLS, AND ABILITIES

The knowledge, skills, and abilities of those in the nursing profession progress along a continuum, with increasing complexity at each practice level. The educational curricula for the LPN/LVN, the RN, and the baccalaureate and higher degree nurse prepare these healthcare providers to perform within the scope of the practice prescribed by law and in the roles identified by professional organizations such as the NLN.

Nursing process, nursing diagnosis, and nursing care plan design require abilities in all six of the **cognitive** learning levels and in the **affective** and **psychomotor** domains of Bloom's Taxonomy (see Chapters 5 and 7). Related to these abilities in the three **learning domains**, LPN/LVNs and RNs demonstrate different competencies within their roles. As stated previously, the *Test Plan for the NCLEX Examination for Practical Nurses* (NCSBN, 2023a) includes test items at the knowledge, comprehension, and application levels, and it includes some analysis questions. The *Test Plan for the NCLEX Examination for Registered Nurses* (NCSBN, 2023b) includes some test items at the knowledge level, but mostly at the comprehension, application, analysis, synthesis, and creating levels. More emphasis is now being placed on the higher-level questions. This reflects the increased complexity inherent in the scope of practice and job analysis study for registered nursing. Chapter 5 describes ADN curricular content and learning activities in each of the three learning domains and in the six achievement levels of the cognitive domain.

CONCLUSION

The roles of the LPN/LVN and the RN are defined by their scopes of practice, which are governed by regulations, policies, and standards tailored to each level of licensure. LPNs/LVNs operate within a more structured framework, guided by regulations that outline their directed practice under the supervision of RNs or providers. RNs have a broader scope of practice, characterized by autonomous and collaborative decision-making. The differentiation between LPN/LVN and RN scopes of practice is further defined by the language used in state nurse practice acts. Whereas LPNs/LVNs are often tasked with providing basic nursing care and assisting with client needs, RNs are entrusted with more complex responsibilities such as medication administration, care coordination, and client education.

Various mechanisms are used to identify the knowledge and roles of LPN/LVNs and RNs, including job analysis studies, licensure examination test plans, licensure requirements, and professional organization standards. The National Council of State Boards of Nursing (NCSBN) test plans describe the content areas and competencies required for both PN and RN licensure examinations and highlight the differences in knowledge and roles between the two levels of nursing practice. Understanding the distinction between the roles is necessary to optimize client care and to ensure the effective utilization of nursing resources across healthcare settings.

STUDENT *Exercises*

Exercise 8.1
Using the following link at the NCSBN (https://www.ncsbn.org/npa.htm), find and analyze the nurse practice acts from your state. What are the differences in permissive and restrictive languages? The many state boards of nursing throughout the United States are easily accessed through the ANA website.

Exercise 8.2
Outline several RN activities that fall within each of the three practice functions: directed, autonomous, and collaborative practice.

Exercise 8.3
Write in your own words a broad definition of the scope of practice of the RN in the United States/Canada.

Exercise 8.4
Develop a chart comparing and contrasting the care provider role competencies in each phase of the nursing process for the LPN/LVN and the associate degree nurse.

Exercise 8.5
Research a nursing organization of your choice. Does it have standards of care? How are they different in scope from the standards of nursing practice?

REFERENCES

American Association of Colleges of Nursing. (2021). *The essentials: Core competencies for professional nursing education.* https://www.aacnnursing.org/Portals/0/PDFs/Publications/Essentials-2021.pdf

American Nurses Association. (2010). *Nursing's social policy statement: The essence of the profession* (3rd ed.).

American Nurses Association. (2021). *Nursing: Scope and standards of practice* (4th ed.).

American Nurses Association. (n.d.). *Three types of nurses and what they do.* https://www.nursingworld.org/practice-policy/workforce/what-is-nursing/types-of-nurses/

Institute of Medicine. (2003). *Health professions education: A bridge to quality.* National Academies Press.

Kansas State Board of Nursing. (2023, July). *Nurse practice act statutes & administrative regulations.* https://ksbn.kansas.gov/wp-content/uploads/NPA/npa.pdf

Licenses, Chapter 21 State Board of Nursing, § 21.23. (2022). *Qualifications of applicant for examination.* https://www.pacodeandbulletin.gov/secure/pacode/data/049/chapter21/049_0021.pdf

National Council of State Boards of Nursing. (2021a). *NCSBN Model act 2021.* https://www.ncsbn.org/public-files/21_Model_Act.pdf

National Council of State Boards of Nursing. (2021b). *NCSBN Model rules 2021.* https://www.ncsbn.org/public-files/21_Model_Rules.pdf

National Council of State Boards of Nursing. (2022a). *2021 PN practice analysis: Linking the NCLEX-PN examination to practice.* https://www.ncsbn.org/public-files/21_NCLEX_PN_PA.pdf

National Council of State Boards of Nursing. (2022b). *2021 RN practice analysis: Linking the NCLEX-RN examination to practice.* https://www.ncsbn.org/public-files/21_NCLEX_RN_PA.pdf

National Council of State Boards of Nursing. (2023a). *2023 NCLEX-PN test plan.* https://www.ncsbn.org/public-files/2023_PN_Test%20Plan_FINAL.pdf

National Council of State Boards of Nursing. (2023b). *2023 NCLEX-RN test plan.* https://www.ncsbn.org/public-files/2023_RN_Test%20Plan_English_FINAL.pdf

National Council of State Boards of Nursing. (n.d.). *Definition of nursing terms.* https://www.ncsbn.org/resources/nursing-terms.page

National League for Nursing. (2012). *Outcomes and competencies for graduates of Practical/Vocational, Diploma, Associate Degree, Baccalaureate, Master's, Practice Doctorate, and Research Doctorate Programs in nursing.*

Potter, P., Perry, A., Stockert, P., & Hall, A. (2023). *Fundamentals of nursing* (11th ed.). Elsevier.

Roux, G., & Halstead, J. (2018). *Issues and trends in nursing: Practice, policy and leadership* (2nd ed.). Jones & Bartlett Learning.

SUGGESTED READING

Bloom, B. S. (Ed.). (1956). *Taxonomy of educational objectives: The classification of educational goals.* David McKay.

Bloom, B. S. (Ed.). (1974). *The taxonomy of educational objectives: Affective and cognitive domains.* David McKay.

On the WEB

California Nurse Practice Act: http://www.rn.ca.gov/npa/title16.htm

National Council of State Boards of Nursing: http://www.ncsbn.org

National Council of State Boards of Nursing, Nurse Licensure Compact: https://www.nursecompact.com/index.page#map

National League for Nursing: http://www.nln.org

Critical Thinking, Clinical Reasoning, and Clinical Judgment in Nursing

CHAPTER 9

LEARNING OUTCOMES

By the end of this chapter, the student will be able to:

1. Describe the importance of critical thinking and clinical judgment for today's registered nurse.
2. Compare and contrast the relationships among evidence-based research, critical thinking, clinical reasoning, and clinical judgment in the profession of nursing.
3. Define critical thinking and describe the role of context in critical thinking.
4. Differentiate between critical thinking and feelings.
5. Describe the role of metacognition and reflective thinking in developing nursing judgment.
6. Compare and contrast the concepts of critical thinking, creative thinking, and reflective thinking.
7. Describe the role of critical thinking in the nursing process.
8. Describe clinical judgment in nursing practice.
9. Analyze and evaluate client situations using a variety of thinking modes, including critical thinking, critical reflection, and clinical reasoning.
10. Describe the role of mindfulness in providing holistic nursing care.

KEY TERMS

background assumptions
clinical imagination
clinical judgment
clinical reasoning
contextual learning
creative thinking
critical reflection
critical thinking
critical thinking abilities
critical thinking dispositions
deductive reasoning
emotional intelligence (EI)
evidence-based practice (EBP)
holistic nursing
inductive reasoning
intuitive decision-making
metacognition
mindfulness
NCSBN Clinical Judgment Measurement Model (NCJMM)
- recognize cues
- analyze cues
- prioritize hypotheses
- generate solutions
- take action
- evaluate outcomes
nursing judgment
nursing process
reflective practitioner
reflective thinking
self-regulation
sociocentric thinking

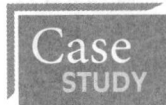

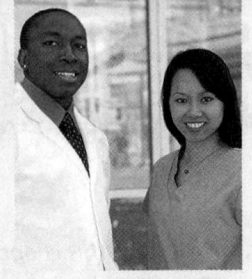

Sally Caruthers is a first-semester LVN returning to school. Tim DeMot is a second-year student.

SALLY: We have a quiz every week, a test every month, and now the instructor says we have to take an ungraded critical thinking test. How do I prepare to critically think? What is critical thinking?

TIM: Boy, I know it sounds like a lot, but you'll be able to do it! This test is not high on the ones you need to be concerned about. This critical thinking test is taken in the first semester and again at the end of the program. Once you get the results from the first test, you can tell what your critical thinking level is when you enter the program. These values are also important to the faculty. They compare our critical thinking entry scores with the ones on the test we will take right before we graduate. Through the assignments given, such as group projects, case studies, threaded discussions, clinical simulations, nursing diagnoses and designing nursing care plans, and many other learning activities, our critical thinking skills should increase as we go through the program. The faculty also needs the information to make adjustments and changes in the program curriculum for continuous improvement.

SALLY: OK, that all makes sense. Even though the test results aren't part of our grade, I can see now why we have to do it. I'll just concentrate and do my best and not worry about it then.

TIM: The tools the instructors use help us prepare to do the complex thinking, problem-solving, analysis, and creative thinking required of a nurse. So, even though we don't get graded, it's all part of the big picture to prepare us professionally. The class content on critical thinking will be coming up with the nursing care planning process in about 2 weeks, if I remember correctly. Would it help for you to go over my notes from last year?

SALLY: I think I'm okay without those for now, but thanks for offering. I have to study for my psychology test. But can we have lunch together around 12:30 in the student center? You've stimulated my curiosity. I like to know what is included in the big picture.

TIM: Great. Yeah, I'll see you then.

THE NEED FOR CRITICAL THINKING

What is critical thinking? When is thinking "critical" rather than just "thinking"? Why is there such a need for critical thinking in today's world? This chapter provides an overview of critical thinking and the use of critical thinking, clinical reasoning, and clinical judgment in nursing. Also included are implications for nursing education and the registered nursing program learning environment you are entering.

Failure to develop critical thinking skills impedes lifelong learning as one enters the workforce, experiences new situations, and is confronted with news articles, media coverage, and ethical dilemmas. Adams and Hamm (1990) stressed the need for critical thinking and collaboration in a democratic society to balance reason, individualism, and community, "Critical thinking involves the ability to raise powerful questions about what's being read, viewed, or listened to" (p. 39). The lifelong tasks of thinking and learning are especially crucial in the global positioning of countries in an era of international competition, continuous and rapid technological and sociologic change, and the increasing ethical dilemmas posed by these changes.

THINKING CRITICALLY
Recall a time in your nursing experience when you were able to solve a problem, answer a question, or work through a situation for which you had not been taught the information. How were you able to solve the problem? What thinking tools had you learned that you were able to modify or adapt to use in this new situation? How did your own culture and values come into play in your analysis?

CRITICAL THINKING DEFINED

Critical thinking as a concept has a rich history, has been defined in a number of ways, and has continued to evolve over time. In the early 1900s, critical thinking was viewed as problem-solving, creative thinking, or what Dewey (1910) termed "reflective thinking." He used this term to refer to "the kind of thinking that consists in turning a subject over in the mind and giving it serious consecutive consideration" (p. 71). He also used such terms as "suspended judgment" and "healthy skepticism" when speaking of what we now call critical thinking.

In the mid-1900s, attempts were made to define critical thinking in a more concrete way. Ennis (1962) developed a comprehensive yet simple approach to the concept. He defined critical thinking as "the correct assessing of statements" and outlined 12 aspects of critical thinking, including grasping the meaning of statements and making judgments about them.

Lists of critical thinking skills—also termed **critical thinking abilities**, or proficiencies—appeared during the next two decades, with the following frequently appearing: "identifying assumptions, both stated and unstated, both one's own and others; clarifying, focusing, and staying relevant to the topic; understanding logic (including inference, deduction, and induction); and judging sources, their reliability and credibility" (Idol & Jones, 1991, p. 14). However, Snook (1974) took exception to this approach, stating, "To imagine that thinking can be broken down into its component parts which are then programmed is to misunderstand the nature of thinking" (p. 154).

The third quarter of the 20th century brought about contributions from the disciplines of mathematics, science, and engineering, with "problem-solving" receiving much attention. Polya (1971) outlined a four-stage approach to problem solving: understanding the problem, devising a plan, carrying out the plan, and looking back. Woods et al. (1975) described an adaptation of Polya's approach for their engineering students, adding a "think about it" step before the devising a plan step.

Continued research in the areas of reasoning and problem-solving by scientists, psychologists, and philosophers provided multiple facets to the evolving concept of critical thinking. Attempts were made to bring together scientific problem-solving and the intuitive, creative aspects rooted in the humanities. Guilford (1967) described critical thinking as "creative problem-solving" in an attempt to merge the two concepts and also incorporated the step of "incubation" into Polya's method to allow for what he called "intuitive leaps."

> ### THINKING CRITICALLY
> As you reflect on these early efforts to define and understand the concept of critical thinking, what concepts do you see as some of the underpinnings of the nursing process we use today in assessing patients' needs and in designing plans of care? What aspects of the aforementioned developments were a surprise to you? At this point in your reading of this chapter, what important concepts related to critical thinking can you think of that have not yet been explored by these early authors and theorists?

In the 1960s, the focus shifted to feelings, challenging beliefs, and using drugs to escape reality and to refute mores of "the establishment." It was a time to "do your own thing" and "go your own way." The extremism led to a lack of critical thinking (Ruggiero, 2024). However, an important contribution was made to the development of the concept of critical thinking. Creativity, challenging background assumptions, and exploring alternatives became important elements in the discussion of critical thinking during the 1970s. Such discussion also gave rise to the importance of dispositions of the thinker. To think critically, one must not only possess the skills and abilities to reason, problem solve, and explore alternatives but also have the disposition, or be so inclined, to do so—to have the desire to engage in such activity. There are a variety of **critical thinking dispositions**, and they received a great deal of attention in the literature during the 1970s and 1980s.

The 1980s witnessed a renewed fervor of discussion about critical thinking. **Contextual learning** became an important topic of discussion, with more fuel added to the fire in the debate regarding whether critical thinking skills could be learned out of context (i.e., on their own, separate from a specific discipline of subject matter). In addition, an emphasis on metacognition (thinking about thinking) emerged as authors examined the thinking process itself and self-regulation—that is, how one assesses and adjusts one's own thinking process. These concepts will be presented later in this chapter. Additionally, Daniel Goleman's work on **emotional intelligence (EI)** in the mid-1990s shed further light on the need for EI along with cognitive skills to engage effectively in critical thinking.

Moving into the 21st century, further exploration was done regarding the relationships among the concepts of problem-solving, reasoning, critical thinking, creative thinking, reflective thinking, and metacognition, and how we teach these. New theory, such as further ponderings on emotional intelligence, was also being examined for its relationship to the construct of critical thinking. Does critical thinking incorporate all the other modes of thinking, or are other ways of thinking each distinct but interrelated concepts? Can thinking be taught, and if so, how can thinking be taught both in and out of a context, such as nursing? Do our current teaching methods teach how to think? What additional teaching methods are needed?

Raingruber and Haffer (2001) emphasized the power of questioning for nurses: Learning to ask "what else?" and "what if?" They defined critical thinking as:

> a multi-faceted process that includes logical, rhetorical, and humanistic skills and attitudes that promote the ability to determine what one should believe and do. Critical thinking requires one to actively process and evaluate information, to validate existing knowledge, and to create new knowledge. It involves reflective thinking. (p. 3)

Once again, as in earlier times, "reflective thinking" was considered an inherent quality of critical thinking. Also, the notion of creativity resurfaced. As the first decade of the new century unfolded, so did the multiple facets of critical thinking. Both standalone coursework in critical thinking and contextualized learning in critical thinking, such as in nursing, continued to evolve. Critical thinking components include insight, intuition, the willingness to take action, and empathy. Nurses implement **intuitive decision-making** based on their experiences, emotional intelligence, and ethical and cultural considerations (Huston, 2023).

The Foundation for Critical Thinking (n.d.) defines critical thinking as

> thinking—about any subject, content, or problem—in which the thinker skillfully analyz[es], assess[es], and reconstruct[s] [their thinking]. Critical thinking is self-directed, self-disciplined, self-monitored, and self-corrective thinking. …It entails effective communication and problem-solving abilities, as well as a commitment to overcome our native egocentrism and sociocentrism. (para. 2)

The Foundation notes that assessing thinking involves clarity, accuracy, precision, consistency, relevance, sound evidence, good reasons, depth, breadth, and fairness.

Increased globalism and the evolving concepts of holism, multiculturalism, and emotional intelligence have all impacted study of the concept of critical thinking. Both "right brain" and "left brain" thinking have come to be considered integral to critical thinking. The reflective process, creativity, and the influence of culture are integral components as well. In addition, there is an increasing emphasis seen in the literature on contextual learning—meaning that the development of critical thinking skills must be done in the context of the discipline—in this case, nursing. The discussion of critical thinking in nursing will be discussed later in this chapter.

For a brief review of some of the essential concepts, the Foundation for Critical Thinking publishes *The Miniature Guide to Critical Thinking Concepts and Tools*, by Paul and Elder (2020). Box 9.1 delineates the essential intellectual traits or virtues they deem essential to critical thinking. Another publication that explores the concept of critical thinking is *Critical Thinking Skills for Dummies* (2015), by Martin Cohen, which includes exercises for developing critical thinking skills.

There is no one modern definition for critical thinking, though most agree that critical thinking is necessary for higher-order thinking, such as that needed by the professional nurse. Hood (2021) identified elements common to most definitions of critical thinking, which include a complex thinking pattern that requires higher-level thinking, examining situations for content and context before making judgments, examining consequences, and applying logical justification for judgments and actions.

> **BOX 9.1**
>
> ### Intellectual Traits or Virtues Essential for Critical Thinking
> Intellectual Integrity
> Intellectual Humility
> Confidence in Reason
> Intellectual Perseverance
> Fair-mindedness
> Intellectual Courage
> Intellectual Empathy
> Intellectual Autonomy

Source: Paul, R., & Elder, L. (2020). *The miniature guide to critical thinking concepts and tools* (8th ed.). The Foundation for Critical Thinking.

> ### The NCLEX-RN *Might Ask* 9.1
> The nursing instructor is explaining critical thinking to a new LVN student. The instructor knows the student needs further clarification when the student incorrectly states the following:
> a. "Critical thinking is acting on how I am feeling about the situation."
> b. "Critical thinking is looking at all possible options."
> c. "Critical thinking involves using new technologies to solve problems."
> d. "Part of critical thinking involves looking at how age, culture, and background influence how nurses think."
>
> • See Appendix A for correct answer and rationale.

CRITICAL THINKING VERSUS FEELING

So when is thinking "critical thinking" and not just "thinking?" Alfaro-LeFevre (2020) explains that thinking is "critical thinking" when it is deliberate, regulated, and uses well-thought-out methods to achieve the desired outcomes. When developing critical thinking skills and abilities, and when thinking critically in context, we cannot, however, avoid confronting issues through our own "lenses." We each carry with us our own biases and "world views," which are composed of our age- and gender-related, cultural, ethnic, religious, and sociologic viewpoints. We rely on feelings, intuitions, and experiential knowledge when posing and selecting solutions for new problems and when confronting issues that arise.

Feelings can be disguised as thinking. Feelings from our past, even childhood, frequently serve as guiding principles in our lives. The thought process developed from past feelings often distorts reasoning and leads to conclusions that feelings have already reached. Making significant decisions based on emotion rather than logic can lead to poor results (Bar-Levav, 1988).

When transitioning to the RN role of independent practice, the LPN/LVN is challenged daily to identify feelings and to discriminate between fact and opinion. When thinking critically, the nurse notes personal beliefs and **background assumptions** based on culture and personal history in order to "bracket" (or set aside) these feelings to confront issues and to approach and solve problems as much as possible in an

TABLE 9.1 Cognitive Skills Used in Critical Thinking

Skill	Definition	Application to Nursing
Interpretation	Clarifying the meaning clustering relevant data	Identifying a nursing diagnosis
Analysis	Examining ideas and analyzing arguments	Making informed decisions based on data and not on assumptions
Evaluation	Looking at the outcomes of one's actions	Determining the outcomes based on nursing actions
Inference	Interpretations or conclusions should logically follow from the evidence looking for alternatives	Looking at relationships between findings and coming up with meaning and relevancy
Explanation	Reasoning behind one's actions based on data presented	Using knowledge and strategies to support your conclusions
Self-regulation	Looking at one's personal professional practice needs	Reflecting on your own performance and experiences; identifying whether you need to get advanced certification or to go back to school

Source: Ignatavicius, D. D. (2001). 6 Critical thinking skills for at-the-bedside success: Key ways to practice, nurture, and reinforce staff members' cognitive skills. *Nursing Management, 32*(1), 37–39; Facione, P. (1990). Critical thinking: A statement of expert consensus for purposes of educational assessment and instruction. *The Delphi report: Research findings and recommendations prepared for the American Philosophical Association* (ERIC Doc No. ED 315-423). Educational Resources Information Center.

unbiased, nonjudgmental manner. A summary of cognitive skills used by nurses in critical thinking is presented in Table 9.1.

Paul and Elder (2020) describe how we all engage in **sociocentric thinking**. We are "culture bound" in our thinking, often unaware of the degree to which we all have internalized the dominant prejudices of our society and culture. Sociocentric thinking can only be diminished by cross-cultural, fair-minded thinking; excellence in thought must be systematically cultivated. Box 9.2 presents Paul and Elder's characteristics of a well-cultivated thinker.

BOX 9.2

Characteristics of a Well-Cultivated Critical Thinker

A well-cultivated critical thinker:

- Clearly and explicitly identifies problems and formulates important questions
- Uses abstract reasoning to assess and interpret relevant information
- Arrives at supportable conclusions and solutions that can be validated against relevant standards
- Considers other points of view with an open mind, understands, and evaluates presumptions, implications, and real-world effects as necessary
- Successfully communicates with others to find answers to challenging issues
- Is cautious not to fabricate or misrepresent facts to support a position or argument and is able to distinguish between fake news and inaccurate information.

Source: Paul, R., & Elder, L. (2020). *The miniature guide to critical thinking concepts and tools* (8th ed.). Foundation for Critical Thinking.

The NCLEX-RN *Might Ask* 9.2

A senior nursing student is being evaluated on critical thinking during client care. Which of the following statements by the student would show the need for additional education on the subject?
a. "It is important to find out if the client is telling me the truth."
b. "It is important to verify evidence to support what the client is saying."
c. "I have a feeling that this is the right thing to do."
d. "I am making this decision based on the facts I have found."

• See Appendix A for correct answer and rationale.

CRITICAL THINKING AND CREATIVE THINKING

Although controversy exists regarding the relationship of creative thinking to critical thinking (namely, whether one encompasses the other or if they are distinct, discrete forms of thinking), there is agreement that they work synergistically to produce "good thinkers." Additionally, reflective thinking, which will be discussed in the next section, is important to both.

Creative thinking involves the generation of new ideas. These can be in the form of new approaches, new solutions to problems nurses encounter, or application of plans to new settings or within new cultures. The interrelatedness of critical thinking and creative thinking is readily apparent. Creative thinking is similar to critical thinking, but when thinking creatively, the focus is more on creating new and original ways of thinking about information rather than thinking critically about the information. Creative thinking requires participating in tasks even when answers or solutions are not immediately evident, challenging the boundaries of one's knowledge and skills, and developing new perspectives on a problem that goes beyond accepted norms (Marzano, 1991). The result of creative thinking is more than mere creativity; three characteristics are typically necessary: the idea must be unique, it must exhibit high quality, and it must be deliberately produced rather than incidental (Smith, 1990).

Creative thinking provides nurses with the ability to think outside what is normally done and can result in novel approaches to client care. However, creative thinking without critical thinking can lead to hazardous solutions (Hood, 2021). Critical thinking requires right-brain thinking, in which new ideas can be generated, along with left-brain thinking, in which the worth each idea is analyzed and evaluated (Alfaro-LeFevre, 2020).

THINKING CRITICALLY

Do any of the creative thinking dispositions just discussed sound familiar? Which dispositions describe you? What implication does this have for you as you transition to the RN role? When might you as an RN need to apply creative thinking to a client situation?

METACOGNITION, REFLECTIVE THINKING, AND SELF-REGULATION

Metacognition is knowledge about our own thinking. It is through metacognition that we come to know and understand our thinking. Have you ever asked yourself, "What was I thinking?!" As you reflected on your actions or decisions, you likely found illogical reasoning, missed steps, or flaws. Perhaps you jumped to conclusions based on your personal biases or did not think through the consequences of your actions. In any case, metacognition, or knowledge about your thinking, caused you to rethink the situation to improve your thinking process and thereby improve your results.

Professional practitioners such as RNs gain insight into their thinking and knowledge of their thinking process through **reflective thinking**—being thoughtful about our decisions and actions—as they critique the thinking that was involved in their decisions. As autonomous practitioners, professional nurses must always be thoughtful about nursing diagnoses made and actions taken in providing high-quality care to patients, clients, and families. **Critical reflection** involves a purposeful process of review, analysis, and evaluation of actions one has already taken, is in the process of taking, or intends to take. When a nurse engages in reflective thinking, nursing care is strengthened.

Another advantage of critical reflection, as a component of critical thinking, is to raise questions about possible approaches to care. The professional nurse who asks, "Is there a better way to do this?" raises prospective research questions, contributing to **evidence-based practice (EBP)** and advancement of the profession of nursing.

Reflection also allows the nurse to check their own background assumptions and biases to be more objective in individualizing care. It is only through reflection and empathic listening that we can imagine alternatives. In registered nursing practice, making accurate nursing diagnoses and designing an individualized plan of care with a client demand that such multiple perspectives be used. Learning activities in the affective domain, and case studies in which problems arise and the nurse is confronted with multifaceted issues, foster critical thinking skills in this mode.

The thoughtful study of decisions and actions or planned actions causes us to think more holistically about the situation, examine all the options available and their possible consequences, and prevents us from making mistakes or errors in judgment. This **self-regulation** is inherent in nursing, as it is in other professions in which independent decision-making is involved and the public is impacted. Practicing evaluation and reflection helps to ensure current and accurate information and allows for any needed corrections (Alfaro-LeFevre, 2020).

Some view reflective thinking as distinct from critical thinking, whereas others view it as part of critical thinking. Regardless, what is important is that nurses engage in critical reflection in conjunction with both critical thinking and creative thinking, as previously described. This is the essence of difference between the directed practice of the LPN/LVN and the independent, autonomous practice of the RN. The old saying "the buck stops here" is applicable, because as an RN *you* will be the one responsible for determining nursing diagnoses and for directing the plan of care based on those nursing diagnoses.

The concept of **mindfulness** is important in the reflective, self-regulatory process; it encompasses:

> a state of awareness ... fostered by the consistent and deliberate effort to take notice of what is occurring in one's inner and outer worlds, with a capacity to be fully engaged in the present ..., rather than distracted by, preoccupied with, or focused on the past or the future. (Raphael-Grimm, 2015, p. 11)

Nurses need to be mindful of both themselves and patients during patient interviews and cautions against habitual, rote responses by the nurse, which can sometimes harm the patient. Through mindfulness, the nurse can become aware of how subjective data gathering during the patient intake process is being influenced by the very nature of the questions, their sometimes unintended implications as seen by the patient, and the patient's responses. Engaging and communicating with patients must be deliberate. Nurses use mindfulness to make adjustments during interactions with patients that ensure therapeutic communication (Raphael-Grimm, 2015).

Mindfulness is part of the metacognitive process. The nurse, through critical reflection, can then ask themselves, "What is this patient not telling me? What else is going on with their health status or home environment? Why am I getting certain nonverbal responses to my questions? What else do I need to ask to obtain a full picture of the human responses of this patient to make correct diagnoses and to develop individualized plans of care?" This mindfulness is also important to seeing the patient holistically, connected to their environment and culture, which will be discussed later in this chapter.

As you embark on the ADN program, you may encounter learning activities that cause you to think about your thinking patterns and process. You may be asked to keep a journal, record verbatim communications you have had in the clinical area, or draw cognitive maps (mind maps) representing your thinking process. All of these activities assist you in becoming a **reflective practitioner**. Teacher role modeling of thinking patterns and processes also assists helps students understand metacognition and self-regulation.

CRITICAL THINKING IN NURSING

As research on the construct of critical thinking evolved, so did its use in the discipline of nursing. Expanding on the Benner (2001) "novice to expert" theory, Benner et al. (2011) examined the development of **clinical reasoning** skills in nurses. Nurses who become skilled at recognizing patterns and themes in patients, reflect on those patterns, think critically, and use clinical judgment provide a more highly skilled clinical practice. Alfaro-LeFevre (2020) emphasized the need for critical thinking and **clinical judgment** as nurses examine outcomes for quality care, engage in EBP, prioritize, and incorporate multiple facets of knowledge to move from novice to expert thinking.

In its most recent publication on outcomes and competencies in nursing programs, the NLN (2012) identified *spirit of inquiry* and *nursing judgment* as two of the four key Nursing Program Outcomes. The NLN (2012) defines **nursing judgment** as encompassing the following three processes:

- **Critical thinking:** Using evidence to logically guide decision-making
- **Clinical judgment:** From the nurse's viewpoint, observing, interpreting, and reflecting
- **Integration of best evidence:** Informing decisions as much as possible by current research

EBP is a fundamental element in healthcare today. It involves integrating the best available research evidence, clinical expertise, and patient preferences and values to guide clinical decision-making. Nurses should stay updated on the latest research findings and use evidence to inform their practice. This ensures that they provide the most effective and up-to-date care to their patients.

The three processes identified by the NLN (2012) are not isolated but are interconnected and interdependent. Nurses use critical thinking to assess and analyze clinical situations, apply clinical judgment to make informed decisions, and integrate evidence into their practice to enhance the quality of care they provide.

Registered nursing programs have integrated critical thinking skills into the curriculum. Accrediting associations examine nursing curriculum for the presence of critical thinking skills. The test plan for the NCLEX-RN has incorporated such skills as well. As discussed in Chapter 7, every 3 years, the National Council of State Boards of Nursing (NCSBN) conducts a job practice analysis of registered nursing practice to ensure that the test plan for the NCLEX-RN is current with the demands of today's practice of nursing. The most recent job practice analysis shows that critical thinking remains a necessary activity of the registered nurse. "Nursing is a dynamic, continuously evolving discipline that employs critical thinking and clinical judgment to integrate increasingly complex knowledge, skills, technologies and client care activities into EBP" (NCSBN, 2023, p. 3).

Practicing RNs employ critical thinking daily in making nursing diagnoses and planning and adjusting nursing care to address changing patient needs. In addition, the need for critical thinking in nursing has never been greater to address the profession's response to bioethical issues and multifaceted changes in the healthcare industry's landscape. As RNs cope with the effects of healthcare reform and changes in the healthcare industry, encounter rapid technological change, experience great demographic shifts and increased globalism, and confront difficult ethical dilemmas, they must bring with them the critical thinking skills to make wise decisions and to collaborate on change that will have a positive impact on future generations. Also, as the opening case study discusses, many schools have opted to assess critical thinking skills of students at entry and upon exit from the nursing program to determine the degree to which critical thinking skills have been strengthened in the program.

THINKING CRITICALLY

Can you think of any teacher's assignment or exercise that caused you to see things differently? What techniques were used that assisted you in interpreting information through a new lens? What were your reactions to the exercise?

CRITICAL THINKING, PROBLEM-SOLVING, AND THE NURSING PROCESS

As discussed at the beginning of this chapter, problem-solving as a mode of critical thinking received a great deal of attention throughout the latter half of the 20th century in the areas of science and mathematics. Polya (1971) outlined a four-stage approach to problem-solving: understand the problem, devise a plan, carry out the plan, and look back. In an effort to incorporate more reasoning and reflection, Guilford (1967) included an incubation step, and Woods et al. (1975) added a "think about it" step before planning.

As a science-based discipline, nursing embraced a problem-solving method at this time. In 1973, the American Nurses Association *Standards of Nursing Practice* adopted a five-step **nursing process** model of assessment, analysis, planning, implementation, and evaluation. After further development, in 1980, the ANA adopted the *Nursing's Social Policy Statement*, incorporating nursing diagnosis into the problem-solving nursing process and thereby establishing nursing as a profession with its own discrete practice. The metaparadigm of nursing (person, environment, health, and nursing) began to be studied by nurse researchers, and nursing education programs adopted conceptual models and curricula based on various nurse theorist' work on understanding these four phenomena. According to the ANA (2015), the nursing process "includes the components of assessment, diagnosis, outcomes identification, planning, implementation, and evaluation. Accordingly, the nursing process encompasses significant actions taken by registered nurses and forms the foundation of the nurse's decision-making" (p. 4).

As the study of critical thinking has evolved, so has nursing's understanding of its value in the nursing process. At its roots, the nursing process as a science-based, problem-solving model is a linear model. Higher-order thinking skills (e.g., analysis, synthesis, evaluation) are incorporated, and reasoning and informal logic can be applied. Professional nurses implement the nursing process to make independent decisions. Inaccurate or inadequate information can cause nurses to act too soon. Insufficient time to process information sabotages critical thinking and clinical judgment. Critical thinking, logical reasoning, and clinical judgment support nursing actions and ensure quality clinical decisions. The effective use of the nursing process requires critical, creative, and reflective thinking (Hood, 2021).

Nursing today is multifaceted and holistic, considering evidence-based research and the multicultural aspects of patients, clients, families, and communities. This holistic approach requires the nurse to effectively employ critical thinking skills.

Research on critical thinking in nursing was concurrent with the energy surrounding critical thinking at the end of the 20th century. In 1984, Benner published her seminal text *From Novice to Expert*, and in 1988, Bandman and Bandman published their seminal text *Critical Thinking in Nursing*. Nursing programs began to structure learning activities for students to develop critical thinking skills and to move them along the continuum from novice toward becoming advanced beginners as they entered practice as a licensed RN. Likewise, the NCLEX-RN strengthened its focus on the higher-order thinking skills inherent to critical thinking.

At the time, nursing education programs, through the use of case studies and other approaches, used problem-solving and the nursing process extensively for developing critical thinking skills in students. Along with the higher-order thinking skills of analysis, synthesis, and evaluation, the nursing process requires clinical reasoning, intuition, and clinical judgment. These will be discussed in the next section.

CLINICAL REASONING, INTUITION, AND CLINICAL JUDGMENT

In their text *Educating Nurses: A Call for Radical Transformation*, Benner et al. (2010) suggest several shifts in the teaching and learning process, one of which is the "shift from an emphasis on critical thinking to an emphasis on clinical reasoning and multiple ways of thinking that include critical thinking" (p. 84). The authors note that many nurse educators have fallen into the habit of using "critical thinking" as a catch-all phrase for the many forms of thinking that nurses use in practice. They advocate, instead, for nursing students to ascertain when critical thinking is needed and when some other form of thinking—such as clinical reasoning, creative thinking, or reflective thinking—is needed.

Unlike critical thinking, clinical reasoning focuses on skills essential for effective problem-solving and decision-making. Clinical reasoning requires identifying and defining problems to systematically generate and assess potential solutions, using inductive and deductive logic to detect and critique fallacies in reasoning, drawing conclusions from various sources of information (written, spoken, tables, graphs), and being able to differentiate between factual information and subjective opinions (Glasman et al., 1984). To increase the effectiveness of the nursing process, nurses must apply logic and scientific reasoning when making nursing decisions (Bandman & Bandman, 1988).

In addition to case studies, nursing programs in the late 1980s and 1990s added learning activities such as **inductive reasoning** and **deductive reasoning** exercises and formal debates to foster reasoning skills. In the last two decades, there has been more emphasis on the variety of thinking skills nurses need to provide high-quality, individualized care to clients and families. Benner et al. (2010) stated that although the nursing process provides a framework for problem-solving and analysis, it does not encompass all thinking; clinical reasoning and intuitive thinking, which are based on tacit knowledge and experience, and skillful nursing judgment are also important. The authors note that nurses must have "the ability to reason as a clinical situation changes, taking into account the context and concerns of the patient and family" (p. 85). Likewise, **clinical imagination** is needed to customize nursing care and patient actions to fit the client's home environment and other unique settings.

Huston (2022) describes the need for nurses to engage in clinical reasoning so they can make adjustments to nursing care as situations change. Knowledge of the patient's clinical data and its trends, and the ability to determine priorities and to understand the rationale of nursing interventions as these trends change, are important to enable clinical reasoning that is consistent with the patient's current status. The outcome of ongoing employment of clinical reasoning by the nurse is improved patient outcomes. As you progress through the ADN program and your instructor provides learning experiences to help you transfer, apply, and individualize nursing knowledge and interventions to a variety of unique patient situations, you will develop your clinical reasoning skills and strengthen your ability to "think like a nurse."

Huston (2022) emphasizes the need for nursing faculty to provide tools and to structure learning experiences to enable students to develop clinical reasoning skills. The nurse must be able to use knowledge, think critically, use clinical reasoning, and integrate nursing processes to consistently make safe and accurate clinical judgments. Box 9.3 is an example of how to provide principles to help a student nurse in the clinical setting develop clinical reasoning skills and establish priorities for which of their assigned patients should be evaluated first.

THINKING CRITICALLY

Review the principles in Box 9.3. How might these principles assist you in organizing your time and approach in the clinical setting? Can you recall a situation in which you would have acted differently had you considered these principles? What would you have done differently, and how might the results have been different?

BOX 9.3 Principles to Guide Clinical Reasoning for Establishing Patient Priorities

Question for Nurse to Consider	Principle for Clinical Reasoning	Patient Priority
How old is the patient?	The older the patient, the higher the risk for developing complications.	Visit and evaluate oldest patient first.
When was the patient admitted?	The more recent the admission, the greater the likelihood of higher acuity and risk for a change in status.	Visit and evaluate most recently admitted patient first.
When did the patient have surgery?	The more recent the day of surgery, the higher the acuity and risk for a change in status.	Visit and evaluate most recent surgical patient first.
How many body systems are involved?	The greater the patient's medical complexity (e.g., renal or cardiac failure), the greater the risk of multiple system derangements.	Visit and evaluate patient with most medical complexity first.

Source: Huston, C. J. (2022). *Professional issues in nursing: Challenges and opportunities* (6th ed.). Wolters Kluwer.

Regardless of whether you believe critical thinking in nursing *encompasses* clinical reasoning or works *as a distinct process in conjunction with* clinical reasoning, your ability to exercise both will result in sound nursing judgment. As Alfaro-LeFevre (2020) notes, clinical judgment is the outcome, or result, of both critical thinking and clinical reasoning. The resulting clinical judgment you exercise as a nurse represents your conclusion, decision, or opinion.

Clinical judgment is the application of critical thinking to clinical situations. It's the process of synthesizing information, drawing conclusions, and making decisions regarding patient care. This includes assessing a patient's condition, recognizing changes or abnormalities, determining the appropriate course of action, and evaluating the outcomes of interventions. Clinical judgment is dynamic and evolves as nurses gain experience and knowledge.

CLINICAL JUDGMENT AND THE NURSING PROCESS

Critical thinking, clinical reasoning, and the nursing process are the foundations of clinical judgment. The **NCSBN Clinical Judgment Measurement Model (NCJMM)** (NCSBN, n.d.) is a systematic framework that describes the series of actions nurses perform when making clinical decisions, as follows:

- **Recognize cues:** The nurse recognizes cues by completing a comprehensive client assessment. The client information is gathered from several sources including observation, current symptoms, physical examination, medical history review, and the environment.

- **Analyze cues:** After gathering client information, the nurse analyzes cues by interpreting the significance of data within the context of the client's health status, recognizing patterns or trends in the data, and identifying potential complications or risks associated with the client's situation. Using critical thinking and evidence-based practice to analyze information, the nurse identifies client needs, formulates problem statements, and constructs potential nursing diagnoses.
- **Prioritize hypotheses:** Once client needs are identified, the nurse considers factors such as client safety and best evaluate and rank hypotheses according to priority.
- **Generate solutions:** After prioritizing hypotheses, the nurse makes decisions and prioritizes care based on the client's needs and the severity of the client's condition. The nurse ensures that interventions are focused on addressing the most critical issues first, thereby minimizing the risk of harm and optimizing client outcomes.
- **Take action:** The nurse takes action by implementing appropriate nursing interventions, which may include administering medications, providing education, or implementing specific nursing procedures.
- **Evaluate outcomes:** After the implementation of interventions, nurses reflect on intervention effectiveness and observe client outcomes. Based on client responses and changes in the client's condition, nurses evaluate the appropriateness of the interventions, identify areas for improvement, identify any emerging issues or complications, and adjust the care plan accordingly.

To provide safe, effective, and client-centered care, nurses apply these actions through a combination of knowledge, skills, and experience to continuously assess clients, gather data, analyze information, and make informed decisions.

The clinical judgment model can be viewed at https://www.nclex.com/clinical-judgment-measurement-model.page. See Table 7-5 in Chapter 7 for a comparison of how the nursing process stages align with the clinical judgment measurement model stages.

CRITICAL THINKING AND HOLISTIC NURSING

Nursing has long been known to be both an art and a science. All registered nursing programs include content from both the arts and the sciences to provide nurses with the foundation needed to employ critical thinking in the design of care plans and nursing interventions. Using the nursing process, nurses are able to apply knowledge from both disciplines to conduct focused patient interviews and to complete comprehensive physical assessments based on subjective and objective data gathered. Although the nursing process is rooted in science, nurses use creativity to individualize nursing care for patients. Nurses apply the nursing process with compassion and sensitivity and take the needs and preferences of each client into account. As a result, nursing is both an aesthetic and a scientific endeavor (Hood, 2021).

The nursing process is rooted in the scientific method, which involves systematic problem-solving and critical thinking. Nurses use EBP and clinical guidelines to assess, diagnose, plan, implement, and evaluate patient care. This scientific aspect ensures that nursing care is based on the best available evidence and promotes safe and effective patient outcomes.

Although the nursing process follows a systematic approach, nurses also infuse sensitivity and caring into their practice. Nursing is a profession that involves working closely with people during vulnerable moments in their lives. Nurses provide emotional support, comfort, and empathy to patients, acknowledging their individual feelings and concerns. This humanistic aspect of nursing helps patients feel valued and respected.

Nurses recognize that every patient is unique. They take into account the individual needs, preferences, and cultural backgrounds of their patients when providing care. This personalized approach fosters trust and enhances the patient's experience and overall well-being.

Nursing often requires creative problem-solving. Nurses must adapt their care plans to meet the specific needs of each patient, especially when faced with complex or unique situations. This creative aspect allows nurses to tailor their interventions and strategies to best support the patient's recovery and overall health.

Combining the scientific method with the humanistic and creative aspects, the nursing process indeed becomes both an art and a science. Nurses blend their clinical knowledge and technical skills with compassion, communication, and creativity to deliver holistic patient care.

Nurses use critical thinking skills in applying sociologic, anthropologic, and transcultural concepts to the care of patients/clients, families, and communities in a **holistic nursing** approach. The unique characteristics of patients and their families must be considered in making nursing diagnoses and in designing culturally relevant plans of care for them that take into account their individual needs, within their unique environments.

A holistic approach to healthcare is one that considers multiple dimensions of human well-being. The ANA (2021) emphasizes the importance of practicing holistic nursing care that integrates "body-mind-emotion-spirit-sexual-cultural-social-energetic-environmental principles and modalities":

- **Body:** This dimension pertains to physical health and well-being. It encompasses aspects such as nutrition, exercise, sleep, and medical care. A holistic approach recognizes the importance of maintaining and optimizing physical health as a foundation for overall well-being.
- **Mind:** Mental health is a critical component of well-being. This dimension involves cognitive functions, emotional regulation, and psychological well-being. It includes practices such as mindfulness, meditation, and therapy to support mental health.
- **Emotion:** Emotional well-being encompasses the ability to recognize, to understand, and to manage one's emotions. Practices such as emotional intelligence training and expressive therapies (e.g., art therapy) can promote emotional health.
- **Spirit:** The spiritual dimension explores a person's sense of purpose, meaning, and connection to something greater than themselves. It can encompass religious or nonreligious beliefs and practices, as well as mindfulness and meditation, to foster a sense of spirituality.
- **Sexual:** Sexual health and well-being involve healthy relationships, sexual education, and addressing issues related to sexuality, including sexual health concerns and relationship dynamics.
- **Cultural:** Cultural competence and sensitivity involve respecting and understanding diverse cultural backgrounds, traditions, and beliefs. It is crucial for providing inclusive and patient-centered care.
- **Social:** Social well-being focuses on the quality of an individual's relationships and support systems. Strong social connections and a sense of belonging are essential for mental and emotional health.
- **Energetic:** This dimension may encompass practices such as acupuncture, energy healing, or yoga, which focus on the flow and balance of energy within the body and its impact on health.

- **Environmental:** Environmental well-being involves recognizing the impact of the environment on health and well-being. This includes promoting clean air and water, sustainable living, and minimizing exposure to environmental toxins.

The integration of these principles and modalities recognizes that health is not just the absence of disease but is a state of overall well-being. It emphasizes that promoting health and actualizing human potential require a comprehensive approach that considers all these interconnected dimensions. Holistic healthcare practitioners include these aspects to help individuals lead healthier, more fulfilling lives.

Equally important in holistic care is cultural competence and the need for nurses to develop cultural assessment skills and critical thinking abilities. Cultural assessment involves systematically gathering information about a patient's individual cultural background, beliefs, values, practices, and preferences, which will enable the nurse to understand how culture influences a patient's health and healthcare choices. Because each person is unique, nurses are encouraged to use assessment skills to tailor meaningful care to each individual's unique cultural context rather than relying on stereotypes or overgeneralizations. Nurses should approach each patient with cultural humility, a sense of openness and respect, and an acknowledgment of their own cultural biases and limitations. (For more information on cultural competence and cultural humility, see Chapter 4.)

Critical thinking is a fundamental skill in nursing that involves analyzing information, considering different perspectives, and making informed decisions. When combined with cultural assessment skills, critical thinking allows nurses to adapt and apply their knowledge in a way that respects and responds to the specific needs of each patient.

THINKING CRITICALLY

Can you remember an occasion when your own culture, beliefs, and background assumptions prevented you from considering alternative solutions to a healthcare problem or additional facets of some patient care issue? How was your ability to provide holistic nursing impeded by these factors? How would you apply a holistic nursing care approach to produce better patient outcomes?

CRITICAL THINKING AND ACCOUNTABILITY

Remember the comment earlier in this chapter, "The buck stops here"? Unlike in your role as an LPN/RN, when you become an RN, if errors occur in nursing judgment or incomplete nursing care is provided based on incomplete or inaccurate nursing diagnoses or nursing interventions, you are accountable for the nursing diagnoses and plans of care for patients/clients assigned to you. Regardless of care given by licensed or assistive personnel who report to you, you are now accountable for high-quality, optimal care.

The ANA *Code of Ethics for Nurses with Interpretive Statements* (2015) outlines nine broad, noncontextual statements of the ethical obligations of nurses. The Code is a dynamic document that is updated every several years as nursing and its social context change. Provision 4 states, "The nurse has authority, accountability, and responsibility for nursing practice; makes decisions; and takes action consistent with the obligation to promote health and to provide optimal care" (p. 15).

The Code's interpretive statements clarify that the nurse is responsible for their own actions as well as those they delegate to others. As you enter registered nursing practice, the accountability for the decisions you make can be overwhelming at times. The better prepared you are to employ the concepts presented in this chapter—critical thinking (all of its aspects discussed in this chapter), creative thinking, reflective thinking, clinical reasoning, holistic nursing, and self-regulation—the more you will be ready to assume accountability for your nursing judgments, the decisions you will make, the actions you will take, and the direction you will provide to others reporting to you and/or carrying out your plans of care.

CRITICAL THINKING AND NURSING EDUCATION

After reading and thinking about the nature of critical thinking, you now have not only a greater understanding of the concept but also a greater appreciation of the need for critical thinking in nursing. Given the need for critical thinking at the RN level, you may be wondering at this point how the ADN educational program will be different from your prior education at the LPN/LVN level.

As has been discussed, the higher-order thinking skills of analysis, synthesis, and evaluation beyond those required of the LPN/LVN but are integral to the practice of registered nursing. Although the NCLEX-RN Test Plan includes questions to test knowledge, comprehension, application, and analysis, most of the questions test at the levels of application, analysis, and above, including evaluation and creation. These higher-order thinking skills are included in the ADN curriculum and are developed through a variety of learning activities that require your active participation and the use of critical thinking. Many authors have cited the knowledge, skills, and abilities (KSAs) required to think critically in the profession of nursing. Box 9.4 highlights some of these KSAs.

Many teaching strategies have been developed in the past few decades to foster critical thinking in students. If it has been some time since you were in school, you may find the classroom setting quite different. There may be many times where you feel uncomfortable that the teacher is not "telling you what you need to know," but rather leaving that role to you. You will likely be asked to be much more active in the teaching and learning process than you were previously in the LPN/LVN program. You may even be asked to take a lead "teaching role" for a case study or ethical debate in the classroom, with the teacher serving as a "guide on the side."

The need for teachers to employ critical thinking methods in the curriculum has never been greater, and yet the challenge has also never been greater. Today's teaching and learning environment exists in an era of increasing diversity among students, larger class sizes, and economic pressures causing both faculty and students to have less time and fewer resources to engage in these new methods. Further complicating the situation is the fact that methods used for critical thinking often vary from discipline to discipline. Strategies used in your psychology class, for example, will differ from those in your nursing class. As you enter the ADN program, some techniques, however, will be universal. Two of these are critical reading and critical writing.

In the 1990s, Paul (1992) described the important roles of critical reading and critical writing. Reading critically is an active, intellectually engaging activity in which the reader engages in an inner dialogue with the author. Most people read without thinking

> **BOX 9.4 Knowledge, Skills, and Abilities Required to Think Critically in the Profession of Nursing**
>
> - Strong knowledge of biological, psychological, and social sciences related to nursing
> - Knowledge of transcultural and holistic nursing concepts
> - Knowledge of nursing therapeutics and approaches for nursing diagnoses
> - Technical skills in nursing, including computer literacy, and how to adjust for client uniquenesses
> - Self-awareness of background assumptions and sociocentric traits and the ability to suspend/"bracket" these in designing care
> - Interviewing techniques; mindfulness; empathic listening to ascertain and understand patient/client/family uniquenesses
> - Skill as a reflective practitioner and self-regulation
> - Strong knowledge of nursing theory and critical thinking behaviors (e.g., critical thinking, creative thinking, clinical reasoning, reflective thinking; imagination; emotional intelligence)
> - Nursing judgment as a care provider, communicator and teacher, and member of the profession
> - Ability to work effectively as an interprofessional practice team member
> - Ability to acquire and apply current theoretical and practice-based research
> - Spirit of inquiry; ability to identify research areas for evidence-based practice
> - Knowledge of and advocacy for the profession of nursing and healthcare reform

critically, so they miss some parts of what is said while misunderstanding other parts. A critical reader recognizes how reading, by definition, involves getting into a point of view other than our own—that is, the writer's point of view. To analyze and judge a written work properly and fairly, a critical reader actively seeks assumptions, important concepts and ideas, explanations and justifications, key conceptions and experiences, implications and repercussions, and any other structural aspects.

The need for critical reading has become increasingly more important with the use of the internet and social media. Nurses must be able to discern fact from opinion in their research, especially when exploring an area for evidence-based research in practice.

Several authors have used the term "strategic teaching." Nursing faculty must construct the learning environment and learning activities so that the student nurse is able to apply higher-order thinking skills (analysis, synthesis, evaluation) and to employ critical thinking, to link theory to practice. Concurrently, nursing students must be "strategic learners" who proactively seek knowledge and experiences that contribute to their ability to "think like a nurse." The purpose of both of these approaches is to enable the student to develop accurate and complete nursing diagnoses and to design individualized patient-centered care plans that promote health, increase well-being, and actualize human potential for clients.

Benner et al. (2010) call for a radical transformation in educating nurses. They suggest that faculty and students make four shifts in their thinking and approach to nursing education, as shown in Table 9.2.

TABLE 9.2 Suggested Shifts in Faculty/Student Approaches to Nursing Education

Previous Thinking	Revised Thinking
A focus on covering contextualized knowledge	An emphasis on teaching for a sense of salience, situated cognition, and action in particular clinical situations
A sharp separation of classroom and clinical teaching	Integrative teaching in all settings
An emphasis on critical thinking	An emphasis on clinical reasoning and multiple ways of thinking that include critical thinking
An emphasis on socialization and role taking	An emphasis on formation

Source: Benner, P., Sutphen, M., Leonard, V., Day, L., & Schulman, L. S. (2010). *Educating nurses: A call for radical transformation.* Jossey-Bass.

THINKING CRITICALLY

Review the four shifts described by Benner et al. Put these into your own words. What do they mean to you? In what ways might the role of nursing faculty as "strategic teachers" and your student nurse role as a "strategic learner" be different in the ADN program than the faculty/student roles in your LPN/LVN program?

Today's teaching and learning environment has changed tremendously in response to research in the area of critical thinking. Additionally, the need for contextual learning has greatly impacted the teaching and learning environment in registered nursing programs. ANA's *Nursing: Scope and Standards of Practice* (2021) and the *NCLEX-RN Test Plan* (2023) demand new content and approaches for nursing education.

Alfaro-Lefevre (2020) argues that, just like technical skills, "thinking like a nurse" takes practice. Huston (2022) advocates using clinical reasoning case studies to contextualize student learning to the bedside, and Benner et al. (2010) note that practicing clinical reasoning in the classroom setting allows nursing students to develop these skills in a safe environment in which mistakes can be made and learning can take place.

To achieve learner-centered education, students must be motivated, self-directed, and capable of making decisions that result in appropriate actions. They must accept responsibility for their own learning outcomes (Bradshaw et al., 2021). Performance-based learning that incorporates interactive, cooperative, and competency-based learning places the responsibility of learning on the learner. This trend—in which the instructor no longer lectures and instead facilitates learning by offering direction for stated objectives—makes the student actively accountable and responsible for gaining competency in the defined knowledge and practice abilities (Cherry & Jacob, 2022).

Advances in technology have been especially supportive of developing critical thinking skills in students in the field of nursing. Today's computer simulations, as well as advanced technology in manikins used in skills laboratory settings, provide students with interactive learning activities that allow them to learn from the case studies, particularly from their errors in nursing actions taken.

The nurse educator must structure the environment so that learning can take place; serve as a facilitator, coach, and guide in the process; and use techniques to stimulate reflection and critical thinking in the student (e.g., they must point out flaws or inconsistencies in thinking, raise opposing views, have students question their background assumptions, and insert transcultural and situational "what if?" questions).

Nurse educators must consider not only the students' cognitive levels but also their learning styles. Using a variety of methods will address the diversity of learning styles of students and thereby promote greater student success in developing critical thinking skills and nursing judgment.

Box 9.5 summarizes a sampling of exercises used in registered nursing programs today to foster critical thinking, strengthen clinical reasoning, and develop nursing judgment. The list represents a variety of approaches that address the multiple learning styles of students and incorporates transcultural and holistic nursing concepts. As you embark upon the ADN program, you may encounter many of these teaching and learning exercises. Be mindful of your strengths and opportunities for growth, and enjoy the journey!

CONCLUSION

The concept of critical thinking has had a lengthy history. Defining critical thinking, distinguishing it from feeling, examining its relationship to creative thinking and reflective thinking, and understanding the need for it in education are all important as one then applies these to the discipline of nursing.

In transitioning from the LPN/LVN to RN role, you will find critical thinking skills essential to your practice. Additionally, with constantly advancing technologies, and

---

BOX 9.5 Teaching and Learning Exercises to Foster Critical Thinking, Strengthen Clinical Reasoning, and Develop Nursing Judgment

- Cognitive mind-mapping and decision trees
- Inductive and deductive reasoning exercises
- Decision-making clinical scenarios
- Interactive clinical simulations with changing patient status
- "What if?" scenarios
- Collaborative work groups
- Clinical reasoning case studies with infused transcultural concepts
- Virtual learning threaded discussions and group work
- Teacher modeling and use of exemplars
- Storytelling
- Teacher-moderated clinical scenarios and debates
- Journaling and clinical reasoning reflective papers
- Self-reflective background assumptions narratives
- Interprofessional collaborative practice role-plays
- Bioethical and policy discussion groups and debates
- Witten position papers and news editorials
- Exercises to stimulate a spirit of inquiry

the accompanying ethical dilemmas the nurse faces, the application of critical thinking skills to EBP becomes imperative for enriching the art and science of nursing for high-quality care.

As you participate in the ADN program, you will likely encounter many new teaching strategies and learning activities to foster critical thinking, strengthen your clinical reasoning, and develop nursing judgment as a professional nurse. View these as an opportunity for growth as you transition to the more autonomous practice of the RN.

STUDENT *Exercises*

Exercise 9.1
Set a timer for 10 minutes. Write as many words or phrases as you can that come to mind when you hear the words "critical thinking."

Exercise 9.2
Using the words or phrases you listed, compose your own definition of critical thinking.

Exercise 9.3
Describe a situation in nursing when you took inappropriate or incomplete actions. What aspect of critical thinking could you have used to strengthen or correct your actions? (Suggestions: bracketing feelings or background assumptions; using reasoning and judgment skills; using analysis, synthesis, and evaluation better; challenging assumptions or exploring alternatives; applying metacognitive or self-regulatory processes.)

REFERENCES

Adams, D. M., & Hamm, M. E. (1990). *Cooperative learning: Critical thinking and collaboration across the curriculum*. Charles C. Thomas Publishing.
Alfaro-LeFevre, R. (2020). *Critical thinking, clinical reasoning, and clinical judgment: A practice approach* (7th ed.). Elsevier.
American Nurses Association. (2015). *Code of ethics for nurses with interpretive statements* (2nd ed.).
American Nurses Association. (2021). *Nursing: Scope and standards of practice* (4th ed.).
Bandman, E. L., & Bandman, B. (1988). *Critical thinking in nursing*. Appleton & Lange.
Bar-Levav, R. (1988). *Thinking in the shadow of feelings*. Simon & Schuster.
Benner, P. (2001). *From novice to expert: Excellence and power in clinical nursing practice* (Commemorative Ed.). Prentice Hall.
Benner, P., Hooper-Kyriakidis, P., & Stannard, D. (2011). *Clinical wisdom and interventions in acute and critical care: A thinking-in-action approach* (2nd ed.). Springer.
Benner, P., Sutphen, M., Leonard, V., Day, L., & Schulman, L. S. (2010). *Educating nurses: A call for radical transformation*. Jossey-Bass.
Bradshaw, M. J., Hultquist, B. L., & Hagler, D. (2021). *Innovative teaching strategies in nursing and related health professions* (8th ed.). Jones and Bartlett.
Cherry, B., & Jacob, S. R. (2022). *Contemporary nursing: Issues, trends, & management* (9th ed.). Elsevier.
Cohen, M. (2015). *Critical thinking skills for dummies*. John Wiley and Sons, Ltd.
Dewey, J. (1910). *How we think*. DC Heath & Company. https://bef632.files.wordpress.com/2015/09/dewey-how-we-think.pdf

Ennis, R. H. (1962). A concept of critical thinking. *Harvard Educational Review, 32*(1), 81–111.

Facione, P. (1990). *Critical thinking: A statement of expert consensus for purposes of educational assessment and instruction. The Delphi report: Research findings and recommendations prepared for the American Philosophical Association (ERIC Doc No. ED 315-423)*. Educational Resources Information Center.

Glasman, N., Koff, R., & Spiers, H. (1984). Preface. *Review of Educational Research, 54*, 461–471.

Guilford, J. P. (1967). Problem solving and creative production. In J. P. Guilford (Ed.), *The nature of human intelligence*. McGraw-Hill.

Hood, L. (2021). *Leddy & Pepper's professional nursing* (10th ed.). Wolters Kluwer.

Huston, C. J. (2022). *Professional issues in nursing: Challenges and opportunities* (6th ed.). Wolters Kluwer.

Huston, C. J. (2023). *Leadership role and management functions in nursing: Theory and application* (11th ed.). Wolters Kluwer.

Idol, L., & Jones, B. F. (Eds.) (1991). *Educational values and cognitive instruction: Implications for reform*. Erlbaum.

Ignatavicius, D. D. (2001). 6 Critical thinking skills for at-the-bedside success: Key ways to practice, nurture, and reinforce staff members' cognitive skills. *Nursing Management, 32*(1), 37–39.

Marzano, R. J. (1991). Creating an educational paradigm centered on learning through teacher-directed, naturalistic inquiry. In L. Idol & B. F. Jones (Eds.), *Educational values and cognitive instruction: Implications for reform* (pp. 411–442). Erlbaum.

National Council of State Boards of Nursing. (2023). *2023 NCLEX-RN test plan*. https://www.ncsbn.org/public-files/2023_RN_Test%20Plan_English_FINAL.pdf

National Council of State Boards of Nursing. (n.d.). *The NCSBN clinical judgment model*. https://www.nclex.com/clinical-judgment-measurement-model.page

National League for Nursing. (2012). *Outcomes and competencies for graduates of Practical/Vocational, Diploma, Associate Degree, Baccalaureate, Master's, Practice Doctorate, and Research Doctorate Programs in nursing*.

Paul, R. W. (1992). *Critical thinking: What every person needs to survive in a rapidly changing world*. Foundation for Critical Thinking.

Paul, R., & Elder, L. (2020). *The miniature guide to critical thinking concepts and tools* (8th ed.). The Foundation for Critical Thinking.

Polya, G. (1971). *How to solve it*. Princeton University Press.

Raingruber, B., & Haffer, A. (2001). *Using your head to land on your feet: A beginning nurse's guide to critical thinking*. F.A. Davis.

Raphael-Grimm, T. (2015). *The art of communication in nursing and health care: An interdisciplinary approach*. Springer Publishing.

Ruggiero, V. R. (2024). *Thinking critically about ethical issues* (11th ed.). McGraw Hill.

Smith, F. (1990). *To think*. Teachers College Press.

Snook, I. A. (1974). Teaching pupils to think. *Studies in Philosophy and Education, 8*(3), 154–155.

The Foundation for Critical Thinking. (n.d.). *Our concept and definition of critical thinking*. Retrieved from https://www.criticalthinking.org/pages/our-conception-of-critical-thinking/411

Woods, D. R., Wright, J. D., Hoffman, T. W., Swartmen, R. K., & Doig, I. D. (1975). Teaching problem-solving skills. *Engineering. Education, 66*(3), 238–243.

SUGGESTED READING

Benner, P. (2001). *From novice to expert: Excellence and power in clinical nursing practice* (Commemorative ed.). Prentice Hall.

Connor, J., Flenady, T., Massey, D., & Dwyer, T. (2023). Clinical judgement in nursing - An evolutionary concept analysis. *Journal of Clinical Nursing, 32*(13/14), 3328–3340. doi: 10.1111/jocn.16469

Goleman, D. (2005). *Emotional intelligence: Why it can matter more than IQ* (10th Anniversary ed.). Bantam Books.

Garmaise-Yee, J., & LeBlanc, R. (2022). Reducing stress and increasing mindfulness in nursing students: An online mindfulness intervention study. *Nursing Education Perspectives, 43*(6), 375–377. doi: 10.1097/01.NEP.0000000000000887

On the WEB

American Nursing Association: http://www.nursingworld.org

The Foundation for Critical Thinking: http://www.criticalthinking.org

National Council of State Boards of Nursing: http://www.ncsbn.org

National League for Nursing: http://www.nln.org

Unit III

Role Concepts Essential for RN Practice

PART A | PROVIDER OF CARE

The Nursing Process: Assessment and Caring Interventions

CHAPTER 10

LEARNING OUTCOMES

By the end of this chapter, the student will be able to:
1. Discuss the development of the nursing process.
2. Explain the rationale for the nursing process development.
3. Discuss the importance of the nursing process in guiding nursing practice.
4. Describe the five components of the nursing process.
5. Formulate an actual nursing diagnostic statement using the PES format.
6. Construct a measurable expected outcome using a case study.
7. Explain the criteria to develop expected outcomes, interventions, and evaluation.
8. Explore the role of EBP in the nursing process.

KEY TERMS

- assessment
- cues
- data collection
- evaluation
- expected outcomes
- focused assessment
- implementation
- nursing diagnosis/ problem
- actual diagnosis
- risk diagnosis
- syndrome diagnosis
- wellness diagnosis
- nursing process
- objective data
- outcome criteria
- PES format
- planning phase
- primary source
- risk diagnosis
- secondary source
- subjective data
- taxonomy
- The Joint Commission (TJC)
- validation

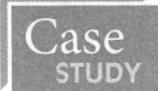

Case STUDY

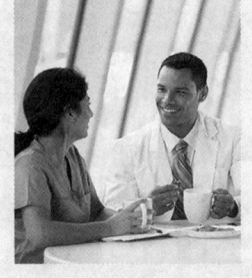

Jane Smith, LPN, and Enrique Martinez, RN, are having lunch at a medical center cafeteria. Jane is a first-semester student at State Community College and Enrique, her friend, suggested she become an RN. Last week, she had her first classroom lesson in planning nursing care and wants to use the process with a difficult client she had.

JANE: Boy, we just had a really difficult class on the nursing process.

ENRIQUE: Oh, yes. I remember the days in school when we had to do those monster care plans and, worse yet, those concept maps.

JANE: Well, we do have to do a concept map later in the semester. But right now, I'm focused on a care plan on an interesting patient I had this week. It sure is a time-consuming process to do the research and to follow the plan through.

ENRIQUE: Yes, and although the hospital doesn't require constructing care plans like the care plans you write in school, we use the nursing process in the hospital to guide our patient care. Care plans are useful when there is a change from the usual things that you do for the client, or a change from the client care paths established by the medical center. Exchanging information verbally isn't good enough when caring for clients. All members of the healthcare team need to communicate to maintain continuity of care and client safety. Client information needs to be documented so all RNs know the plan. It can't stay just in here (he points to his head).

JANE: Our instructor says care planning and concept mapping are ways to learn a disciplined approach involving critical thinking and clinical decision-making so I don't overlook anything. He also says that care plans are a way to communicate the client's many complex problems and should be partnered with the patient. But you're right—care plans are also a learning tool to help me think critically. And besides ... I need all the help I can get learning how to put it all in here! [She points to her head and laughs.]

FROM LICENSED PRACTICAL NURSE TO PROFESSIONAL NURSING PRACTICE

In the case study, Jane Smith and Enrique Martinez are discussing learning and using the nursing process in clinical practice. As an LPN, you learned about and are using the nursing process, or some form of it, to assess and to intervene in client care. At your present job, you assist with parts of the nursing process, but it is quite different when you must develop the plan of care.

Practicing LPNs continue to perform—and to have input into—many vital functions in the nursing process. As an RN, you will be in a leadership role with designing, implementing, and evaluating the entire process. You will be implementing the process from beginning to end and thus, as Jane stated, will be using a disciplined approach to think critically, problem solve, set safe priorities of care, test the efficacy of interventions, and evaluate your nursing interventions.

AN HISTORICAL OVERVIEW OF THE NURSING PROCESS AND NURSING LANGUAGE

The nursing profession is in its infancy. Although nursing in various forms has existed throughout history, it was not until the profession defined what nurses were and what nursing did that the nursing process was first established. Many of the interventions that nurses did in the past were based on trial and error, intuitive problem-solving, and scientific methods. Although Hall first used the term "nursing process" in 1955, it was not until 1967 that Yura and Walsh first published what they described as the steps in the nursing process (Taylor et al., 2023). In the beginning, the steps of the nursing process were assessment, planning, intervention, and evaluation. In 1974, Gebbie and Lavin established nursing diagnosis as a step in the process.

NURSING DIAGNOSIS TAXONOMIES

As discussed in Chapter 4, the first national conference on nursing diagnosis was held in 1973. In 1982, the North American Nursing Diagnosis Association (NANDA) was born, and it evolved into the North American Nursing Diagnosis Association International, or NANDA-I, in 2002. There are currently over 200 NANDA-I diagnostic statements, and the organization continues to accept and test new and existing nursing diagnoses.

Similar to the numeric classification system used in biology that includes kingdom, phylum, class, order, family, genus, and species, the nursing classification **taxonomy** system classifies and categorizes nursing areas of concern (Herdman et al., 2024). Taxonomies of nursing diagnoses other than NANDA-I exist, established by other organizations (such as the International Classification for Nursing Practice [ICNP]).

The language of patient care in today's healthcare environment is rapidly changing. The introduction of interdisciplinary teams (groups of professionals from several different specialties who work together to treat client conditions) has created the need for common language that all disciplines can interpret and understand. The gap between medical language and nursing language can lead to poor client care and compromise client safety. Many healthcare organizations have sought out language that is universal to all healthcare providers. The International Health Terminology Standards Development Organization (SNOMED International), a not-for-profit organization, is the developer of a worldwide comprehensive clinical terminology. The terminology, used in 75 counties, is an enhanced common vocabulary that enables healthcare providers to exchange accurate health information across all specialties and disciplines.

As nursing continues to evolve and nurses provide care in increasingly complex environments, the profession continues to develop organizing structures to facilitate communication, enhance standardization, teach new nurses, develop curricula, promote research, use nursing information systems, and promote a reimbursement system. It is important to note that although nursing language continues to evolve, nursing actions remain much the same today through the nursing process.

THE NURSING PROCESS AS THE ORGANIZER OF PATIENT CARE

Many nursing organizations have espoused the nursing process as the organizer of nursing care. The American Nurses Association (ANA, 2021) addressed the steps of the nursing process in their *Nursing: Scope and Standards of Practice*, and the National League for Nursing requires that all educational programs incorporate the steps of the nursing process into the curriculum. The National Council of State Boards of Nursing has rewritten the NCLEX-RN to relate to the steps of the clinical judgment measurement model, which are based on the steps of the nursing process (NCSBN, 2023). (For more on the clinical judgment measurement model, see Chapter 9.)

Other healthcare organizations also use the nursing process. **The Joint Commission (TJC)** mandates that documentation must be made according to the nursing process. Thus, the nursing process is used widely throughout nursing and other healthcare arenas. The next section gives an overview of the steps in the nursing process.

THE NURSING PROCESS: OVERVIEW AND STEPS

So, what is the **nursing process**? It "provides a framework for independent nursing action; promotes a consistent structure for professional practice; and helps bring focus more precisely on each patient's health care needs" (Phelps, 2023, p. vii). The nursing process is a systematic, clinically oriented, problem-solving method that guides nurses in giving client-centered, reality outcomes–oriented, effective, prioritized nursing care. The process is systematic, and it consists of sequential steps or phases similar to the steps of the scientific method used in laboratory studies and the general problem-solving process. Table 10.1 shows a comparison of these three processes. (See Table 7.5 to see how the steps of the nursing process map to the steps of the NCSBN Clinical Judgment Measurement Model.)

The nursing process is circular, dynamic, and flexible, with a great deal of interaction and overlap, as depicted in Figure 10.1. In uncomplicated situations, the nursing process can be followed sequentially, with each step relying on the accuracy of the one preceding it and influencing the one that follows it. In complicated or emergency situations, all five phases may occur simultaneously. In any event, the various elements of the process enable the nurse to do the following:

- Collect client data.
- Think critically about the data.

TABLE 10.1 Comparison of the Scientific Method, Problem-Solving Method, and Nursing Process

Scientific Method	Problem-Solving Method	Nursing Process
1. Define problem. 2. Collect data. 3. Formulate hypothesis. 4. Design plan to test hypothesis. 5. Test hypothesis. 6. Interpret results. 7. Evaluate for study conclusion or revision.	1. Encounter problem. 2. Collect data. 3. Analyze data to specify problem. 4. Determine plan of action to resolve problem. 5. Execute action plan. 6. Evaluate plan for effectiveness in problem resolution.	1. Assess the healthcare need or problem. 2. Diagnose. 3. Plan. 4. Implement. 5. Evaluate.

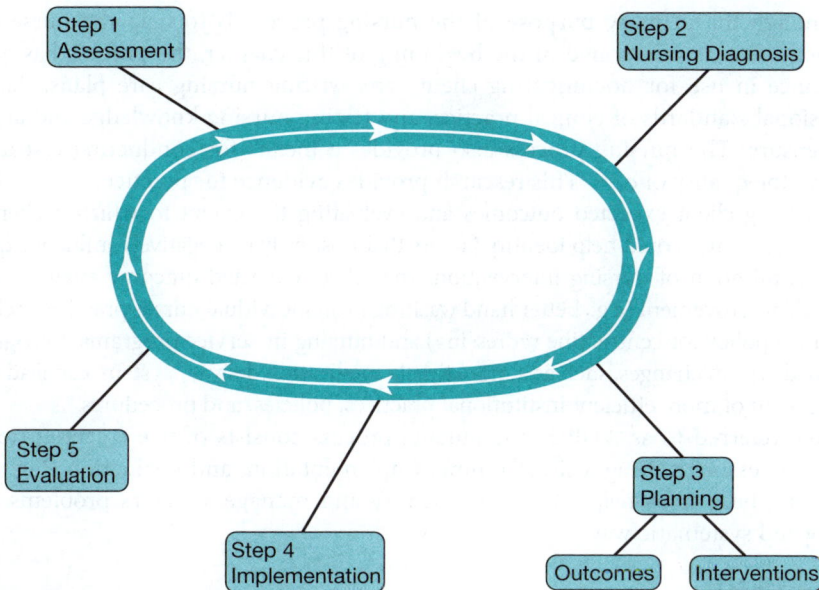

FIGURE 10.1. The nursing process.

- Collaborate with the client to identify strengths, needs, or problems.
- Establish priorities and expected outcomes with the client.
- Develop an individualized plan of care with written interventions based on EBP.
- Provide client-centered individual care.
- Evaluate the effectiveness of care and the attainment of client expected outcomes.

Table 10.2 shows the steps and activities of the nursing process.

The nursing process is recognized as client centered because it involves the nurse and client interacting in each phase to ensure that an individualized plan is developed. The plan focuses on client strengths and specifies the client's desired expected outcomes with nursing actions needed to meet those outcomes. If the client is unable to participate in the process because of age or health condition, a legally empowered person participates in the process.

TABLE 10.2 Activities Performed During Each Step of the Nursing Process

Assessment	Diagnosis	Planning	Implementation	Evaluation
• Collect data. • Validate data. • Organize data. • Report data.	• Identify patterns. • Validate diagnosis. • Formulate nursing diagnostic statement.	• Establish priorities. • Establish outcomes. • Plan nursing care. • Write plan of care.	• Reassess. • Set priorities. • Perform or delegate nursing care. • Document actions.	• Review outcomes. • Collect data. • Determine goal attainment. • Terminate or modify plan of care. Evaluate quality of care provided.

Although the primary purpose of the nursing process is to help the nurse manage client care, as mentioned in the beginning of this chapter, the process has gained acceptance in use for documenting client care, writing nursing care plans, defining professional standards of clinical practice, and testing nursing knowledge and abilities for licensure. The nursing process also provides a means for conducting research to improve the quality of care. This research provides evidence for practice.

Reviewing client expected outcomes and evaluating the extent to which a client has achieved outcomes could help identify factors that positively or negatively influence quality care. Identification of nursing interventions that affect expected outcome attainment can guide self-improvement (e.g., better hand washing in an individual nurse's practice or change in hospital policy for central line redressing) and nursing in-service programs. Recognition of needed system changes, such as a more timely medication delivery system, can lead to the development of more efficient institutional practices, policies, and procedures.

Often referred to as ADPIE, the nursing process consists of five essential steps or phases: **A**ssessment, **D**iagnosis, **P**lanning, **I**mplementation, and **E**valuation (Fig. 10.1). Following these steps helps the nurse identify and manage a client's problems in an orderly and systematic way.

ASSESSMENT

The first phase of the nursing process, **assessment**, is the continuous and systematic collection, validation, and communication of client data. During the assessment phase, the nurse establishes and develops a comprehensive database by observing, interviewing, and performing physical assessments with the client. The objective is to gain insight and information about the client's condition/situation. For example, as an LPN, you have been asked to help with data collection, such as obtaining vital signs, weight, or allergies. The RN then used that information to make sound clinical nursing judgments in the diagnostic and planning phases.

Assessment activities that are necessary for a greater understanding of the client's situation are as follows:

- Collect data: Gather client information.
- Validate data: Determine the accuracy of the information.
- Organize data: Cluster cues into related groups that show illness or health patterns.
- Report data: Document and report findings.

The NCLEX-RN *Might Ask* 10.1

The primary nurse is providing orientation to a new nurse. Together they are reviewing the nursing plan of care for an older adult client. The primary nurse knows that the new nurse needs additional help with the nursing process when the new nurse states the nursing process is:
a. an extension of the medical plan.
b. developed with the client.
c. comprehensive.
d. a systematic problem-solving method.

• See Appendix A for correct answer and rationale.

Collecting Data

Because nursing is a holistic profession, **data collection** involves gathering information about the client, family, or even the community. Information is gathered about physiologic, psychosocial, cultural, developmental, spiritual, and environmental aspects of the client. Data collection involves making general observations, obtaining a health history or admission nursing database, reviewing diagnostic studies, and performing a physical examination. The nurse must keep in mind that the single most important source of information is the interview with the client. The significant others are also excellent sources, but because of privacy laws (HIPAA), the client should always be consulted to confirm they approve the use of others as a data source (see Chapter 16). Additional information can be gained from secondary sources, such as reviewing client records and consulting with the client's family members and other healthcare professionals. The nurse would use these modes of data collection to supplement findings rather than to duplicate other previous assessments (Hood, 2021).

The focus of a nursing assessment is getting to know the person. Nurses should attempt to gain as much information as possible directly from the client. The client is considered the **primary source** of information. **Secondary sources**, such as medical records and other healthcare providers, are useful for supplementing and validating the information obtained from the client. Good interviewing skills are essential to obtain the required client data and to communicate concern for the client (see Chapter 11). The physical examination should be accomplished in a thorough and organized way using a consistent and systematic approach, such as head to toe or by body systems.

The nurse should use evidence-based assessment techniques and standardized tools for collecting data. In emergency situations, the nurse may base interventions on a partial assessment; however, as soon as the emergency has passed, the nurse should finish the assessment or delegate it to a nurse continuing with the care of the client. As an LPN, you assisted the RN with assessments and learned much by observing nurses and providers perform physical assessment. As the RN student nurse, you will learn to conduct the entire admission assessment as well as a more in-depth physical assessment and will add to that skill throughout your nursing career. The history/database and physical assessment should be obtained as soon as possible after a client presents for care (hospital admission, home health visit, or clinic appointment).

Evidence-Based Use of Assessment Tools

Communication with providers is paramount in today's fast-paced healthcare environment. Evidence from research proves that communication tools facilitate and improve the quality of care. Tools such as the Fall Risk Assessment, Risk Factors for Surgical Site Infection, and the Braden Scale are known for their evidence-based use in preventing the associated negative events. One widely used communication tool is SBAR (**S**ituation, **B**ackground, **A**ssessment, and **R**ecommendation), which promotes clear communication that promotes client safety and fosters quality care that leads to positive client outcomes.

The nursing assessment should be comprehensive and include data concerning all aspects of the client's health. Most healthcare facilities and nursing schools have developed assessment tools (forms) to collect and report assessment data (Table 10.3).

Use of an assessment tool helps prevent omissions in data collection and improves data analysis in the diagnostic phase. Tools are extremely important during data collection, but it takes practice and experience to determine areas of need that are particularly troubling and to follow **cues** related to those areas.

TABLE 10.3 Body Systems Assessment Tool (Quick Physical Assessment Tool)

Appearance Overall	Head/Neck	Thorax/Lungs	Heart/Vascular
Demeanor	Eyes	Respiratory pattern/regularity	Heart sounds (rubs/murmurs)
Grooming	Symmetry	Tracheal midline	Pulses
Posture	Speech	Symmetry of chest wall movement (Retractions)	Capillary refill (brisk/sluggish) Peripheral edema
Response to nurse	Mouth/lips (dry/moist, color)	Breath sounds	JVD
VS	Skin	Abdomen	Equipment/Invasive Lines
T: _____	Color	Configuration	IV type, drip rate
P: _____	Temperature	Bowel sounds	O_2 type, flow
R: _____	Texture	Percussion	Foley catheter
BP: _____	Turgor	Palpation	Drainage tubes
SaO_2: _____	Pressure ulcers/injuries	Pulsations	Tube feedings
			Dressings
Pain Assessment: Onset: Provocation: Quality: Radiation: Severity: Location: Timing			
Neurologic	Extremities	Safety	Psychosocial
Orientation	Strength	Bed position	Strengths
GCS	Symmetry	Call bell	Needs
Follows commands	Positioning	Bed rails	Family
Cranial nerve check		Bed check	Religion
Pupils/direct/consensual		Assistance	Coping skills
		OOB order	Education level
		Level of activity	

JVD, jugular venous distension; VS, vital signs/temperature, pulse, respirations; BP, blood pressure; SaO_2, peripheral oxygenation; O_2, oxygen; GCS, Glasgow Coma Scale; OOB, out of bed.

A comprehensive database should include both subjective information (client's and family verbal information) and objective information (observable, measurable data) about the client (Table 10.4).

The depth and breadth of data collected in assessment depend on the purpose for the assessment as determined by the client's developmental stage, nursing care needs, and urgency of the situation. Once the nurse establishes a comprehensive database determining priorities for ongoing assessment, a more focused assessment can be used to update and evaluate specific problems or needs that have been identified. A focused assessment is done to concentrate on one area, specifically the client's primary problem, gathering as much information as possible. A comprehensive assessment is obtained

TABLE 10.4 Subjective Data Associated With Objective Data

Objective*	Subjective*
Pulse 120/min, respiration 36/min; sweating profusely	"I have pain."
Absent bowel sounds; abdomen distended; eats <25% of breakfast tray contents	"I'm not hungry."
Urine foul smelling, cloudy; urinary output 100 mL in 8 h	"I have difficulty urinating."

*Objective data are what the nurse observes; subjective data are what the client says.

during initial contact with the client (admission to hospital, home health, or clinic). To strengthen and update the information, ongoing focused assessments of the client's problem areas are conducted during each client–nurse contact.

Validating Data

Validation is the act of verifying the truth. It is important to validate data to ensure that it is accurate and free from bias. Incomplete or inaccurate assessment data might lead to false assumptions. Validation ensures that information is accurate and complete. The nurse must confirm subjective data by asking the client more questions, eliciting confirmation from a reliable secondary source, or confirming the data with objective information. For example, a nurse might infer that a child is not hungry because they did not eat the pork chop and squash served at dinner. The nurse should seek validation of the observed behavior by asking, "You didn't eat much; aren't you hungry tonight?" This could lead the nurse to discover that the child just did not like the food or was in pain. Inconsistency in a client's behavior and verbal responses should always be double-checked to avoid misunderstandings or incorrect inferences. Using inaccurate or incomplete information can result in errors of problem identification in the diagnostic phase of the nursing process. Validating data prevents missing information, misunderstanding situations, jumping to conclusions, and focusing in the wrong direction.

The nurse collects and validates subjective and objective data (Table 10.4). **Subjective data** are what the client says; for example, they indicate "I'm in pain," "I'm not hungry," or "I have difficulty urinating." **Objective data** are information the nurse gathers on what the nurse feels, smells, sees, or hears and which can be confirmed by another nurse.

Organizing Data

It is necessary to organize collected data to identify problems and to formulate nursing diagnoses. Use of an assessment tool facilitates some organization of the data during collection, but it does not always bring related information together for a more holistic view of the client. Clustering relevant data into established categories for interpretation can produce a better clinical picture of the client's strengths and problems. A nursing model is more effective for establishing nursing diagnoses because it reveals the functional health or human response patterns that nursing interventions are most effective in managing. Other models may be helpful at times. For example, in an emergency situation, using the airway, breathing, circulation (ABC) model approach, rather than the functional health patterns approach, helps the nurse set priorities (Box 10.1). Nurses may cluster data according to body systems. The nurse who thinks critically may want to look at a particular healthcare problem by using one model and look at the same problem by using a different model. Each model may give the nurse a different perspective from which they can discern different patterns.

> **BOX 10.1 Data Organization According to Gordon's Functional Health Patterns**
>
> **Client Data Bill Akins**
> 1. A 69-year-old man
> 2. Widowed 2 years: two children
> 3. Occupation: retired economics professor
> 4. Religion: Baptist
> 5. Height: 5 ft, 11 in.; weight 170 lb
> 6. Temperature: 98°F; pulse: 62/min, irregular; respiratory rate: 16/min
> 7. Blood pressure: 112/64 mm Hg
> 8. Alert and oriented
> 9. Swims 4 days a week at college pool
> 10. Walks a 3-mi. course 3 days a week
> 11. Smoked cigars and pipe for 30 years; quit 8 years ago
> 12. Lungs clear
> 13. Episodic mild–moderate chest pain, activity controlled with nitroglycerin SL
> 14. Voiding clear urine; 250 to 300 mL every 3 to 4 hours
> 15. No bowel movement in 3 days
> 16. Son states hospitals terrify him
> 17. Son asks many questions about father's condition
> 18. Son and daughter visit frequently
> 19. Allergic to ampicillin
> 20. Patient states he likes to take care of himself; does not want to be a burden to children
> 21. Awakens frequently during night
> 22. Wants to know what kind of activity restrictions he will have
> 23. Likes to barbecue and picnic in summer with family members
> 24. Intermittent headaches relieved with acetaminophen
> 25. Abdominal cramping; passing gas
> 26. Bed rest
>
> **Data Organization by Functional Health Patterns**
> Health promotion—health management pattern: 9, 10, 20
> Nutritional metabolic pattern: 5, 6, 7, 11, 12, 14, 15, 19, 23, 25
> Elimination pattern: 14, 15, 24, 25, 26
> Activity–exercise pattern: 9, 10, 13, 22, 23, 26
> Cognitive–perceptual pattern: 8
> Sleep–rest pattern: 13, 21, 24
> Self-perception–self-concept pattern: 20
> Role–relationship pattern: 1, 2, 3, 4, 17, 18
> Sexuality–reproductive pattern: 2
> Coping–stress tolerance pattern: 11, 13, 22, 24
> Value–belief pattern: 4, 20

As a student, it is important to find out the model or system used by the school you are attending or the institution where you are caring for clients and to follow that system. For example, you might have a conceptual-based nursing program that links nursing diagnoses with concepts. When you become comfortable with this system, under guidance from an instructor or clinical mentor, you may want to try other systems.

Reporting and Documenting Data

The final activities in the assessment phase are reporting abnormalities to expedite treatment and documenting all collected data in a clear, concise, and timely manner to facilitate continuity of care by other members of the healthcare team. Record specific objective observations of client status and avoid use of nonspecific terms, such as good, average, normal, and poor, which are subject to interpretation. Documented information should be written legibly and according to legal and professional standards. Most institutions have implemented electronic nursing plans of care and documentation in standardized computerized forms. One of the challenges with implementation of these standardized forms is that space is needed for the nurse to individualize and tailor the plan of care to the client (Hood, 2021).

Read the following case study. Then, look at Box 10.1. The client data on Bill Akins is organized according to Gordon's (2014) functional health patterns. We will ask questions throughout the remaining portion of this chapter about the story of Bill and Roy Akins and their nurse, Gloria Linquist.

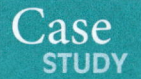

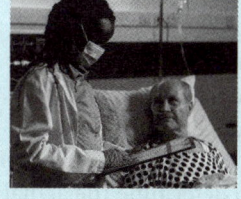

Bill Akins, age 69, was admitted to the local hospital yesterday after experiencing a heart attack. Today, Roy Akins, age 35, enters his father's room to visit for the first time. Gloria Linquist, RN, is standing at the bedside talking to Bill about the heart medications he just took for the first time. As Roy quickly and briefly touches his father's outstretched hand, he looks nervously at the IV bags and sites, the monitors, and the oxygen tubing attached to his father's nose.

ROY: How's it going, Dad?

BILL: Not too well. They say I've had a heart attack.

Gloria notices Roy's pale color, shaky voice, and trembling hands, and offers him a chair.

GLORIA: Your father has had a heart attack, but his condition is stabilizing.

ROY: How long does he have to stay here? I'd like to take him home as soon as possible.

GLORIA: It usually takes a few days. We are getting his medications regulated, and his condition is remaining stable. This must be overwhelming for you.

BILL: Could you help me get comfortable in this bed, Gloria? This is the hardest mattress I've ever laid on. I could use some cooler air and something to drink too.

GLORIA: Sure thing.

Gloria assists Bill to turn, arranges the pillow more comfortably under his head and shoulders, and turns up the air conditioning.

GLORIA: I'll get that cool drink; you two visit for a while. I'll go see about getting a foam mattress pad for your bed. We'll go for a short walk in about an hour, Bill. Ring if you need anything.

Later, Roy comes to the nurses' station to speak with Gloria.

ROY: I'd like to leave my cell number so that you can get in touch with me if necessary. I'm glad my Dad's OK. I sure was scared when my sister called and told me he had a heart attack. I wasn't sure I could come visit him. I do appreciate all those things you're doing for him.

THINKING CRITICALLY

1. List the subjective data the nurse would obtain from Bill and Roy.
2. What objective data would Gloria collect about Bill and Roy?

DIAGNOSIS

When the nurse has completed the collection, validation, and organization of client data, it is time to begin the second phase of the nursing process: analyzing and synthesizing the data to determine what the client needs. The purpose of the second phase is to determine the actual problem—that is, the human response condition for which the client is at risk.

The use of the **nursing diagnosis/problem** to describe what nurses can do for clients experiencing a human response to injury or illness may be inconsistently applied in clinical nursing practice. Resistance may arise from reluctance to devote the time it takes to develop a nursing diagnosis, confusion about the difference between nursing and medical diagnoses, or confusion about the changing terminology.

Organizations such as NANDA-I and ICNP recognize the nursing diagnosis as a clinical judgment about individual, family, or community responses to actual or potential health problems or life processes. The nursing diagnosis identifies a client problem for which a nurse can legally manage. You can better grasp how nursing practice differs from medical practice by becoming familiar with nursing diagnoses and problem statements. Nursing and medicine practices frequently identify the same problems, but they approach treatment in different ways. Nursing places a greater emphasis on providing holistic care that includes comfort, whereas medicine places a greater emphasis on treating disease.

Activities in the diagnostic phase include the following:
- Identifying patterns or clustering data
- Validating diagnosis
- Formulating diagnostic statements

Identifying Patterns or Clustering Data

The interrelationship of the assessment phase and the diagnosis phase occurs when the nurse analyzes data obtained in the assessment and identifies patterns to determine the client's nursing diagnosis.

The ability to cluster data and identify problems takes time to develop. It is sometimes helpful to list client problems and begin to match problems that have similar symptoms or focus. Generating a list using a conceptual model or an accepted set of criterion norms, such as normal physical and psychological development and Gordon's functional health patterns, helps in organization and clustering. Nursing students and beginning practitioners should expect to follow guides and use resources to accomplish this diagnostic activity. Caution should be taken to avoid making decisions about client strengths and problems with insufficient, inaccurate, or inconsistent information. If cues do not match or seem inadequate for the category, additional information should be gathered (by a **focused assessment**) to validate the diagnosis.

Box 10.2 provides an example of data analysis for the clinical example of Bill Akins.

BOX 10.2

Data Analysis for Clinical Example of Bill Akins

Gloria has a concern about Bill Akins' level of rest and reviews the clustered cues for his sleep–rest pattern category:

1. Episodic mild–moderate chest pain with activity; controlled with nitroglycerin SL
2. Awakens frequently during night
3. Intermittent headaches relieved with acetaminophen

Before drawing any conclusions about Bill's inability to achieve a restful sleep at night, Gloria questions the completeness and accuracy of the existing information and conducts a focused assessment. Although she knows that he awakens frequently during the night, no information indicates the reason for this. Gloria further evaluates the physiologic, psychological, and environmental factors that might be contributing to Bill's inability to get a good night's rest.

Gloria's focused assessment includes the following:

1. Frequency of voiding secondary to increase in diuretics
2. His tolerance for unit noise, lights, and presence of staff in the room; noise and activities concerning other patients in the unit
3. Bill's concern about his condition, fear of dying, and lifestyle changes after discharge
4. Bill's level of comfort and the frequency of chest pain during the night
5. Bill's ability to obtain rest during other periods during the day

Validating Diagnosis

When the client's information has been analyzed and a nursing diagnosis selected, the diagnosis needs to be validated with the client and/or family. Validation provides an opportunity to examine the client's perception of the problem and to determine whether there is a willingness to participate in its resolution. Through validation, the client's motivation and desires regarding care can be realized. Some clients are not ready or motivated to resolve problems that are clearly evident to healthcare providers. Use of client validation allows the client to be an aware, informed, and willing participant in their care. Validation also closely links the client's diagnosis with the client, allowing the nurse to focus on the client and not the disease, which helps to ensure client-focused care.

Formulating Diagnostic Statements

When you have completed the assessment phase clustering the data, it is time to determine whether the client's situation is normal, altered, or at risk for altered functioning and to name the problem by using the problem label that most closely matches your client's cues. Clients can have the following types of nursing problems: **actual diagnosis**, **risk diagnosis**, **syndrome diagnosis**, and **wellness diagnosis** (Box 10.3).

When writing problem statements, nurses and students use the diagnostic labels and titles developed by NANDA-I or ICNP. Each organization updates their lists periodically to ensure reflection and relevance to current practice. A nurse formulating a nursing diagnostic statement must use a diagnostic label or title from the organizational lists and not create a label or title of their own, unless they are researching a new diagnosis.

Actual Diagnosis

If the client has signs or symptoms of an active illness or problem, you will formulate an actual nursing diagnostic statement. Actual problem diagnostic statements are the only problem statements that are written in three parts using the proper components of the **PES format**, as outlined in Box 10.4.

Link the diagnostic label/title (problem) and etiology (cause) with the words "related to" or "associated with," and state the signs/symptoms (assessment data) that support the diagnosis with the phrase "as evidenced by" or "as indicated by."

EXAMPLE 10.1 Actual Diagnosis

Here is an example of an actual nursing diagnostic statement that might be applied to Bill Akins. Because it is an "actual" nursing diagnostic statement, it has three parts.

Constipation (problem) related to (or associated with) **bed rest and lack of exercise** (etiology), as evidenced (or indicated) by **decreased frequency of bowel movements, headache, abdominal cramping, and passing flatus** (signs and symptoms).

BOX 10.3

Types of Nursing Diagnostic Statements
Actual: Three-part nursing diagnostic statement
Risk: Two-part nursing statement
Syndrome: One-part nursing statement
Wellness: One-part nursing statement

> **BOX 10.4**
>
> **PES Format for Writing Actual Nursing Diagnostic Statements**
> P = Problem statement (diagnostic label or diagnostic title)
> E = Etiology or causes/risk factors
> S = Signs/symptoms: supporting data

Risk Diagnosis

Risk diagnostic labels are used when the client's database shows no evidence of current signs or symptoms but indicates a vulnerability to developing this problem. Risk diagnostic statements are written in two parts: the label/title (problem) and etiology (cause).

EXAMPLE 10.2 Risk Diagnosis
Risk for pressure ulcer (problem) related to **bed rest and pressure over bony prominences** (etiology).

Risk nursing diagnostic statements are extremely important in a healthcare environment that has shifted to predicting, preventing, and managing. In certain circumstances, risk diagnosis might be prioritized higher than actual diagnoses. For example, for a client such as Bill Akins, risk for pressure ulcer would be prioritized higher than his discomfort due to bed rest. As an LPN/LVN, an advantage you bring is your background knowledge and experience of seeing complications in your previous care.

Syndrome Diagnosis

A syndrome diagnosis consists of a group of actual and/or risk nursing diagnoses that are likely to be present because of a certain event or situation (Taylor et al., 2023). Syndrome diagnoses have one part: the diagnostic label itself.

EXAMPLE 10.3 Syndrome Diagnosis
For Bill Akins, a syndrome diagnosis could be:
  Disuse syndrome (problem).

Wellness Diagnosis

A wellness diagnosis is formulated when a healthy client wants to attain a higher level of function in a specific area. Wellness diagnoses are written as one-part statements and may begin with the term(s) "readiness" or "readiness for" followed by the listed problem label.

EXAMPLE 10.4 Wellness Diagnosis
After his acute stage settles, the following are examples of wellness diagnoses that could apply to Bill Akins.
- Readiness for discharge
- Ready to learn

Students and nurses must refer frequently to the defining characteristics or supporting data for the nursing diagnostic label. Defining characteristics and supporting data are the signs/symptoms or cues that support the decision to use a specific nursing diagnosis.

> **THINKING CRITICALLY**
>
> Review the database for Bill Akins in Box 10.1, and write actual and risk nursing diagnoses, not used in the previous examples, using the PES format.
> 1. Actual nursing diagnosis
>   Stem: _____
>   Etiology: _____
>   Signs/symptoms: _____
> 2. Risk nursing diagnosis
>   Stem: _____
>   Etiology: _____

Medical Versus Nursing Diagnoses

Medical diagnoses and nursing diagnoses differ in several ways. Whereas medical diagnoses identify disease and organ dysfunctions, nursing diagnoses describe the client's response to actual or potential health problems or conditions. A second major difference is that medical diagnoses do not change as long as the disease is present, whereas nursing diagnoses can change from day to day as the client's response to illness changes. Also medical diagnoses do not provide nurses with enough detail to plan nursing care. Because the nursing diagnosis reflects the client's response to the illness or disease, the nursing diagnosis is fluid and ever changing (Phelps, 2023), and the nursing care can also change over the course of treatment.

Most significantly, medical diagnoses require medical intervention and treatment, whereas nursing diagnoses are within the legal scope of independent nursing practice. Therefore, the use of medical diagnoses in nursing diagnostic statements should be avoided (see Table 10.5).

TABLE 10.5 Comparison of Nursing Diagnoses Versus Medical Diagnoses for Bill Akins

Medical Diagnoses	Nursing Diagnoses
Myocardial infarction	Impaired cardiac output
Bowel obstruction	Constipation
Anxiety	Impaired sleep
	Risk for difficulty with coping

PLANNING

The **planning phase** of the nursing process involves developing strategies to resolve the client's identified problems and to help the client achieve an optimal level of functioning. When possible, client strengths identified in the diagnostic phase should be used to resolve health issues. Planning and implementation activities often occur concurrently in simple or complex situations. The written plan of care is a major outcome for this step in the nursing process. Planning phase activities include the following:

- Establishing priorities
- Establishing expected outcomes
- Planning nursing interventions
- Writing an individualized plan of care

The NCLEX-RN *Might Ask* 10.2

The nurse is formulating a nursing diagnostic statement for a client with an *actual* healthcare problem. Which of the following statements is *correct* regarding an actual nursing problem? (Select all that apply.)

a. Impaired airway clearance related to thick sputum
b. Risk for fall related to weakness and orthostatic hypotension
c. Impaired sleep related to death of spouse as indicated by inability to get to sleep and excess sleepiness during the day
d. Impaired cardiac output related to ineffective heart pumping and death of myocardial tissue
e. Relocation stress

- See Appendix A for correct answer and rationale.

Establishing Priorities

The initial step in developing a nursing care plan is to examine the identified needs and set priorities. The ABCs of cardiopulmonary resuscitation can be used when setting priorities because they allow quick and easy screening for problems that require immediate. Maslow's (1968) hierarchy of needs may be used with problems that are not life threatening (mobility, pain, nutrition), need referral to others (diet consultation), or require ongoing attention (wound care, counseling). Priorities are set by considering the severity of the situation (life-threatening conditions take priority over personal enrichment) and recognizing the differences between clients. A plan is tailored to meet the client's individualized needs. One client may be ready and willing to perform their own dressing change after watching the nurse one or two times, whereas another may need a supportive family member to perform the task. Box 10.5 shows a few suggestions on how to establish priorities for client nursing diagnoses.

The NCLEX-RN *Might Ask* 10.3

The nurse has identified the following problems list for a client who has been admitted to a long-term care facility. Which of the following would be a *top* priority nursing diagnosis?

a. Chronic low self-esteem
b. Activity intolerance
c. Risk for impaired cardiac function
d. Impaired airway clearance

- See Appendix A for correct answer and rationale.

BOX 10.5 Establishing Priorities for Nursing Diagnoses: Questions the RN Should Ask

1. Does it involve the ABCs of emergency care?
2. Can Maslow's hierarchy of needs be used?
3. How many symptoms does the client exhibit?
4. Do the symptoms appear in clusters?
5. What priority does the client place on the problem?
6. Is there a simple solution that can be performed immediately?

Establishing Expected Outcomes

The terms goals, objectives, and expected outcomes are often used interchangeably in practice, references, and educational situations. In the 1990s, the NOC group initiated the use of outcomes to determine the effectiveness of nursing actions. The NOC group developed a list of research-based interventions that encompasses nursing activities for each intervention (Herdman et al., 2024). Students are encouraged to visit the website for this group and the NIC (see the end of this chapter).

Expected outcomes are written statements of specific, measurable, achievable, realistic, and timed statements of goal attainment. Because outcomes describe actions and behaviors, all outcome statements should be written using action verbs. Outcomes present criteria that facilitate evaluation. Expected outcomes help all nurses involved in a client's care identify specifically what the planned care is trying to accomplish.

Verbs used in outcome statements should be behavioral, measurable, and specific. Choose action verbs that measure success. Verbs such as know, understand, think, accept, and feel should be avoided because they are not measurable. (See Table 10.6 for examples of appropriate action verbs to use.)

The ANA's (2021) *Scope and Standards of Practice* specifically states that expected outcomes must be individually tailored to clients. The standards identify six criteria that must be achieved when planning outcomes. Box 10.6 lists the ANA's measurable **outcome criteria**.

Alfaro-LeFevre (2014) recommends a five-part outcome statement: subject, verb, condition, criteria, and specific time. If the subject is assumed to be the client for whom the nursing care plan is written, the outcome statement begins with the verb. The following are examples using Bill Akins.

EXAMPLE 10.5 Five-Part Outcome Statements

For the nursing problem "impaired cardiac function related to irregular pulse," the expected outcome would be:

> Client will have a systolic BP greater than 100 mm Hg systolic but less than 150 within 2 hours. (That is, subject [client], verb [will have], condition [BP], criteria [greater than 100 mm Hg systolic but less than 150], and specific time [within 2 hours].)

For the nursing diagnostic statement "constipation related to bed rest as manifested by decreased frequency of bowel movements, abdominal distention, and passing flatus," the expected outcome would be:

> (Client) will report the passage of soft, formed stool within 1 day. (That is, subject [assumed to be the client], verb [will report], condition [passage of], criteria [soft, formed stool], and specific time [within 1 day].)

TABLE 10.6 Measurable and Unmeasurable Action Verbs

Measurable	Unmeasurable
List/Label	Know
Describe	Understand
Explain	Feel
Discuss	Experience
Assemble	Accept
Report	
Calculate	
Has an increase or decrease in	

> **BOX 10.6** Measurable Outcome Criteria According to the ANA
> 1. Expected outcomes must be related to the nursing diagnosis.
> 2. When appropriate, expected outcomes must be formulated with the target population (i.e., patient, family, community).
> 3. Expected outcomes must address the current and potential capabilities of the client and be culturally sensitive.
> 4. Expected outcomes need to take into consideration the resources available to the client.
> 5. Expected outcomes need to provide direction for continuity of care and be evidence-based.
> 6. Expected outcomes must be documented as measurable goals with a time estimate.

Source: American Nurses Association. (2021). *Nursing: Scope and standards of practice* (4th ed.).

Expected outcomes may be short or long term, depending on the specific problem being addressed. Short-term outcomes have target dates that can be achieved in a few hours, a day, or a week. Long-term outcomes require more time, perhaps several weeks or months. Care should be taken to sequence large objectives into smaller increments to prevent discouragement and to ensure reasonable attainment of the care plan. For example, a client who wants to lose 150 lb may become discouraged when facing a weight-reduction outcome of such magnitude. A more realistic approach may be an outcome of 5 lb per month.

> **The NCLEX-RN *Might Ask* 10.4**
> The nurse is designing expected outcomes for a client with the nursing diagnosis of fluid imbalance related to excess oral fluid intake as indicated by S3 heart sounds and crackles in the lungs. Which of the following would be a properly written expected outcome for this client?
> a. The client will list foods high in cholesterol.
> b. The client will have clear lung sounds within the next 4 hours.
> c. The client will lose 5 lb within the next week.
> d. The client will have their lung sounds assessed every 4 hours.
>
> • See Appendix A for correct answer and rationale.

> **THINKING CRITICALLY**
> Write goal or client outcome statements for the nursing diagnoses you developed for Bill Akins in the previous Thinking Critically activity that do not duplicate examples in the text.

Planning Nursing Interventions

In the planning phase, it is important to identify specific nursing measures that can resolve the issues and problems identified in the diagnostic phase. Nursing interventions are treatments based on evidence-based practice (EBP) and clinical judgment that a nurse performs to create a successful outcome. (For more about EBP and clinical judgment, see Chapter 9.) Interventions consist of nursing ongoing assessments for possible

> **BOX 10.7**
>
> **Nursing Interventions: The AMT Method**
> A = Assessments: What ongoing assessments do I need to perform?
> M = Measures: What nursing actions (measures) or physical tasks do I need to do?
> T = Teaching: What kinds of teaching do I need to do with this client?

complications, teaching, counseling, consulting, giving referrals, and performing direct client care tasks, such as bathing, dressing, toileting, and ambulating. A way to comprehensively cover the necessary nursing activities is referred to as the "AMT method." See Box 10.7 for the components of the AMT method of writing nursing interventions.

Nursing interventions should be selected based on practice literature, scientific evidence from research, and client preference (Box 10.8). Evidence-based research is key for nursing growth because it translates nursing research into improved delivery of care. Resource materials that a nurse could use include the NIC system, research-based nursing literature, national standards, and academic textbooks.

First published in 1992, the NIC system was developed in Iowa to standardize nursing interventions and continues to add to this collection of knowledge every 5 years. The NIC system defines 614 interventions, 30 classes, and 7 domains that have unique codes and activities (Wagner et al., 2024).

Nurses must develop both collaborative and independent actions. Collaborative actions are nursing interventions that engage other healthcare professionals such as providers, social workers, dieticians, pharmacists, and physical therapists. The nurse must also use time wisely and delegate interventions when appropriate.

Standardized planning guides are usually available in nursing schools and clinical practice settings to make the work of planning care easier. However, these need to be adapted and individualized to each client situation. When using standard plans such as computerized plans, standard care plans, and critical pathways, it is important to screen the material and to use only information that applies to a particular client. Not all information given in a standard plan is applicable to every client. In addition, the nurse must use scientific rationale for the selected interventions, as well as be creative and willing to add alternative activities and actions so that no interventions are missed. When used correctly by nursing students and clinical nurses, standard plans can provide valuable direction for developing an individualized nursing care plan. If used incorrectly or relied upon without changes or revision, standard plans may block professional growth, decrease critical communication, and bring harm to a client.

Writing an Individualized Plan of Care

Once the interventions are identified, it is time to write a nursing care plan (nursing orders) so that all nursing personnel involved in the client's care have clear direction for

> **BOX 10.8**
>
> **How to Perform EBP**
> 1. Identify the problem or issue from the client, family, or community.
> 2. Search the literature for data supporting the problem or issue.
> 3. Evaluate the research using the scientific method.
> 4. Choose interventions justified by the evidence.
> 5. Evaluate the outcome: Is it the same, improved, or worsened?
> 6. If the change is positive, incorporate it into practice.

BOX 10.9 Sample Individualization of Standard Nursing Care Plan

NURSING DIAGNOSIS: Risk for impaired thermoregulation related to limited metabolic compensatory regulation secondary to age (neonate)

Client-Centered Outcomes:
1. Infant will maintain temperature between 36.4°C and 37°C (target date).
2. Caregivers will explain/demonstrate techniques that keep infant's temperature stable/normal (add target date).

Standardized Care Plan	Individualized Care Plan
Monitor infant's temperature.	Assess axillary temperature every hour until stable after birth; check once per shift thereafter.
Teach caregivers how to protect infant from hypothermia and hyperthermia.	Show caregivers how to dress and bundle infant for home and outings, and how to conserve heat during bathing. Explain how to protect infant from drafts and heat loss in the environment.
Reduce/eliminate sources of heat loss; prevent hyperthermia.	Wrap infant in one or two blankets; use that and booties if appropriate to keep temperature between 37.4°C and 37°C; protect from dampness, drafts, and cold surfaces. Keep room temperature at 70°F. Place infant in crib away from windows, doors, and walls.
Make referrals to community resources for infant care.	Offer free public health/neonatal nursing home visit(s) after discharge. Offer name, address, and telephone number, of a well-baby clinic or pediatrician (and/or make an appointment for the client and baby there).

implementing the plan of care. The written plan needs to include the nursing orders, which clearly reflect the three intervention types that organize nursing interventions—that is, assessment, measures (acting), and teaching. In Box 10.9, the nursing orders include these types of interventions.

Written nursing orders should be specific and clear. They must always contain the date the order was written, the action to be performed, who is to do it, and a descriptive phrase that includes the specifics needed for the activity (how, when, where, how much, how long); see the below example.

EXAMPLE 10.6 A Nursing Order

04/02/2024: Assist Kate to walk to the end of hall with walker 10 a.m., 1 p.m., 4 p.m., and 7 p.m. daily. M. Wilson, RN

Written nursing care plans come in a variety of designs, including portable cards, Kardex, and multiple-page forms but are now usually computer-generated documents. No matter the format, the basic components for written care plans are the nursing diagnosis, client-centered outcomes, and specific nursing interventions. Nurses and nursing students need to become competent in the use of the required documentation type in their clinical practice and/or educational program settings to implement and document a client's care properly. Student plans of care that you will complete during school are used as a teaching/learning tool and are much more detailed than those required by institutions. Student care plans often require a column for scientific rationales to foster student learning of WHAT to do and also WHY to do it.

THINKING CRITICALLY

Write nursing interventions for the expected outcomes you developed for Bill Akins in the previous Thinking Critically activity. Be sure to include the three intervention types appropriate for ongoing assessment, measures (actions), and teaching activities of nursing care.

IMPLEMENTATION

Implementation is the action phase of the nursing process. During this phase, the written nursing care plan is followed, and the nursing orders are executed to move the client toward achievement of their established goals. Implementation activities include the following:

- Reassessing
- Setting priorities
- Performing or delegating nursing interventions
- Documenting actions

Reassessing

Implementation requires more than just doing; it requires revisiting some of the activities used in previous phases to ensure that new events and changes in the client's situation are identified and incorporated into the client's care. In each client encounter, the nurse gathers information on the client's condition to identify changing problems. The data obtained are used to document the client's condition and to evaluate whether nursing interventions are effective and client outcomes are being met.

Setting Priorities

Just as priorities were established during the diagnostic phase, priorities need to be reestablished on a daily and sometimes hourly basis to ensure that the client's immediate needs are met.

Performing or Delegating Nursing Interventions

The RN carries the primary authority and responsibility for directing client care in institutional and community settings. When implementing the plan, the nurse either performs the interventions personally or delegates them to another member of the nursing team (nursing assistant or LPN). Chapter 11 provides more detail on delegation. When a group of clients is under the care of a nurse, the nurse is responsible for assessing and reviewing the plan of care with each client and communicating the needs and schedule of planned interventions with the other members of the nursing care team. The nurse generally reserves direct performance of nursing interventions for educating, communicating, and providing complex technical skills and procedures.

Documenting Actions

Nurses must accurately document actions and interventions to ensure comprehensive and individualized client care. Documentation serves as a baseline and as a record of care for healthcare team members, ensuring continuity and consistency in treatment. Detailed documentation allows nurses to monitor the effectiveness of interventions, track client progress, and make informed adjustments to care plans as needed.

EVALUATION

Evaluation is the final step in the nursing process. Evaluation is recognized as a separate, distinct phase and an ongoing process (Alfaro-LeFevre, 2014). Evaluation can be described as using the nursing process within nursing the process. Activities include doubling back on all the steps of the process: reassessing, rediagnosing, replanning, and—in some situations—reimplementation. Remember the following:

- Expected outcomes are evaluated.
- Interventions are *not* evaluated.

When possible, the client and the family (with the consent of the client) should participate in the evaluation of the outcome.

Nurses begin evaluation by reviewing client goals/expected outcomes to determine whether they were measurable, realistic, and appropriate for resolving the client's problems. It is then necessary to collect data about the client's condition, being alert for changes and unknown factors that have positively or negatively influenced goal achievement.

Barriers and facilitators to outcome achievement may be unknown factors, such as client reactions, worsening condition, cultural beliefs, moral values, and religious beliefs of the family. Reviewing how the nursing team applied the interventions is equally important when developing a comprehensive database on which to make a judgment about goal attainment.

After collecting subjective and objective data, the nurse analyzes the information to formulate a conclusion about the client's behavioral responses to the implemented nursing interventions. Some nursing diagnoses will be resolved, whereas others will be completely or partially unmet. It is also possible for new problems and new diagnoses to develop. If a nursing diagnosis is resolved, it can be eliminated from the plan. Partially met nursing diagnoses should be additionally assessed, and necessary modifications should be made to the plan of care. If new problems have developed, new nursing diagnoses should be identified and a new plan of treatment written.

CONCLUSION

The nurse uses the nursing process in a variety of settings with clients of all ages to identify actual and potential health issues and problems, as well as to design strategies for resolving them. By providing individualized care through a combination of independent and collaborative actions, nurses are valued contributors to the healthcare system in providing holistic, comprehensive care.

REFERENCES

Alfaro-LeFevre, R. (2014). *Applying nursing process: A tool for critical thinking* (8th ed.). Lippincott Williams & Wilkins.
American Nurses Association. (2021). *Nursing: Scope and standards of practice* (4th ed.).

Gordon, M. (2014). *Manual of nursing diagnosis* (13th ed.). Jones and Bartlett Learning.
Herdman, T. H., Kamitsuru, S., & Lopes, C. (Eds.). (2024). *Nursing diagnoses: Definitions and classification 2024-2026* (13th ed.). NANDA International, Inc.
Hood, L. (2021). *Leddy & Pepper's professional nursing* (10th ed.). Wolters Kluwer.
Maslow, A. (1968). *Toward a psychology of being* (2nd ed.). Van Nostrand Reinhold.
National Council of State Boards of Nursing. (2023). *2023 NCLEX-RN test plan.* https://www.ncsbn.org/public-files/2023_RN_Test%20Plan_English_FINAL.pdf
Phelps, L. L. (2023). *Phelps' nursing diagnosis reference manual* (12th ed.). Wolters Kluwer.
Taylor, C., Lynn, P., & Bartlett, J. L. (2023). *Fundamentals of nursing: The art and science of person-centered nursing care* (108th ed.). Wolters Kluwer.
Wagner, C., Butcher, H., & Clarke, M. F. (Eds.). (2024). *Nursing interventions classification (NIC)* (8th ed.). Elsevier.

SUGGESTED READING

Brown, S. (2023). *Evidence-based nursing: The research-practice connection* (5th ed.). Jones and Bartlett Learning.
International Council of Nurses. (n.d.). *About ICNP.* https://www.icn.ch/how-we-do-it/projects/ehealth-icnptm/about-icnp
Makic, M. B. F., & Martinez-Kratz, M. R. (Eds.). (2023). *Nursing diagnosis handbook: An evidence based guide to planning care* (13th ed.). Elsevier.
World Health Organization. (2021). *Global patient safety action plan 2021–2030: Towards eliminating avoidable harm in health care.*

On the WEB

Rosalinda Alfaro-LeFevre, RN, MSN. A great reference for critical thinking and care planning: http://www.AlfaroTeachSmart.com

Institute for Healthcare Improvement—SBAR Tool: http://www.ihi.org/resources/Pages/Tools/SBARToolkit.aspx

International Council of Nurses: https://www.icn.ch/

The Joint Commission SBAR Communications: https://www.jointcommissionjournal.com/article/S1553-7250(06)32022-3/fulltext

North American Nursing Diagnosis Association International: http://www.nanda.org/

Nursing Outcomes Committee at Iowa State University: https://www.nursing.uiowa.edu/cncce/nursing-outcomes-classification-overview

Website for flash cards/review of Gordon's Functional Health Patterns: https://www.quizlet.com/6177850/gordons-functional-health-patterns-flash-cards/

The Nurse as Communicator

CHAPTER 11

LEARNING OUTCOMES

By the end of this chapter, the student will be able to:
1. Describe the importance of effective communication to quality nursing care.
2. Describe the characteristics of effective therapeutic, caring nurses.
3. List ways a nurse can judiciously use communication skills to prevent a malpractice claim.
4. Discuss the two forms of communication.
5. Identify factors that promote effective communication.
6. Describe blocks to communication.
7. Discuss the techniques used in therapeutic communication.
8. Evaluate therapeutic communications by using a checklist or process recording.
9. Describe effective communication techniques applicable across the lifespan.
10. Describe the importance of stopping bullying in the professional context.
11. Identify key factors that enhance or detract from collegial communication.
12. List the five rights of delegation according to the NCSBN.

KEY TERMS

accountability
active listening
assertiveness
blocks in communication
bullying
caring behaviors
clarification
collaboration
collegial communication
decode
de-escalation
delegation
empathy
encode
false reassurances
general leads
incivility
judgmental
mindfulness
negative humor
nonverbal communication
paralanguage
posture of involvement
privileged communication
process recording
receiver
responsibility
restating
SBAR (situation, background, assessment, recommendation)
self-awareness
sender
silence
summarization
sympathy
therapeutic communication
therapeutic humor
trust
verbal communication

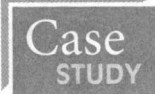

James Clancy, a 68-year-old retired Irish American firefighter, has severe bilateral arterial occlusive disease. Conservative treatment with diet, exercise, and medication has failed. Tomorrow, he will be admitted to the hospital for bilateral above-the-knee amputations. Nurse Charles Seymour, RN, and student nurse Marie Laurent, LPN, are entering Mr. Clancy's room for his morning assessment.

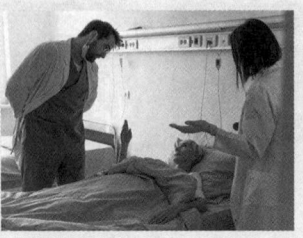

Mr. Clancy is disheveled and unshaven, with puffy eyes. He is difficult to wake.

MARIE: Hello, Mr. Clancy. My name is Marie Laurent. I am a student nurse and will be caring for you today.

MR. CLANCY: Why do you always have to be doing something with me? Leave me alone! I just want to sleep.

MARIE: Mr. Clancy, you look tired. Did you sleep well last night?

Mr. Clancy's legs are painful with the slightest movement; he grimaces when moving them back and forth.

MR. CLANCY: What do you think? I'm losing my legs tomorrow! Why don't you just let me die? I'm no good to anyone this way!

Marie looks at Charles helplessly and backs away from Mr. Clancy. She remains silent, sad, and thoughtful-looking.

CHARLES: Did the pain keep you awake last night or worrying about the surgery?

MR. CLANCY: Both! What do you think? You are always doing things with me. Don't you understand how much pain I'm in? It's agony when I move the tiniest bit, and now I hear I need to go for more tests today. Just let me die!

CHARLES: *(Moves closer to Mr. Clancy, drops to eye level, pauses, and looks directly at him.)* I can give you something stronger for the pain, and we can use your bed to transport you.

MR. CLANCY: All I'm asking for is peace. I really don't want to have this surgery; I'm in more pain when I'm moved.

CHARLES: This is a difficult decision for you. *(Charles pauses, stays close to Mr. Clancy, and has a look of genuine concern on his face but remains silent and picks up his hand.)*

MR. CLANCY: *Mr. Clancy is sobbing openly now.* I don't deserve this! What will I do with the rest of my life? How will I get anywhere without help? I hate relying on anyone!

CHARLES: *(Responds in a mindful and dramatically quieter voice.)* It sounds as if you have not made up your mind completely yet … about this surgery?

MR. CLANCY: I still think my legs can get better.

CHARLES: Let's talk about what the doctor said yesterday and review the information some of those tests are telling us. Then, we can call the doctor and ask if they can spend some time with you …. However, this is your decision, and you have the right to refuse surgery. But let me get those pain meds; I will be back in 5 minutes.

MR. CLANCY: Yeah, thanks… I could use that, and staying in the bed in a good plan.

Later, Charles and Marie are discussing Mr. Clancy's case.

MARIE: I never know what to say when patients get angry and upset. The same approach doesn't work with everyone. I melt when they start to cry.

CHARLES: It's hard to know what to say when someone is so upset and writhing in pain. But there are some good principles of communication that I always remember. First, focus and stay in the moment. I believe it's called mindfulness. Second, talk less and listen more. Third, be human and try to get at the root of the problem from the client's perspective. Then, I also review what has worked well and what hasn't.

MARIE: Yes, I remember some of those skills from my LPN training. I remember starting off wanting to give patients that kind of attention. It takes ongoing education and working on it … doesn't it?

CHARLES: Yes, communication is complex. Concerned healthcare professionals go to seminars to enhance their skills. With reminders and education, everyone listens better. The patient is happier, the staff feels satisfaction, and the quality of care is better.

Scenarios such as the one involving Charles, Marie, and their client Mr. Clancy are repeated every day in healthcare settings. To be effective in delivering quality nursing care, nurses not only need to be good communicators but also need to be able to skillfully defuse situations such as Mr. Clancy's. Communication is the key to human relationships and the glue that binds caring human interaction; it is an essential need of humans, a universal characteristic of life and living. When learning communication techniques, it is beneficial to determine what is helpful or not helpful, what is detrimental, what promotes growth and satisfaction, and what blocks understanding. Continuing education and working at it are the keys to improving communication.

The skill of communication was introduced in your previous nursing studies. It is one you continue to use in your clinical practice and everyday life. Many seasoned nurses say that they, like Marie, feel helpless in certain circumstances. Like Charles, the entire healthcare system is realizing the need to brush up on clear communication, study exemplary mentors, and practice communication techniques for worthwhile client interactions.

This chapter is divided into two sections. The first section reviews concepts of communication (verbal and nonverbal) and provides strategies for effective communication with clients. The second section addresses the subjects of effective team building, assertiveness skills, and delegation.

BASIC COMMUNICATION REVISITED

The process of communication is complex. It is helpful to review the linear two-person communication model developed by Berlo (1960). This model involves many variables that affect the sender, the message, and the receiver. Communication begins with a message and the sender's desire to be understood. The sender communicates the message by encoding verbal and nonverbal signals to the receiver. The receiver **decodes** the message—that is, tries to understand the meaning of the message (see Fig. 11.1). Feedback is given to the sender from the receiver, and the process continues. Although this model is simple, it does not take into account many preexisting factors that influence communication, including the physiologic, biologic, cultural, and gender-specific characteristics of the participants. The choice of words and terminology of the communicators, as well as a common shared experience, are essential (Boggs, 2022). These variables can also alter the clarity of communication. Anywhere in this model, a breakdown in the message can occur, causing miscommunication or an inaccurate message to be conveyed between the two participants. **Therapeutic communication** is important in the healthcare sciences, particularly nursing. Therapeutic communication fosters healing by conveying caring and understanding for the client. An additional benefit for nurses is the confidence that the interaction is helpful (Rosdahl, 2022).

TWO FORMS OF COMMUNICATION: NONVERBAL AND VERBAL

In the simplistic model of communication in Figure 11.1, there is a **sender** (who **encodes**) and **receiver** (who decodes); these individuals impart nonverbal and verbal messages (or cues). Nonverbal behaviors can support, emphasize, confuse, or contradict what the verbal part of the message implies. Although **verbal communication** is important, most communication is nonverbal. Understanding that both parties' participation, perceptions, and emotions are interactive and affect how the message is conveyed is necessary for effective communication (Catalano, 2020). There needs to be congruency and consistency between the verbal message the nurse is trying to express and the **nonverbal communication** cues; otherwise, the patient may not develop trust in the

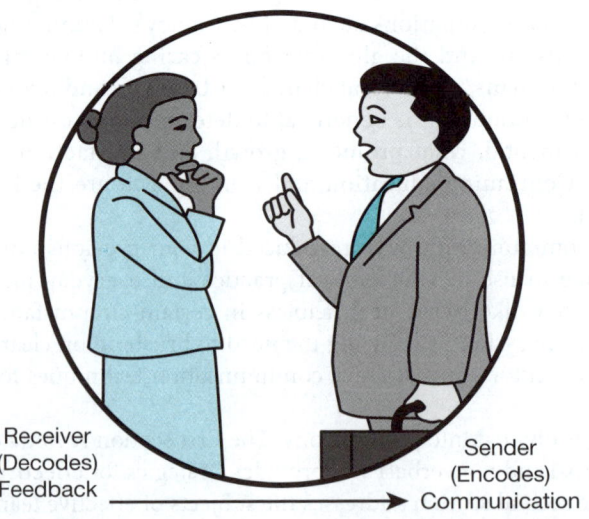

FIGURE 11.1. The Transactional Communication Model.

BOX 11.1 Factors That Promote Nonverbal Communication

- Focus undivided attention on active listening skills.
- Sit down to listen whenever possible.
- Use silence judiciously.
- Moderate your voice tone and pace.
- Use good eye contact.
- Minimize gesturing.
- Smile appropriately.
- Simplify your language.
- Use proper touching techniques.
- Respect cultural diversity.
- Try to mirror the client's positive nonverbal communication.
- Identify and explore inconsistencies/contradictions.

nurse. Techniques that can be successful in promoting effective communication include active listening, judicious use of silence, speaking clearly and distinctly, maintaining eye contact, and using open body gestures, simple words, and a caring touch (Box 11.1). Nurses are usually aware of their verbal statements but may be unaware of what they "telegraph" or tell the client with nonverbal cues. If nonverbal and verbal communication is not consistent, it is generally accepted that the nonverbal cues sent will be taken as the true meaning; therefore, nurses must be aware to observe and convey congruency (Taylor et al., 2023).

Nonverbal Communication

Active Listening: Being Mindful

Effective communication occurs when you observe verbal and nonverbal cues and messages. **Mindfulness** is being present in the moment and noticing attentively (Chen et al., 2023). Being mindful helps with active listening skills. Mindfulness is actively staying focused in the present; in other words, the mind is not on autopilot or falling into a habit. Mindfulness allows the listener to think more, react less, and seek meaning in the relationship. Necessary in the helping relationship, mindfulness enhances and fosters maintaining trust, rapport, and genuineness. It is one of the most caring aspects of a therapeutic relationship. The nurse's attitude is paramount for active listening. The nurse needs to convey readiness to hear and understand what the client wants to say without argument, judgment, or interruption. Although silence is passive, **active listening** is not. As the term implies, active listening requires intense concentration on the part of the nurse. Nonverbal and verbal information are processed and understood. A student nurse can observe listening behaviors while learning from a seasoned nurse mentor but must actively practice them to instill their effectiveness.

Behaviors a nurse can perform to enhance attentive listening are called the **posture of involvement**. The nurse should turn toward the client and lean slightly forward. To convey an open and less threatening position, the nurse should make an attempt to be at the client's eye level when possible. This will make the client feel less like they are being talked "down to" or being "talked at" and more like they are an equal partner in the communication. Moving closer to the client without violating their body space will help lessen the distance from formal to therapeutic. Sit down whenever possible, even if it's only for a moment. This communicates that you are taking the time to listen, and the client perceives that you are there for longer than you actually are.

Timing is critical with active listening. Every effort should be made to decrease interruptions. In the home and hospital settings, with the client's permission turn off televisions, radios, or electronic devices. In the hospital, draw the curtain and pull up a chair. Decreasing interruptions allows both nurse and client to focus on emotions, facts, and problem-solving. As a rule, the nurse should listen more and speak less.

Silence
Silence can be both a verbal technique and a nonverbal technique of enhancing quality discussion. Silence allows the nurse to fully concentrate on the client. The proper use of silence decreases the pace, allowing the nurse to observe and to interpret the client's meaning. The nurse may miss valuable information and cues if the sometimes uncomfortable void of silence is filled with meaningless conversation. In times of severe distress, the simple gesture of sitting with the client can be seen as an empathetic gesture by the nurse. Be patient and don't fill in words for the client.

Paralanguage
Clarity, quality, pitch, tone, and tempo of the spoken word are called paralanguages. **Paralanguage** deals with *how* a word or words are said, independent of *what* is said. Speak to the client in a clear, moderate voice at a medium rate of speed. Mumbled, indistinct, fast communication by the nurse can be misinterpreted as the nurse not having the time to spend with the client and may contradict caring behaviors that the nurse wants to convey. Speaking clearly presents a clear message. Use verbal checks—such as asking the client whether you are speaking clearly enough or speaking too fast—periodically throughout the conversation to determine whether your intentions have been understood by the client.

Eye Contact, Body Postures, and Gestures
Eye contact and moderate body gestures can enhance the quality of effective nurse–client interaction. Friendly eye contact by the nurse promotes interest and caring. Comfortable eye contact does not include glancing, darting, shifting, or fixed gazes. An inability by the nurse or client to maintain eye contact may convey anger, mistrust, or even suspicion.

The nurse must exercise cultural sensitivity when using eye contact. Clients from some cultures may not look at the nurse directly and may give the impression that they are not sincere or not listening. The nurse be culturally sensitive when dealing with nonverbal messages of clients from other cultures. (For more information on cultural competence and cultural humility, see Chapter 13.)

Although eye contact is dictated by cultural norms, facial expressions are not. Charles Darwin (1872) noted that facial expressions have universal meanings. Laughing, smiling, frowning, and crying convey universal emotions. The nurse needs to adopt a friendly, open facial expression. The nurse who frowns or nervously paces the room indicates nonverbally that they have terminated the interaction. Warmth and caring can be displayed by a relaxed stance and posture, with shoulders level and flexible, and hands unclenched.

Gestures made with the body and hands may have culturally defined meanings. Although in one culture uplifted hands with the head tilted may mean the communicator is not sure, in another culture, this gesture may mean something vastly differently. The nurse should use a minimum of gestures when they are not sure of the audience's cultural heritage. Avoid crossing arms and legs; these are sometimes interpreted as closed postures and do not convey openness.

Appearance

Clients and nurses can communicate much about grooming, hygiene, and emotional and mental status by their appearance. An adage relevant to this situation is "Looks can be deceiving." A nurse should not make snap judgments about a client's status based on appearance alone; they should ask the client questions, as needed. A client who enters a community clinic with untrimmed hair and dressed in worn clothes but who is essentially clean and has no body odor may, at first glance, convey the impression of a person experiencing homelessness. However, during an assessment interview, the nurse may discover that this client is employed but barely making ends meet or is financially well off.

The nurse also needs to be conscious of their own dress and behavior and how it affects those around them. A nurse who has clean, neatly tailored and pressed clothes, neatly manicured nails, and a prominently worn name badge conveys a strong professional self-concept upon entering the room.

Touch

Although touch is listed last, it is an important form of nonverbal communication because it involves sensory input from the body's largest organ—the skin. Touch can be a powerful communicator of caring, respect, and acceptance. Touch is a basic human need and part of every nursing procedure. How the nurse performs a vital signs assessment, gives a bed bath, or administers medication conveys the nurse's basic philosophy about caring. Touch should be used only after an introduction and should be done with close observation paid to the client's verbal and nonverbal reactions. If the nurse encounters a negative response to touch by the client, the nurse needs to step back, increasing physical distance to restore respect and comfort.

Using nonverbal communication takes practice, guidance from mentors, and **self-awareness**.

THINKING CRITICALLY

Referring to the example in the Case Study, visualize Mr. Clancy and the nurses. Write down the nonverbal communication Mr. Clancy is conveying to the nurses.

Verbal Communication

Therapeutic verbal communication encompasses the content of *what* is said during a therapeutic interaction. To enhance your professional effectiveness, you need to revisit the many techniques you were introduced to in your previous training and refine them periodically. Verbal communication is a lifelong learning skill. The nurse should keep conversation simple and use general leads, open-ended questions, share observations, restatement, clarification, silence (as discussed in the

TABLE 11.1 Summary of Verbal Therapeutic Communication Techniques

Technique	Examples
1. General leads	"I see …" "Go on …" "I hear what you are saying."
2. Open-ended relevant questions	"Where would you like to begin?" "Tell me more about what happened to you." "Can you describe what you were feeling?"
3. Sharing observations	"Are you uncomfortable when you …?" "I noticed that you have a hard time when you …" "You seem to be in more pain today …"
4. Restating	*Client*: "I'm sorry about doing that." *Nurse*: "You're sorry." *Client*: "I'm angry I have to take all of these pills!" *Nurse*: "You're angry that you have to take so many pills."
5. Clarification	"I'm not sure I understood …" "I didn't follow that part about …" "Did I understand you to say …" "Could you give me an example of how this affects you?"
6. Silence	*Client*: "I'm afraid of losing both of my legs." *Nurse: Stops, sits down in a chair by the bed, leans close to the client, and takes an offered hand.*
7. Summarization	"So far we have talked about …" "I think the main ideas you have told me are …" "Do I have this straight about your problem with …"

above section), and **summarization** in promoting effective interaction. A summary of these techniques is included in Table 11.1.

Keeping It Simple

In the medical setting, clients are not unlike strangers in a land in which a foreign language is being spoken. As the client advocate, the nurse is in an excellent position to simplify medical terminology in words that the client, family, or community can understand. Use of complex words to describe treatment, medications, or complications can confuse the client, leading to feelings of anger and frustration. The nurse should use simple terms or concrete layman's examples when describing the more complex medical protocols.

General Leads

General leads are brief words or phrases to tell the listener that reception is occurring; these leads encourage the client to communicate further. Phrases such as "I see," "Oh, then what happened?" "Tell me more," and "I follow what you are saying" are useful when trying to promote more information exchange from the client.

Open-Ended Questions

Open-ended questions encourage the client to elaborate on a subject; they require more than a "yes" or "no" answer. Open-ended questions may be useful in situations in which the client is guarded or resistant to talking. Questions may begin with "who," "what," "when," or "where." "Why" questions are usually avoided because requiring an explanation tends to place the client on the defensive. Open-ended questions add depth and relevance to the communication.

Sharing an Observation

When using this technique, the nurse shares the observation of something significant with the client, such as a client behavior or a client event. Refer to the below examples.

EXAMPLE 11.1 Sharing an Observation
- "I haven't seen you drink anything today. Am I wrong?"
- "You seem sleepier today."

Such questions or statements are neutral and allow the client to confirm or deny the nurse's observation. Observations can often be used to initiate a conversation.

Restating

When using the **restating** technique, the nurse uses a verbatim segment of what the client has said. See the below example.

EXAMPLE 11.2 Restating Technique
Client: "I'm afraid to put on this dressing at home."
Nurse: "You are afraid to do this at home?"

As with general leads, this technique lets the client know that the nurse is following the intent of the interaction. This technique should not be relied on frequently because the client may start to believe that the nurse is mocking or making fun by parroting back what the client has said.

Clarification

Clarification is essential to ensure effective communication. An individual may make a statement that is unclear to the interviewer; in such a situation, the interviewer must clarify the meaning of the statement.

EXAMPLE 11.3 Leads That Seek Clarification
- "I don't quite understand."
- "Could you explain that again?"
- "I think what you are saying is …. Am I wrong?"

It is tempting for the novice interviewer to pretend to understand and hope the meaning will become clear later in the interaction. However, such an approach is usually not effective and could compromise client safety.

Summarization

A helpful way to conclude a therapeutic interaction is to summarize the ideas developed, clarify expected outcomes, and list the actions to be taken by the individual. Although mutually acceptable outcomes are important in some situations, in other circumstances, the nurse must be able to accept client actions and decisions with which they do not agree. See below for examples of conversation closures.

EXAMPLE 11.4 Conversation Closure
- "Taking everything we talked about under consideration, I believe what we have agreed on is …"
- "We have discussed …; are there any other concerns you have before we move forward?"

The NCLEX-RN *Might Ask* 11.1

The nurse is interviewing a client. Effective therapeutic techniques a nurse can use in the communication process are (Select all that apply):

a. general leads.
b. active listening.
c. using close-ended questions.
d. a professional appearance.
e. changing the subject.

• See Appendix A for correct answer and rationale.

VERBAL BLOCKS IN THERAPEUTIC COMMUNICATION

Blocks in therapeutic communication are techniques used by the nurse that decrease their ability to identify client needs. Verbal blocks are words or phrases that are frequently used in the social setting, may be habitual, and may be used out of sympathy. Verbal **blocks in communication** include providing false reassurances, giving advice, being judgmental, and changing the subject.

False Reassurances

One of the most frequently used blocks in therapeutic communication is providing **false reassurances** to the client. "It's okay; everyone feels that way" or "You'll see, everything will be just fine" are phrases the nurse might say after a client reveals a major problem or concern. Unintentionally, the nurse has belittled the individuality of the client's fears and concerns. The client may perceive that the nurse does not take them seriously, because these statements trivialize what the client is experiencing. Each client is unique and wants the nurse to recognize their unique experiences.

Instead of false reassurances, the nurse should respond with neutral statements, such as "Tell me more about …" or "You sound worried or fearful about …."

Giving Advice

Although clients frequently ask the nurse what the nurse would do, giving advice may prematurely end the interaction with the client. Clients are really not asking for advice; they are working through the decision-making process verbally. The client might feel as though the nurse is dictating what they should do, thereby dominating them. Giving advice also fosters a feeling of dependency in the client and leads the client to believe that only the nurse knows what is best. Statements by the nurse that indicate advice-giving include: "The best thing for you to do is …," "Why don't you …," and "If I were you, I'd …."

The best way to eliminate giving advice is for the nurse to be self-aware. Another technique a student could use is asking for feedback from the clinical instructor. Alternatives to giving advice include: "I wonder if you've considered …" and "Maybe we should look at …. Let's talk about all of the options you might have." In this way, instead of imposing their will, the nurse is asking the client to explore options.

Being Judgmental

When a nurse responds with a moralistic statement, they are adopting a **judgmental** attitude (Taylor et al., 2023). Similar to giving advice, judgmental statements negate the client's right to choose and belittle the feelings the client may express. Because personal values and attitudes can affect client interaction, the nurse needs to overcome their personal ideals to allow the client the respect and right to make decisions. Moralistic statements, such as "I'm glad you have come to your senses" and "You should never feel that way," should be revised to be more neutral in tone—for example, "You sound confused" or "Tell me more about how you feel."

Changing the Subject

Changing the subject involves introducing an unrelated topic into the discussion that diverts the client from revealing feelings and thoughts. When the content of the client's communication is sudden and surprising or when the subject is too painful for the nurse to discuss, the nurse may react by changing the subject. This block in communication tells the client that the nurse is no longer listening and quickly ends the interaction. See the below example.

EXAMPLE 11.5 Changing the Subject

Client: "I want to kill myself right now."
Nurse: "Did you have any visitors today?"

One of the easiest ways to deal with surprise revelations is the use of silence. The adage, "If you don't know what to say, don't say anything," may be helpful for the nurse to keep in mind when confronted with a surprising or disturbing situation. A few moments of silence allow the nurse to gather their thoughts and respond in a meaningful way.

A summary of types of blocks in communication is included in Table 11.2.

TABLE 11.2 Summary of Blocks in Communication

Technique	Examples
1. False assurances	"Don t worry." "Things will all work out for the best."
2. Giving advice	"I think you should …" "Everyone I know does this when this happens …"
3. Being moralistic	"You should be ashamed of your behavior." "Someone your age should …"
4. Changing the subject	*Client:* "I have been very depressed for about a week." *Nurse:* "Come, let's play a nice game of checkers." *Client:* "When my baby died, I thought I couldn't go on." *Nurse:* "How many other children do you have?"

PROCESS RECORDINGS

Newer technologies provide ways for nurses to practice and improve their therapeutic communications. Interactive videotape, role playing, clinical simulation, and computerized learning scenarios can safely simulate the proper use of therapeutic techniques until the student gains comfort. In your class work, you may be asked to video- or audiotape your interaction with another student and then analyze that conversation. It may be helpful to use a checklist (Box 11.2) to fine-tune your use of therapeutic techniques.

BOX 11.2 Therapeutic Communications Performance Checklist

The following checklist can be used by a student to evaluate the use of therapeutic interventions during a client interaction or when viewing a videotape of a client interaction.

	Yes	No
1. Introduces self and states the purpose of the visit.		
2. Asks the client how they would like to be addressed.		
3. Identifies expected outcomes for the day and for the termination time of the therapeutic relationship.		
4. Maintains eye contact and minimizes gestures.		
5. Maintains consistency between verbal and nonverbal communication.		
6. Subtly mirrors the verbal/nonverbal client behaviors.		
7. Avoids rushing or forcing the conversation (sits, if possible).		
8. Avoids dominating the conversation with personal details.		
9. Asks open-ended questions.		
10. Promotes expression of client feelings.		
11. Clarifies and restates main ideas.		
12. Offers alternatives to the plan of care.		
13. Avoids the use of blocks in communication.		
14. Summarizes the content of the exchange.		
15. Terminates the relationship by identifying: • Outcomes accomplished • Needs to work on		

Comments

_____
_____
_____

A common teaching tool used in nursing programs to refine therapeutic communication is a process recording. A **process recording** is a written record of a therapeutic conversation with a client that displays oral and written information as well as an analysis of the interaction by the student (Fosbre & Varcarolis, 2023). See Box 11.3 for a sample of a process recording.

BOX 11.3 Sample Process Recording

Client initials: _____   Student name: _____

Client diagnosis: _____   Date: _____

Setting: _____   Instructor: _____

Clinical site: _____

Nonverbal and Verbal Data	Thoughts/Feelings	Analysis of Client/Student Communication Techniques

The NCLEX-RN *Might Ask* 11.2

The use of therapeutic communication by the nurse in client interaction is primarily done to (Select all that apply):
a. foster dependence on the nurse.
b. discuss the client's inner secrets.
c. lay a framework for a trusting relationship.
d. obtain information required for outcome-oriented nursing care.
e. give the client an opportunity to verbalize and clarify fears and frustrations.

- See Appendix A for correct answer and rationale.

CHARACTERISTICS OF AN EFFECTIVE, THERAPEUTIC, CARING NURSE

Therapeutic relationships are more effective if the nurse demonstrates caring behaviors and characteristics, both verbal and nonverbal, to establish, promote, and terminate the relationship. The subsections that follow describe these traits. See also Box 11.4 and Table 11.3 for caring characteristics used by successful nurses to help clients solve problems.

Engenders Trust

The nurse must establish **trust** with the client to be an effective communicator and change agent. Keeping promises, being there for the client, and using therapeutic communication that accepts the client's feelings as valid can establish trust. Providing and interpreting information with the client and their family and offering reassurance are important in laying a foundation for and perpetuating **caring behaviors** (Zalon, 2023).

The client has the right to confidentiality and to trust that their information is protected. With the enactment of the Health Insurance Portability and Accountability Act in 1996, all client healthcare information is considered **privileged communication**. Healthcare providers should only share client information with other healthcare professionals and covered entities who have a legitimate need to know. When disclosing client information, healthcare providers should only share the minimum amount of information necessary to accomplish an intended purpose (Boggs, 2022). Communicable diseases, child/older adult abuse, and gunshot and/or knife wounds are the exception and are reportable under the law. Some tips to prevent malpractice claims against the nurse, provider, and hospital for divulging confidential information are listed in Table 11.3. Legal issues are explored in more depth in Chapter 16.

Is Empathetic

It is important for the nurse to understand the difference between sympathy and empathy. **Sympathy**, common in social relationships, is described as feeling sorry for a client, reacting

BOX 11.4 Characteristics of Therapeutic Communication by Nurses

Focused on client
Respectful, sincere, patient
Empathetic
Clear
Outcomes oriented
Confidential
Acknowledges client feelings and emotional content
Promotes effective problem-solving/coping

TABLE 11.3 Caring Characteristics of the Nurse and Tips to Prevent Malpractice Claims

Caring Characteristics	Tips to Prevent Malpractice Claims
Trustworthy Knowledgeable Nonjudgmental Empathetic	Involve the client in the informed consent process.
Genuine Accepting	Be available and accessible to the client.
Warm Patient	Do not make promises you cannot keep.
Authentic Respectful	If you say you are going to do something, do it.
Understanding Use of humor	Strive to understand the client's emotions by listening and looking for cues.
Confidential	Share information on a "need-to-know" basis.

to the situation as a friend would under the same circumstance. In contrast, **empathy** is defined as understanding the client by mentally placing themselves in the client's situation (Boggs, 2022). Attentiveness, timeliness, soothing voice tones, active listening, and overall empathetic demeanor and attitude assist in establishing a caring relationship.

Uses Therapeutic Humor

Therapeutic humor means using the power of laughter and smiling to improve healing. Therapeutic humor can be a powerful tool, physiologically and psychologically, when used in both client and staff communication. Much like other forms of physical exercise, laughter creates predictable physical and psychological responses that reduce stress, anxiety, worry, and frustration (Horowitz & Kellogg, 2022). Done with common sense and in good taste considering the individual, laughter and humor have been known to stimulate the immune system, increase pulmonary volumes, promote coughing, and boost cardiac exercise by increasing the heart rate (Cousins, 1983). Psychologically, well-timed humor can diminish anger and frustration, leading to the release of tension, creating a human connection.

Initially, a smile and a relaxed attitude by the nurse are easy to exhibit; they help set an initial positive tone to the conversation and show care early in the relationship. However, during busy or stressful times, smiling may be difficult to achieve. However, there are many other ways to enhance humor appropriately. Cartoons, toys and props, joke books, music, DVDs, and CDs can be provided to promote therapeutic humor. Many hospitals encourage the use of clowns and volunteers to cheer clients and to provide diversion from pain. Many websites promote the use of professional, therapeutic humor in the workplace (see the "On the Web" section at the end of this chapter for a few examples).

Whereas laughter and humor can have a positive influence on client outcomes, **negative humor** can be harmful or offensive to the client. Box 11.5 lists times when humor and laughter are inappropriate and may be perceived as unprofessional. There are no hard-and-fast rules in applying laughter and humor, but considering individual variations in taste, humor is best approached in a test-the-waters manner. Go slowly and try a few light comments, noting the client's verbal and nonverbal reactions. If the client is open to the approach, more techniques may be added—but always observe the client's reaction and adjust your approach as needed.

> **BOX 11.5 Inappropriate Situations for the Use of Humor**
>
> Timing is important for the effect of humor to be positive. The nurse should use caution when engaging in humorous, playful behavior when the client:
> - Is trying to communicate something serious
> - Is receiving unexpected and unwelcome test/diagnostic results
> - Is in the same room with a client who is very ill
> - Is unfamiliar, and the nurse has not yet established a trusting relationship
> - Is offended by the content of the humor
> - Seems "put down" by the nurse's use of sarcasm
> - Shows nonverbal signs of wanting a relationship that is more serious in tone
> - Experiences pain from the act of laughter (abdominal or chest sutures)

COMPETENCE IN COMMUNICATION ACROSS THE LIFESPAN

The general communication skills covered so far in this chapter are useful in communicating with all types of clients, families, coworkers, or groups. However, sometimes specific techniques are useful, such as when caring for children, adolescents, or older adults.

Infants and Children

Infants and children are sensitive to nonverbal communication. Tone of voice and gesture can startle or frighten a small child. Comforting techniques such as cuddling, patting, or rocking in the presence of the primary caregiver are important to adopt. (When children are very young, the caregiver may be their only trusted source of needed information.) Using simple words, short sentences, and talking to the child at eye level are important tips to remember. Toys, games, and dolls can help young children relate to situations and should be used frequently to communicate with this age group. When caring for older children, it is important to talk to the primary caregiver and to the child in conversations; information must be provided in language and terms that are appropriate for the child's developmental level.

Adolescents

One of the most important communication techniques in conversations with adolescents is to listen first and remain nonjudgmental. Every effort should be made to give the adolescent a sense of modesty and privacy. A give and take strategy is important and should be maintained with thoughtful, creative, firm limit setting. Encouraging the adolescent's self-expression shows tolerance and respect for their developing individuality.

Older Adults

In communicating with the older adult, assessment of the client is important. Sensory needs, such as hearing and vision difficulties, can accentuate the need for face-to-face interaction; when talking with the client, face the client and use simple nonverbal gestures to help facilitate clear interaction. Establishing priorities with the client can assist in retaining needed information. The nurse should focus on one topic at a time, allowing time for the client to respond with an answer. Selecting a time in which the client is less fatigued or stressed helps facilitate communication. Asking about the client's previous experiences with health-related issues can help the nurse to understand the client's present experience. Consistent thought and consideration for the dignity of the older client is paramount. The nurse should address such clients in the manner they request; always ask about preference to use a first name or to use Mr., Mrs., Ms., etc. Include a significant other in care to help verify and clarify important facts only if permission is granted by the client.

COMMUNICATION IN THE HEALTHCARE SETTING

Social and therapeutic communications are important aspects of an RN's practice. Effective communication and interprofessional teamwork are essential for the delivery of safe, high-quality client care (Potter et al., 2023). Nurses need to develop and maintain strong team building skills with other healthcare colleagues, acquire assertiveness skills to act in the client's best interest, refrain from incivility and bullying, learn how to de-escalate high-stress situations, and delegate appropriate tasks clearly, appropriately, and concisely. As an LPN transiting into the role of an RN, you will need to communicate persuasively as a colleague as your scope of **responsibility** and **accountability** broadens.

TEAM BUILDING

The nurse needs to foster **collegial communication** and team building. *Collegial communication* is skillful verbal, nonverbal, and written communication that results in enhanced relationships with colleagues and safer, quality care. Communication between colleagues is known as **collaboration** or *interprofessional practice*. Interprofessional collaboration strengthens health systems and improves client outcomes (NLN Board of Governors, 2015).

Nurses provide valuable input in interprofessional teams and function as leaders in healthcare. Nurses provide leadership during staff meetings, care conferences, project teams, and client support groups. For teams to work well, there must be a sense of trust, a mature way of handling individual and group conflict, group identity, and synergy (Albert et al., 2022). Similar to therapeutic communication, team members need to be clear and brief in their verbal/written communication. RNs need to:

- Assume all members have best intentions
- Use active listening skills
- Praise and inspire
- Be mindful and respectful in interactions
- Know when to speak and when to be silent
- Use open body language
- Be sensitive to nonverbal communication cues of self and others
- Be factual, not emotional

In the common mission to provide individualized, quality care, a team of colleagues may progress through stages. According to Tuckman (1965), these are forming, storming, norming, and performing. Many of the same attributes for the stages of a therapeutic relationship learned as an LPN are similar to these stages (see Table 11.4). A team of

TABLE 11.4 Stages of Team Development Compared to Stages of a Therapeutic Relationship

Stage of Team Development	Stage of a Therapeutic Relationship
Forming—polite but informal; figuring out players and goals	Preinteraction—gathering patient data and planning for a meeting
Storming—power struggles and conflict occur	Orientation—establishing trust, needs determination; identifying problems and suggested outcomes
Norming—getting organized; figuring out rules and confronting problems	Working—stressors analyzed; resistance behaviors explored
Performing—open, honest confrontation and collaboration; respect and quality work	Termination—reviews outcomes and determines effectiveness

Source: Tuckman, B. (1965). Developmental sequences of groups. *Psychology Bulletin, 63*, 384.

BOX 11.6 Qualities of Effective Team Members

- Assume responsibility for their actions.
- Respect and trust others.
- Listen completely to others.
- Provide consistent positive and negative feedback (even when difficult).
- Commit to the goals of the team.
- Build winning alliances.
- Recognize, support, and reward success.

colleagues may dissolve in the storming stage if they do not recognize that conflict is healthy in team building. Box 11.6 lists the necessary qualities of effective team members.

Interaction With Administrators and Providers

Although they are great listeners, today's nurses need skills to effectively communicate in larger interdisciplinary settings. Many agencies now recognize the special contributions that nurses make in safety during client care and the need to provide input into client-centered care (NLN Board of Governors, 2015). Change, in this aspect, should be viewed as an opportunity for nurses rather than an imposition. To continue to develop as leaders in client care, nurses need to:

- Suggest solutions for problems, especially evidence-based ones
- Be self-confident, with high self-esteem
- Be visionary
- Become actively involved

Clear communication with all members of the healthcare team fosters collaboration and continuity of care. Miscommunication is often the root cause of client injury.

TeamSTEPPS Strategies

Nurses can learn, practice, refine assertiveness communication skills, and take part in developing effective teams by participating in TeamSTEPPS. TeamSTEPPS (Team Strategies and Tools to Enhance Performance and Patient Safety) is a teamwork and communication training program designed to improve patient safety and healthcare quality. The program was developed by the Agency for Healthcare Research and Quality (AHRQ) in collaboration with the Department of Defense. The overall goals of TeamSTEPPS are to improve teamwork, enhance communication, promote a culture of safety, and reduce medical errors. TeamSTEPPS training can be customized to fit the specific needs of healthcare organizations and may be delivered through workshops, online courses, or a combination of both (AHRQ, n.d.-a).

SBAR

A widely used strategy to enhance communication included in TeamSTEPPS training is "SBAR." **SBAR**—which stands for situation, background, assessment, and recommendation—is a structured format that can be used to share client information with members of the healthcare team (AHRQ, n.d.-d).

- **S**ituation: Identify yourself, the client, room number, and change in status.
- **B**ackground: Provide relevant background information that relates to the situation.
- **A**ssessment: Offer the nurse's analysis of the source of the problem (critical thinking).
- **R**ecommendation: What would help resolve the situation or problem?

Closed-Loop Communication

Closed-loop communication is another of the strategies included in TeamSTEPPS. Closed loop communication is a method of verifying the sender's verbal message. Closed-loop communication is valuable in situations in which miscommunication can have serious consequences, such as during a code-blue. The strategy is helpful in preventing medical errors and ensuring that orders and procedures are carried out accurately. Closed-loop communications begin with one individual sending a message or instruction to another individual. The message should be clear, concise, and use language that is appropriate for the situation. Upon receiving the message, the receiver acknowledges its receipt. Acknowledgment by nurses includes stating, "I heard you say …" or "I hear the order as …." After receiving acknowledgment from the receiver, the sender confirms that the acknowledgment of the message is the intended message. This important step ensures that there are no misunderstandings or misinterpretations (AHRQ, n.d.-b).

CUS

Another tool included in TeamSTEPPS training that is highly useful for nurses in building communication skills is CUS—I am **C**oncerned, I am **U**ncomfortable, This is a **S**afety Issue. The CUS technique provides a tool for advocacy, assertion, and mutual support. Using CUS phrasing provides members of the healthcare team with a clear message about a concern (AHRQ, n.d.-c). See the below for an example.

EXAMPLE 11.6 CUS

"I'm **C**oncerned that Mr. M is deteriorating. I'm **U**ncomfortable that he is behaving strangely. I believe he is not **S**afe and that he may have something serious happening that is being missed."

ASSERTIVENESS IN COMMUNICATION

Assertiveness is the ability to advocate for oneself and others using direct, honest, and open dialogue. Assertiveness behaviors have many of the same attributes as caring communication. An assertive communication style is open, honest, direct, and confident. Strong assertiveness skills enable the nurse to express emotions, including anger and frustration, in a positive manner that focuses on cooperation and problem resolution. Nurses that use an avoidance style in resolution of conflict have a higher level of personal stress, which can undermine quality care (Folse, 2023).

Assertive communication fosters a win/win situation where both parties mediate for a positive outcome.

Although there can be negative results from aggressive behaviors in communication, when nurses learn assertive behaviors, there are positive outcomes (Table 11.5).

TABLE 11.5 Benefits of Assertive Behavior

Benefit	Explanation
Decreases stress and anxiety	Because your needs are openly expressed
Decreases the use of brain power	Because you do not ruminate over problems
Increases respect	Because colleagues and other workers engage in open and transparent communication
Withdraws the invitation for aggression	Because you are standing up for your needs
Increases achievement	Because your needs are clear
Promotes team spirit	Because you are enhancing win/win situations

Assertiveness can be learned through observation of skilled mentors and leaders, workshops, and reading. To promote assertive behaviors in communication, you, as a nurse, can:

- Describe the specific instance that violated your sense of "fair play"
- Express your feelings
- Specify the action or change needed
- Concentrate on the desired results

Assertiveness Versus Aggressiveness

Many nurses do not differentiate between assertive and aggressive behaviors and mistakenly define assertiveness as being pushy. Aggressive communication focuses more on the selfish needs of an individual. There is an "I want … I deserve" underlying communication. In aggressive communication, there is a winner and a loser. An aggressive individual dominates the discussion and rarely strives to understand the position or emotions of anyone other than themselves. Aggressive behaviors result in angry, hostile, or offended colleagues and coworkers. For a comparison of aggressive and assertive behaviors, see Table 11.6.

BULLYING AND INCIVILITY

Bullying (also referred to as horizontal violence) and **incivility** can have a severe negative impact upon the care of clients. According to Folse (2023), the disruptive and rude behavior that occurs with incivility may include gossiping, disrespectful behaviors, refusal to assist colleagues, intimidation, omitting information, and negative nonverbal actions (eye-rolling, arm-crossing). Incivility and bullying can take place between many different roles and relationships in healthcare. Lateral or horizontal violence between healthcare staff can create a toxic environment that damages staff morale, increases staff turnover, and eventually leads to poor client outcomes. Those in leadership roles may misuse their authority by removing or adding responsibilities and/or patient assignments unfairly, using threats of retaliation, and accommodating some staff but not others due to personal bias.

If not addressed, *bullying*—the harmful offensive actions intended to humiliate another—may escalate into dangerous or threatening circumstances, causing psychological or emotional distress. There is a willful intent to deprive an individual of their dignity. Although uncivil behaviors can be habitual in nature and nurses are sometimes

TABLE 11.6 Comparison of Aggressive and Assertive Behaviors

Aggressive	Assertive
"I want …"	"We need …"
"I win, you lose."	"I win, you win."
Dominates the discussion	Listens to others
Says one thing verbally and conveys the opposite nonverbally	Congruency between verbal and nonverbal behaviors
Controlling	Cooperating
Fault finding	Nonaccusatory focus (focuses on behavior, not personality)
Only strives to be understood	Strives for mutual understanding
Focuses on blaming the other person	Focuses on problem resolution

reluctant to speak up, nurses have the power to turn a toxic environment into a healthy workplace by following the six standards established by the American Association of Critical Care Nurses (n.d.):

- Skilled communication
- True collaboration
- Effective decision-making
- Appropriate staffing
- Meaningful recognition
- Authentic leadership

Nurses must recognize horizontal violence and take action on behalf of colleagues who are experiencing it. A solid base for fostering a positive workplace culture includes orientation programs that provide examples of appropriate behaviors and information about how to identify harmful behaviors in themselves and in colleagues. To establish a healthy working environment, conflict management training including instruction on how to identify and defend against horizontal violence, should be regular content in continuing staff education. Although one-on-one conflict resolution is encouraged for instances of bullying, healthcare organizations must also provide a mechanism for nurses to confidentially report bullying (Folse, 2023).

The American Nurses Association (ANA) Position Statement on Incivility, Bullying, and Workplace Violence (ANA, 2015) is still relevant today. It states that all nurses across the healthcare continuum are responsible for creating healthy and safe work environments for all members of the healthcare team.

DE-ESCALATION OF HIGH-STRESS SITUATIONS

Strong protocols have been in place for a long time in hospitals and health systems to identify and to prevent violence against team members. Unfortunately, workplace violence has increased in the healthcare setting since the start of the COVID-19 outbreak. The pandemic strained the healthcare system as a whole, and in some cases, patients, guests, and family members attacked medical workers, endangering their capacity to offer care. When nurses and doctors are concerned for their own safety, preoccupied with disruptive patients and family members, or traumatized by earlier violent encounters, they are unable to give focused treatment. Violent encounters at medical facilities also waste resources and delay other patients' desperately needed care (American Hospital Association, 2023).

Despite the prevalence of workplace violence and its negative impacts on healthcare systems, no federal laws shield workers in the healthcare industry from harassment or assault on the job. In response to the growing trend of violence in medical facilities, nurses may want to be trained in **de-escalation**, which is the application of methods and tactics to lessen or stop the escalation of a potentially violent situation.

The goals of de-escalation are to defuse tension, encourage communication, and protect everyone involved without resorting to physical force or violence. Because it can be difficult to remain composed and productive in high-stress situations, violence de-escalation requires training and practice. The Cybersecurity and Infrastructure Security Agency (n.d.) lists the following key principles and strategies for violence de-escalation:

- Maintain calm and composure.
- Actively listen.
- Practice empathetic communication.

- Use nonthreatening body language.
- Respect personal space.
- Offer options.
- Stay patient.
- Know your limits.
- Call for assistance.

Different situations may require different tactics. The ultimate goal is to settle disputes peacefully and to safeguard the well-being of everyone involved.

DELEGATION

Delegation is the transfer of responsibility for the performance of an activity from one individual to another, while retaining accountability for the outcome (National council of State Boards of Nursing [NCSBN] and American Nurses Association [ANA], 2019). Nurses must use all communication skills, team building concepts, and assertiveness when delegating to others in the healthcare team. In today's environment of cost cutting and nurse shortages, the nurse must be able to (1) delegate to the appropriate personnel, (2) delegate tasks that those personnel have been trained to perform, (3) identify routine circumstances for delegation, (4) provide the delegate with appropriate direction and communication regarding the task at hand, and (5) provide suitable supervision in accordance with state law. See Box 11.7 for definitions of terms associated with delegation.

As an LPN, by law, you are a dependent practitioner supervised by an RN, advanced practice nurse, or other independent healthcare practitioner. That is, you are delegated work by your supervisory healthcare professional, who is ultimately accountable for your actions. In your role transition, you will delegate but remain accountable for the outcomes of the actions of UAPs or other licensed personnel. Therefore, your scope and responsibilities will be much broader, greater, and more complex.

The steps of delegation (NCSBN, 2016) closely resemble the steps of the nursing process (see Table 11.7).

The first step in the delegation process is to determine (assess) the correct person for a task. Depending on the place of employment, the person who helps the nurse can be called a nurse's aide, a support technician, or a care partner. Regardless of the terminology used, nursing organizations clearly outline that the UAPs are in place to support the RN's or LPN's practice but are not a substitute for their professional scope of practice or judgment.

BOX 11.7

Terms Associated With Delegation

Accountability: Being responsible for the actions and/or lack of actions of oneself and others

Assignment: Task or skill for which a UAP, LPN/LVN, or RN is responsible

Delegation: Assignment of responsibility for a task from one person to another; the delegator is responsible for the outcome of this assignment

Unlicensed assisted personnel (UAP): Any unlicensed person to whom a task is delegated

Responsible: Liable to be called to answer for the actions of oneself or others

Supervision: Directing, watching, evaluating, and correcting the actions of others

TABLE 11.7 The Nursing Process and the Five Rights of Delegation

Nursing Process	Five Rights of Delegation
Assessment	Person (Who)
Plan	Task (What)
	Circumstance (When)
Implementation	Direction/Communication (Where)
Evaluation	Supervision

Source: The National Council of State Boards of Nursing and American Nurses Association. (2019). *National guidelines for nursing delegation.* Retrieved from https://www.ncsbn.org/public-files/NGND-PosPaper_06.pdf

For wise delegation, the nurse must link the right person to the right task. In assigning a task, the RN must be aware that it is the task, not the responsibility and accountability for the outcome, that is being delegated. Matching the appropriate person to the task is critical for quality care.

The nurse must be sensitive to the needs of the UAP when creating a delegated assignment. Evidence demonstrates that effective communication promotes successful delegation (NCSBN, 2016). Applying the same principles of communication discussed previously, the RN must take the time to give CLEAR direction to that individual. CLEAR is an acronym that may help you remember the steps for promoting clear communication (see Box 11.8).

The nurse may not delegate to a UAP, student, or licensed person who lacks training or the ability to perform a skill safely. This becomes a real concern when there are float personnel or unfamiliar personnel working with the RN or when staffing is inadequate. As the nurse, you should always take the time to assess the level of training of an individual you do not know, having them restate the assignment and their ability to do that task. Not all tasks should be delegated. If the task has the potential for harm, involves complex assessments and skills, requires critical thinking or problem-solving, and has an unpredictable outcome, the nurse should not delegate the task.

There may be circumstances that dictate that delegation is inappropriate. The RN can delegate only those tasks that are within the realm of agency policies and job descriptions. Tasks must be routine and must be within the UAP's educational training and experience level. An example of how a circumstance would change a routine task that is usually delegated to a UAP would be that of a glucose finger stick for a client with diabetes. Routinely, in many healthcare institutions, finger stick glucose testing is delegated to UAPs. However, for many clients with diabetes, glucose finger stick results are unpredictable and can frequently be out of acceptable range, making it necessary for the RN to immediately intervene. Because of the unpredictability of glucose finger sticks for such clients, the task of finger stick glucose testing should be done by RNs. UAPs do

---

BOX 11.8

CLEAR Communication With a UAP

C: Clearly and simply outline the task.
L: Legally know what is within the UAP's job description.
E: Eagerly praise positive behaviors.
A: Acknowledge contributions and confidentially resolve differences.
R: Respect the individual's individuality.

not have the scope of practice to be assigned tasks that produce unpredictable outcomes, and therefore, the RN must assume responsibility for the client.

The final step in the five elements of delegation is supervision and evaluation. Although the nurse delegates an appropriate task to the right person using the correct communication style, it is also the nurse's responsibility to confirm that the task has been completed and evaluated. When delegation is successful, tasks are completed safely, in a timely manner, and satisfactorily to everyone involved. When delegation is unsuccessful and the outcome is different from the one predicted, then—similar to the nursing process—the delegation process needs to be evaluated, and the process starts over from the beginning. The nurse must frequently and periodically ask for feedback from the UAP and/or LPN/LVN. More frequent feedback is required when the UAP has limited experience and/or the UAP is unfamiliar to the nurse. It is important to remember that to provide efficient and safe care, tasks can and should be delegated; however, the responsibility to ensure that tasks are assigned appropriately lies in the scope of the RN's practice.

CONCLUSION

Nursing communication is a multifaceted skill that involves verbal and nonverbal communication, empathy, cultural sensitivity, and the ability to collaborate with a diverse team of healthcare professionals. Effective communication is vital for providing high-quality client care, promoting client safety, and enhancing the overall client experience.

STUDENT *Exercises*

Exercise 11.1
Consider the following scenario:
Jane Frederick, RN, is caring for Mr. N., a client who recently received a diagnosis of acute leukemia. As Jane enters the room, Mr. N. is sitting on the side of the bed, staring vacantly into space. His bathwater and his washcloth are unused. When she says "Hello," he does not respond. She stands by his bedside looking at her assignment sheet. Without looking at Mr. N., she asks, "How's the appetite?" A soft "Okay" in a monotone voice is the reply. "Have you had a BM?" The nurse is still not looking at him. "Yes." Mr. N.'s low monotone voice and vacant stare continue. Jane Frederick asks to listen to heart and breath sounds, quickly glancing at him. She documents her findings on the room's computer. "Looks good," she says and leaves the room.

1. Describe the nonverbal communication of nurse and client.
2. Identify the barriers to communication demonstrated by the nurse.
3. Suggest some verbal and nonverbal techniques the nurse could have used to encourage Mr. N. to verbalize his concerns.

Exercise 11.2
Consider the following scenario:
Student nurse Coletta Reese reports to her charge nurse before going off duty. Coletta states, "Mrs. Jones slept a little. She had chest pain twice, and ate very little lunch. She received a PRN medication and weighed 110 lb."

1. Using an SBAR approach, discuss some areas the nursing student omitted in her report. Why do you think these areas were omitted?
2. Suggest some therapeutic techniques the nursing student might have used to elicit the needed data from Mrs. Jones.
3. Write the response you would use if you were the charge nurse to help the nursing student elicit the needed information.

Exercise 11.3
Consider the following scenario:
You have been working hard on a new cost-cutting measure to reduce lost client charges on your unit. You have presented many good ideas to the nurse manager. Your nurse manager asks you to volunteer for a committee forming in the hospital composed of administrators and providers. She wants you to share your ideas in this committee.

1. You are really afraid of making a fool of yourself but want to share your proposal. Using the information in this chapter about interactions with administrators, outline a plan of how you will present your proposals.
2. During the meeting, one of the providers challenges you on your ideas. You feel yourself getting red and angry. Using assertiveness techniques, how can you change this to a win/win situation?

Exercise 11.4
Consider the following scenario:
A new UAP has had 3 weeks of hospital orientation and had previously been coassigned with an experienced UAP. Now assigned to your unit, she seems shy but eager to learn. For four stable clients, you assign her the vital signs, glucose sticks, and morning care. Midway through the morning, she comes to you in tears stating that she is having a bad day and wants to quit.

1. Using communication skills, explain how you can find out what is happening to this UAP and suggest ways to help you both manage the day.
2. Applying the five steps of delegation, what measures could you have taken to ensure that the UAP had a positive experience?

REFERENCES

Agency for Healthcare Research and Quality. (n.d.-a). *TeamSTEPPS*. U.S. Department of Health & Human Services. Retrieved from https://www.ahrq.gov/teamstepps-program/index.html

Agency for Healthcare Research and Quality. (n.d.-b). *Tool: Closed-loop communication*. U.S. Department of Health & Human Services. Retrieved from https://www.ahrq.gov/teamstepps-program/curriculum/communication/tools/loop.html

Agency for Healthcare Research and Quality. (n.d.-c). *Tool: CUS*. U.S. Department of Health & Human Services. Retrieved from https://www.ahrq.gov/teamstepps-program/curriculum/mutual/tools/cus.html

Agency for Healthcare Research and Quality. (n.d.-d). *Tools: SBAR*. U.S. Department of Health & Human Services. Retrieved from https://www.ahrq.gov/teamstepps-program/curriculum/communication/tools/sbar.html

Albert, N. M., Pappas, S. H., O'Grady, T. P., & Malloch, K. (2022). *Quantum leadership: Creating sustainable value in health care* (6th ed.).

American Association of Critical Care Nurses. (n.d.). *Healthy work environments*. https://www.aacn.org/nursing-excellence/healthy-work-environments

American Hospital Association. (2023). *Fact sheet: Workplace violence and intimidation, and the need for a federal legislative response.* https://www.aha.org/system/files/media/file/2022/09/Fact-Sheet-Workplace-Violence-and-Intimidation-and-the-Need-for-a-Federal-Legislative-Response.pdf
American Nurses Association. (2015). *American Nurses Association position statement on incivility, bullying, and workplace violence.* https://www.nursingworld.org/~49d6e3/globalassets/practiceandpolicy/nursing-excellence/incivility-bullying-and-workplace-violence--ana-position-statement.pdf
Berlo, D. (1960). *The process of communication: An introduction to theory and practice.* Holt, Reinhart and Winston.
Boggs, K. U. (2022). *Interpersonal relationships: Professional communication skills for nurses* (9th ed.). Elsevier.
Catalano, J. (2020). *Nursing now: Today's issues, tomorrow's trends* (8th ed.). F. A. Davis.
Chen, J., Peng, W., & Han, L. (2023). The trickle-down effect of leader mindfulness on employee creative deviance behavior: A moderated mediation model. *Social Behavior and Personality, 51*(9), 1–13. 10.2224/sbp.12574
Cousins, N. (1983). *Anatomy of an illness: As perceived by the patient.* Norton.
Cybersecurity & Infrastructure Security Agency. (n.d.). *De-Escalation: How you can help defuse potentially violent situations.* U.S. Department of Homeland Security. https://www.cisa.gov/sites/default/files/2022-11/De-Escalation_Final%20508%20%2809.21.21%29.pdf
Darwin, C. (1872). *The expression of emotions in man and animals.* John Murray.
Folse, V. N. (2023). Communication and conflict. In P. S. Yoder-Wise & S. Sportsman (Eds.), *Leading and managing in nursing* (8th ed., pp. 178–197). Elsevier.
Fosbre, C. D., & Varcarolis, E. M. (2023). *Varcarolis' essentials of psychiatric mental health nursing: A communication approach to evidence-based care* (5th ed.). Elsevier.
Horowitz, J. A., & Kellogg, M. B. (2022). Stress management. In C. L. Edelman & C. L. Mandle (Eds.), *Health promotion throughout the life span* (10th ed., pp. 330–353). Elsevier.
National Council of State Boards of Nursing and American Nurses Association. (2019). *National guidelines for nursing delegation.* Retrieved from https://www.ncsbn.org/public-files/NGND-PosPaper_06.pdf
National League for Nursing Board of Governors. (2015). *Interprofessional collaboration in education and practice: A living document from the National League for Nursing.* Retrieved from https://www.nln.org/docs/default-source/uploadedfiles/default-document-library/ipe-ipp-vision.pdf?sfvrsn=70c8d10d_0
Potter, P., Perry, A., Stockert, P., & Hall, A. (2023). *Fundamentals of nursing* (11th ed.). Elsevier.
Rosdahl, C. (2022). *Rosdahl's textbook of basic nursing* (12th ed.). Wolters Kluwer.
Taylor, C., Lynn, P., & Bartlett, J. L. (2023). *Fundamentals of nursing: The art and science of nursing care* (10th ed.). Wolters Kluwer.
Tuckman, B. (1965). Developmental sequences of groups. *Psychology Bulletin, 63,* 384.
Zalon, M. L. (2023). Person-centered care. In P. S. Yoder-Wise & S. Sportsman (Eds.), *Leading and managing in nursing* (8th ed., pp. 217–243). Elsevier.

SUGGESTED READING

Riley, J. (2024). *Communication in nursing* (10th ed.). Elsevier.

On the WEB

Agency for Healthcare Research and Quality (AHRQ)—Team building information and resources for healthcare professionals: https://www.ahrq.gov/teamstepps/index.html

Association for Applied and Therapeutic Humor: https://www.aath.org/humoracademy

Institute for Healthcare Improvement—SBAR Toolkit: http://www.ihi.org/resources/Pages/Tools/sbartoolkit.aspx

National League for Nursing—Interprofessional Education Resources Page: https://www.nln.org/education/teaching-resources/professional-development-programsteaching-resources/interprofessional-education-ipe-e0e2b35c-7836-6c70-9642-ff00005f0421

Nursinghelp—An example of a student process recording on the web: https://nursinghelp.wordpress.com/med-surg/process-recording/

Quizlet—flash cards that students can make to study therapeutic relationships: https://www.quizlet.com/88556367/nur-131-therapeutic-relationships-varcarolis-flash-cards/

U.S. Department of Veterans Affairs—The Healing Benefits of Humor and Laughter: https://www.va.gov/WHOLEHEALTHLIBRARY/tools/healing-benefits-humor-laughter.asp

Wiki—How to talk to patients: http://www.wikihow.com/Talk-to-Patients

The Nurse as Teacher

CHAPTER 12

LEARNING OUTCOMES

By the end of this chapter, the student will be able to:
1. Explain the challenge of client education as a nursing responsibility.
2. Describe the differences between teaching and learning.
3. Apply principles of teaching to client education.
4. Describe internal and external influences that affect client learning.
5. Identify teaching methods appropriate for cognitive, affective, and psychomotor learning.
6. Compare and contrast the teaching–learning process to the nursing process.
7. Identify assessment data necessary to determine client learning needs.
8. Formulate nursing diagnoses for identified client learning needs.
9. Outline the essential components of a teaching plan.
10. Describe how to implement client education.
11. Explain how to evaluate client education.
12. Discuss the essential elements of documenting client education.

KEY TERMS

affective learning objectives	learning	pedagogy
andragogy	learning style:	psychomotor learning objectives
cognitive learning objectives	• auditory	reinforcement
functional literacy	• kinesthetic	teaching
health literacy	• visual	
	motivation	
	partnering	

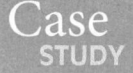

Case STUDY

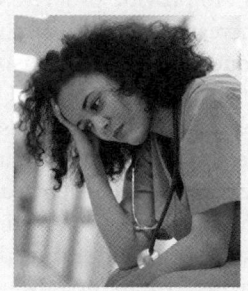

Mary has been an LVN for 2 years and has just graduated from an ADN program. She is working on a busy medical-surgical unit with an LPN and two UAPs. Mary enters the nursing station at 10 AM and sits down, looking tired and overwhelmed.

MARY: How am I going to teach my patients anything when there isn't enough time?

ALICE (PATIENT CARE COORDINATOR): You look frustrated; how can I help?

287

MARY: Mr. Martinez in 203 isn't doing well with his insulin injections because he doesn't understand English. And he's going home today. Mrs. Duncan is going into surgery in 1 hour, and I haven't taught her how to deep breathe and cough yet. Mr. James is upset about the medication changes Dr. Lotte made and won't take his new BP medications until he knows why they've been changed. Mr. Willis is afraid to take his wife home tomorrow because he can't move her himself. I need to change Mrs. Lewis's dressing, but Dr. Craig has ordered a new IV antibiotic, and her IV is infiltrated. Sometime this morning, I have to irrigate Mr. Martin's colostomy! Teaching was one of my strong points in school. Now, dashing from room to room, I barely have time to explain things to patients. My LPN and my UAPs can't help with patient teaching.

ALICE: Yes, it's hard to make time when busy, and the importance of teaching is getting greater. Teaching begins on admission and should be thought of as a process. We will be getting electronic tools to help everyone next week; they'll help personalize education and documentation.

However, you still will have to evaluate the outcomes of your teaching.

MARY: That sounds good—I definitely need something to help!

ALICE: Yes, you do. As for today: Mr. Lewis is your priority. I have time, so I'll restart that IV and hang the antibiotic. We can use the phone interpreter service for Mr. Martinez, but I know his wife has been partnering in his care, so we can use her help with the diabetic educator. Dr. Lotte will be rounding soon; we can make him aware of Mr. James's issue. PT will be helping Mr. Willis within the hour. This will leave you free to help Mrs. Duncan and then irrigate that colostomy.

MARY: Thanks, Alice. I sure appreciate the help.

THE CHALLENGE OF CLIENT EDUCATION

Mary is correct to be concerned about her client teaching. **Partnering** with the client is an expectation of the role of the RN in helping and empowering clients to assume self-care (Hood, 2021). Teaching is such an important legal and professional nursing role that teaching responsibilities are included in most state nurse practice acts, in professional organization standards, and may also be required for reimbursement. Nurses who fail to provide proper client education are negligent in their nursing practice; they also increase their risk of civil liability. Another challenge to completing competent client education is the downsizing of professional nursing staff positions and the substitution of such positions with UAP staff. Although UAPs help with basic physical care, there is less client contact for assessment, and clients can be confused about the roles of their healthcare providers. Nurses are challenged daily by the increasing demands of the work setting to meet their teaching responsibilities. Patients and families are presented with the challenge of managing more complex health problems at home. Learning must now occur in a shorter time than previously was the case, as well as in situations and environments that are not always ideal for learning (Bastable, 2017).

New professionals must have superior communication and documentation skills to make the transition from the healthcare setting to home safer and more efficient for clients like Mr. Martinez and Mr. Duncan. In cases such as that of Mr. Martinez, the nurse must be flexible and open to clients' learning needs, especially needs not previously encountered by the nurse. Nurses like Mary are duty bound to protect client confidentiality; so when clients do not speak English, family members should not be used as interpreters unless the family member is a caregiver and the nurse has the client's consent. Teaching is an intangible part of caring that stays with the client long after the client is discharged.

Research has shown how valuable health teaching is for the healthcare recipient. Health teaching shortens hospital stays, minimizes complications, and reduces symptoms of illness and surgery (Kopec et al., 2023; Ng et al., 2022). Given a partnering client, the extent of client education that can be accomplished is limited only by the depth and breadth of the nurse's knowledge, the constraints of the setting, and the circumstances in which the nurse–client interaction occurs. In each teaching interaction, there is a shared learning experience; although learning is mostly geared toward and designed for the individual client, learning also occurs for the nurse.

TEACHING, LEARNING, AND FUNCTIONAL LITERACY DEFINED

Teaching "is a plan of action to bring about learning" (Miles, 2017, p. 124). Patient education is an ongoing process whereby the nurse organizes experiences in varied ways to facilitate client learning. Clients are partners in their healthcare and are experts in how health issues affect them. When patients can make informed decisions about their care, they feel empowered, increasing feelings of control and hopefulness. Client teaching can be a powerful means of achieving positive nursing outcomes to prevent illness, to promote or restore health, and to facilitate coping with chronic and terminal illness.

Learning is the process in which someone gains knowledge, develops new skills, or measurably modifies their behavior as a result of lived experiences or an event (Taylor et al., 2023). To promote learning, the nurse must apply teaching–learning principles. Learning does not help only the client; with each teaching experience, the nurse enhances their own ability to teach, bringing increased satisfaction to the nursing role.

Functional literacy is the ability to obtain, process, and understand basic information. **Health literacy** is the ability of someone to read and act upon health information. Many healthcare agencies report that a decrease in health literacy is associated with poorer patient outcomes and an increase in healthcare costs (Kopec et al., 2023; Ng et al., 2022).

PRINCIPLES OF TEACHING AND LEARNING

The purpose of client teaching is to ensure safety and optimal quality of life. Principles of teaching and learning provide basic guidelines for the nurse assuming the role of a teacher. The teaching process and principles require the high-quality communication skills presented in Chapter 11. Teaching and learning principles are necessary for planning individualized patient education so that the nurse can select teaching materials and methods that best meet client education needs. The teaching and learning principles are explained in the below subsections and are listed in Box 12.1.

> **BOX 12.1**
>
> **Principles of Teaching and Learning**
> 1. Establish trust.
> 2. Partner with the learner.
> 3. Motivate the client; motivation signifies readiness to learn.
> 4. Customize teaching style to the client's learning style and needs.
> 5. Individualize strategies and materials.
> 6. Capitalize on client strengths and resources.
> 7. Simplify language.
> 8. Consider developmental stage.
> 9. Modify the environment.
> 10. Consider content sequencing.
> 11. Provide repetition and practice.
> 12. Relate new learning experiences to client's past.
> 13. Reinforce newly learned behaviors.

ESTABLISH TRUST

People learn best when they are accepted, understood, and connected to the healthcare provider. For the teaching–learning process to succeed, clients must trust their nurse, and nurses must respect the client's ability to learn. Client attitudes toward teaching vary from pleasant and accepting to hostile, bitter, or rejecting. Also, keep in mind that some clients have learning disabilities.

Nurses must also be aware of their own personal biases and how these affect the teaching–learning process. They must be sensitive to personal attitudes and adapt their teaching approach so that learning can occur (Bastable, 2017).

PARTNER WITH THE LEARNER

The teaching–learning process will be more effective and empowering to the client if the nurse partners with the client in as many aspects of the process as possible. Including the client in the teaching–learning process informs the nurse of what the client is willing and unwilling to do. Partnering is best attained when the nurse and the client agree on outcomes and an action plan. Unless the learning outcomes are centered on what the client values and is willing to achieve, little learning will take place. It is important to assess the client's understanding of the benefits of treatment, the risks for failure to follow healthcare teaching recommendations, and the severity of their condition. The use of active listening techniques and clear, simple language help to establish trust.

MOTIVATE THE CLIENT

Motivation is the internal urge that prompts an individual to act or to modify their behavior (Taylor et al., 2023). Motivation is individualistic; what motivates one individual may not motivate another. One of the principles of adult learning is that of relevancy (Knowles et al., 2020). The client will have less motivation to learn if they believe inapplicable information is being taught. The best-laid plans of the nurse may be ineffective if the targeted learner lacks the motivation to learn.

The nurse needs to identify emotional, physical, and experiential factors that signal a client is able, motivated, and willing to learn. The emotional state of the client can be a motivator to learn or inhibit learning. Emotions such as anxiety, depression, denial, and fear can require a great deal of the client's energy, distracting from learning. However, anxious caregivers of a sick child, for example, may be receptive to learning special techniques that allow them to participate in their child's care, because the immediate need for this information may override the emotions they are feeling.

Assess for physical barriers to learning such as pain, acuity of illness, or prognosis of illness. A client who is in pain, weak, or preoccupied with thoughts about dying may be unable to concentrate on instructions and attend to learning.

A client's experiences, background, skills, knowledge, and attitudes regarding a health situation provide the necessary foundation for developing the teaching plan. Learning is more successful if a client builds upon previous knowledge. A client who has successfully cared for a homebound, frail relative after a stroke may be better able to cope with a spouse convalescing from a heart attack than a client who has always depended on others to care for ill family members.

The NCLEX-RN *Might Ask* 12.1

The nurse is assessing a client's motivation to learn. Which of the following factors could block that client's motivation to learn? (Select all that apply.)

a. Severe pain
b. Successful past experiences
c. Strong family support system
d. A positive attitude
e. Anxiety due to cost of illness

• See Appendix A for correct answer and rationale.

Client attitudes and values can facilitate or inhibit the learning that can be achieved. A client who values independence and is recovering from knee replacement surgery will be more motivated to use a walker and accept direction and help than a person who does not value independence.

CUSTOMIZE TEACHING BASED ON CLIENT'S LEARNING STYLE

A **learning style** is a complex process affected by how individuals respond to varied sensory input and how they perceive, process, and retain information. The nurse must recognize that because each individual has a preferred and effective learning style, learning materials should be presented in varied ways (see Table 12.1). Learning styles include the following (Miles, 2017):

- **Kinesthetic:** Individuals learn by performing tasks or by manipulating new information.
- **Auditory:** Individuals learn by hearing new information.
- **Visual:** Individuals learn by seeing a pictorial presentation of new ideas.

TABLE 12.1 Learning Styles and Effective Methods

Style of Learning	Sense	Example
Kinesthetic	Feeling, touching, and manipulating	Touching ostomy supplies Redressing a wound
Auditory	Listening	Listening to a tape player Listening to a lecture
Visual	Seeing	Reading a booklet or information from the internet
Auditory and visual	Seeing and listening	Watching a video with commentary

A combination of styles addresses diverse learning needs. Nurses are more effective teachers if they ask their client learners how they learn best before teaching begins.

Another aspect of learning style to consider is the client's way of understanding the situation. Some prefer to look at the big picture and then learn about its segments, whereas others like to look at one piece at a time to learn about the whole situation. A client who prefers to see the whole may respond to segmental teaching with the plea, "Would you get to the point; what does all this mean?" A client who likes to consider things segmentally might respond to an explanation of the big picture by saying, "This is very confusing. Can you explain it one step at a time?"

INDIVIDUALIZE TEACHING MATERIALS

Use charts, models, pictures, diagrams, television programs, CDs, DVDs, podcasts, and the internet to enhance learning. Self-study modules, along with small group sessions, can be used effectively in the outpatient setting (Kopec et al., 2023; Ng et al., 2022). However, be careful not to use resources as a substitute for the nurse–client interaction. With less time and fewer resources available, it is common to see instructional pamphlets, CDs, or computer programs used to teach about medical conditions such as diabetes and heart failure, or other topics, such as breast-feeding. Clients such as Mr. Martinez in this chapter's opening case study may not understand written instructions because of language differences or functional illiteracy. Thus, it is important to assess the client's reading ability and fluency in the English language at the onset of a client teaching relationship. If the client is not fluent in English, there are other ways to enhance learning, such as by using patient education materials written in the client's native language.

Some clients are unable to read or write; this can be true of individuals of all ethnicities and socioeconomic levels. U.S. government data from 2017 reveal that 19% of the U.S. population may be considered functionally illiterate in English; they lack the ability to comprehend simple phrases, scan brief texts for specific information, or finish basic forms (National Center for Education Statistics, n.d.-a; National Center for Eduction Statistics, n.d.-c). More than half (54%) of Americans between the ages of 16 and 74 read below the equivalent of a sixth-grade level (National Center for Education Statistics, n.d.-b). Teaching materials need to be developed for people who do not speak English and to people who read at a sixth- to eighth grade reading level.

Nurses should never assume that an individual, even if literate, can read and comprehend translated health literature; the nurse should always assess the client's literacy level when teaching. Direct testing is the best method for assessing client literacy but is not practical in clinical settings. Screening tools, such as the Newest Vital Sign by Pfizer, Inc., are evidence based, can be tactfully used in about 3 minutes to determine literacy, and are available in English and Spanish (see the "On the Web" section at the end of this chapter). A less accurate but more tactful and expedient method might be to observe how the client interacts with paperwork during intake or consent processes; valuable insight can be gained if the client struggles with filling out forms or with reading written instructions. Assess the client for an inability to focus on reading materials, a tendency to focus on detail, a consistent tendency to interpret literature literally, and a lack of ability to concentrate on dominant themes. These are common assessments found in clients who have difficulty reading. In addition, a functionally illiterate client may be slow to return demonstrate skills. Careful, tactful assessment is the key.

Monitor the client's understanding frequently by asking them to return demonstrate or by asking them to verbalize the steps of a task. The teach-back method (see the "On the Web" section at the end of this chapter) is a quick and easy tool for the nurse to use to evaluate teaching methods.

> **The NCLEX-RN *Might Ask* 12.2**
>
> In the home care setting, the nurse is assessing the reading skills of a client with newly diagnosed diabetes. The best way the nurse could assess this skill is by:
> a. asking the client to take a literacy test.
> b. checking the client's type of pleasure reading.
> c. making the client read a complex instruction sheet.
> d. asking the client's husband the last year of school the client completed.
>
> • See Appendix A for correct answer and rationale.

CAPITALIZE ON CLIENT LEARNING STRENGTHS AND RESOURCES

Determine the client's learning strengths and resources to facilitate learning. Client strengths are the internal physical, psychological, social, and spiritual resources a person mobilizes to cope with problems. See Box 12.2 for examples of strengths that nurses can use to develop a teaching plan.

Resources are external forces such as support systems, housing, income, transportation, and education that influence a person's ability to meet their needs. These resources must be considered for teaching to be effective. For example, if Mr. Martinez, the Spanish-speaking client with diabetes from the chapter-opening scenario, has a language barrier and vision loss, he may never achieve a degree of independence in self-injection unless Mary teaches him with these issues in mind. The client Mr. James with hypertension has a limited income and a lack of housing, so he may not be able to comply with the medication regimens and diet modifications that would most effectively control the disease. Because discharge planning begins on admission, nurses would be working as a team to meet the needs of most of the clients in the chapter-opening case study. For example, Mr. Willis will have help from physical therapy if coordinated correctly, and Mr. Martinez and his wife should have regularly scheduled visits by a diabetes educator and translator. Education may need to be carried into the home setting by a bilingual, culturally sensitive community nurse.

> **THINKING CRITICALLY**
>
> Select three clients mentioned in the chapter-opening case study other than Mr. Martinez and Mr. Willis. What resources should you identify that would be useful for these clients?

SIMPLIFY LANGUAGE

Take into consideration the client's fluency with the English language, level of education, learning style, and emotional state when deciding what vocabulary to use in teaching. Be sensitive to the client's unfamiliarity with medical terms and jargon. Simplify terms

BOX 12.2 Examples of Client Strengths

Physical Strengths
Maintains good health through daily exercise
Moves about with ease
Maintains skin integrity
Sleeps well
Eats a nutritional diet
Breathes effectively
Has stable blood pressure
Is independent in activities of daily living

Psychological Strengths
Resolves developmental tasks favorably
Demonstrates positive problem-solving skills
Verbalizes confidence in philosophy of life
Expresses knowledge about health condition
Uses humor appropriately
Shows insight into personal situations
Communicates willingness to learn
Reports ability to cope with health concerns
Verbalizes positive feelings of self-esteem

Spiritual Strengths
Actively participates in religious or spiritual rituals
Expresses spiritual peace
Verbalizes confidence in religion or spirituality

Social Strengths
Relates well with spouse, significant other, children, and others
Has a strong support system
Uses personal/family resources appropriately
Seeks out appropriate healthcare resources (e.g., online resources, support groups, health club)
Accepts help from family and friends
Is a dedicated employee
Contributes to financial security of family

---

you normally use, such as say "walk" instead of "ambulation," and try to use terminology with which the client is familiar. If a client does not speak English well, the nurse should obtain a translator to assist with the instruction. A family members or a friend should not be used as an interpreter unless the patient has given specific permission for this arrangement.

Use analogies, comparisons, examples, and illustrations to promote understanding. Common analogies include comparison of the heart to a pump, the bladder to a reservoir tank, the eyes to a camera lens, a heart valve anomaly to a leaking washer, and a joint to a hinge.

Healthcare literacy for patients with limited English proficiency can be improved by providing written materials in the client's native language and interpreters, as needed, to facilitate effective communication. Teaching materials and methods should be inclusive, using diverse images, examples, and stories to reflect the varied patient population. Ensure that all patients have access to educational resources, including printed materials, online resources, and tools that are affordable and easy to understand.

Promoting diversity and equity in patient teaching is essential to ensure that all patients receive high-quality healthcare education and information, regardless of their background, identity, or socioeconomic status. Nurses should work to recognize and to mitigate implicit biases that may affect their interactions with patients from diverse backgrounds. (For more on cultural competence and cultural humility, see Chapter 13.)

CONSIDER DEVELOPMENTAL STAGE AND GENDER

To individualize teaching and to ensure optimum learning, consider the client's developmental level and gender when planning client teaching.

Developmental Stage

Pedagogy is the art and science of teaching methods. Children and adolescents have varying limitations in attention, concentration, and cognitive and psychomotor skills related to developmental level (Table 12.2).

Andragogy is the study of how adults learn (Knowles et al., 2020). Adults are generally motivated learners but often lead busy lives and/or lack the self-confidence to try something new. Adults also learn best when they see a clear and immediate need for information to be integrated into their lifestyle.

The process of aging changes many neurosensory body systems. The older adult may have hearing and visual impairments and reduced motor abilities. If the client has difficulty understanding you, shorten the length of the teaching session, establish priorities for teaching the information, and repeat the material as necessary. Box 12.3 provides techniques for promoting learning when teaching the older adult.

TABLE 12.2 Learning Aids for Children, Adolescents, and Adults

Children	Adolescents	Adults
• Work at the eye level of the child. • Check the child's developmental level, which may differ from their age. • Assess self-care abilities. • Use dolls, dress-up, or imitation. • Use video, video games, and computer interactives. • Use simple terms. • Use frequent and consistent repetition and reinforcement. • Use short sessions because children have short attention spans.	• Earn respect by matching words with actions. • Seek input and opinion, and engage the adolescent in problem-solving. • Explore the feelings of the adolescent. • Assess how health problems affect the adolescent's interactions with peers. • Assess and accentuate positive qualities. • Make language clear and health related. • Encourage independence and informed choice. • Use reputable social media to help learning.	• Motivated by what is needed to know to function. • Come with experience and knowledge to build upon. • Are problem oriented rather than subject oriented. • Need to know why they are learning something. • May like to socialize and learn in groups. • Assess use of internet and social media for learning.

> **BOX 12.3** **Tips for Enhanced Learning in Older Adults**
> 1. Make client comfortable.
> 2. Assess developmental level, motivation, readiness to learn, anxiety, depression, and motor abilities.
> 3. Present materials at learner's pace.
> 4. Give frequent feedback.
> 5. Shorten sentences.
> 6. Use gestures.
> 7. Ensure adequate lighting.
> 8. Decrease distractions.

For people with a learning disability, nurses should use visual aids and gestures, simplify information, and speak in short sentences. It may be necessary to ask family members to carry out more complicated regimens and to reinforce provided information.

Gender

When planning patient education, consider possible gender-specific differences. There is a need to be more focused on health promotional initiatives when addressing men's health challenges (Ballering et al., 2023; Petrie et al., 2022). Men may not access healthcare systems as frequently as women; the social stigma of seeking assistance along with the stereotypical male-fostered "man as protector" image may contribute to a lack of important education on subjects such as prostate and testicular cancers and other men's health issues (Mursa et al., 2022). It is important that health education be accessible yet confidential. An outreach program or clinic attempting to reach out to men may be more successful if it is conducted at a sporting event or another type of event traditionally attended by men.

MODIFY THE ENVIRONMENT

Determine environmental factors that influence client learning. Careful attention should be paid to time constraints, the physical environment, client activity schedules, and client privacy. For example, during the morning medication period, it may be unrealistic for a nurse to give instructions for self-injection to a patient with diabetes. Like Mary, when the nurse is rushed and responsible for so many tasks, teaching becomes rushed. Closing doors and turning off distractions help the nurse and client focus on the needed learning.

If a client's learning needs can be anticipated, such as relaxation techniques for childbirth or preoperative instructions, the nurse could arrange for the client to come in for more focused instruction in advance of their time in the hospital. Or perhaps home care visitation could be scheduled at a time when the client is free to meet the care provider, who can then be an additional resource for the client. The nurse uses multiple resources to skillfully enhance teaching and learning.

SEQUENCE THE SERIES OF INSTRUCTIONS

Plan a series of instructions that builds on previous knowledge and lays the groundwork for future learning. Teach from easy to difficult, known to unknown, well to ill, normal to abnormal, and step by step for complicated topics.

Instruction in self-injection of insulin and then about routine glucose monitoring at home is an example of sequential instruction. Clients are first taught about the insulin and then the steps in preparing the injection, and finally, they are taught the injection technique.

When teaching a client to perform blood glucose testing, set up a sequence that begins with the purpose of testing and then progresses through equipment operation and maintenance, the testing procedure, and finally quality assurance and troubleshooting problems. Similar to your training as a student, such sequencing of complex procedural steps leads to optimal learning. Access to computerized teaching plans and training tools that can be adapted for uniqueness, such as the one Mary's unit will be implementing, will help nurses clearly document progress and communicate with everyone on the healthcare team.

PROVIDE REPETITION AND PRACTICE

Repeat, summarize, and ask questions after each segment of instruction. Reviewing material covered in previous teaching sessions or during an earlier segment of the teaching period reinforces the learning, rewards the client, and helps the nurse evaluate learning. To provide motivation and to enhance incentive, reinforce small successes.

Provide frequent and repeated opportunities to practice new skills, especially with adults, because adult learners learn by doing. Generally, several practice sessions spaced over a period of time are more effective than one long practice session, during which client fatigue may impede performance. Also, having the client review self-paced computerized modules or booklets will not replace nursing education but can make learning more effective, consistent, and efficient.

RELATE NEW LEARNING TO PAST EXPERIENCES

At all developmental levels, keep in mind that, new learning is affected by a client's previous life experiences. Use the knowledge of the client or family as a base on which to build. For example, you may use a garden hose as an analogy for blood pressure if the client is a gardener or the analogy of flushing a radiator to describe how to prime an intravenous line if the client works on cars.

Be alert for the client who mentioned they had a previous bad experience in the healthcare setting. In this event, the entire team will have to work harder to win trust and to accomplish outcomes.

REINFORCE NEWLY LEARNED BEHAVIORS

Reinforcement is a reward that strengthens the possibility that the behavior will occur again (Bastable, 2017). A smile, a kind gesture, or words of encouragement when the client achieves the desired learning objective are all examples of reinforces. The type of reward should be appropriate to the client and should immediately follow the desired behavioral response. For example, a nurse might provide reinforcement for a child with diabetes who correctly self-administering an insulin injection by providing them with a favorite computer game, whereas verbal praise and a smile would be more appropriate for an older adult client who has diabetes.

THINKING CRITICALLY

Access the websites on teach-back training and the newest vital sign mentioned in the "On the Web" section at the end of this chapter. Write down how you would apply these and the principles of teaching–learning to the patients Mary is assigned in the chapter-opening case study, discuss in small groups with your classmates, and formulate an ideal approach for these clients.

TEACHING INTERVENTIONS

The nurse uses a variety of teaching strategies to meet the client's learning needs (Box 12.4). Choosing the right strategy, based on a thorough assessment of the client's learning style and mutually acceptable goals, will make the experience enjoyable and effective for both the client and the nurse. The nurse should incorporate teaching methods that actively engage the client in learning and that continuously assess the patient's understanding and progress throughout the teaching process. The method or strategy chosen depends not only on the setting in which teaching will occur but also the type of learning that needs to take place. Encourage questions, discussion, and hands-on activities to promote active participation and to enhance understanding. Use feedback from the client to adjust the teaching strategy as necessary and to address any areas of confusion or misunderstanding. If the use of one learning domain (cognitive, affective, or psychomotor) is unsuccessful, changing or combining modalities—such as seeing, doing, and hearing—may achieve the desired learning outcome. The following subsections discuss these strategies.

COGNITIVE (KNOWLEDGE)

Lecture

Lectures are an effective and efficient way to teach groups. The lecture approach works well with people who are seeking information on common healthcare issues such as diabetes management, prenatal care, and infant care. Lectures with audience participation can draw on the diversity of members of the healthcare team, providing the listener with new perspectives and interests.

One of the problems inherent in the lecture format is that it does not usually promote active participation. The nurse should not confuse telling with learning. When using the lecture technique, the nurse cannot be sure that learning is taking place unless the group is actively engaged or some evaluation occurs. Lectures are less effective in most acute care hospital settings, in which the ill client needs shorter and more individualized instruction.

BOX 12.4

Teaching Strategies for the Clinical Setting

Cognitive (Knowledge)
Lecture
Independent study (reading, CD viewing, self-paced modules, computerized learning)

Affective (Values)
Discussion
Values clarification
Role-playing
Role modeling
Simulation

Psychomotor (Skill)
Demonstration/return demonstration
Guided practice
Independent practice

Independent Study

Many adults are independent learners and prefer self-paced learning through independent study of printed, audiovisual, or online resource materials. The internet has become a popular resource for health information. Although there are many excellent resources online, there is also much misinformation regarding healthcare. It would be helpful for the nurse to show the client the more reputable sites as well as showing them which unreputable sites to avoid.

Independent study should not be used in isolation but as a stimulus or a precursor to a nurse–client learning interaction and evaluation of outcomes. Allowing a client to view a program on breast-feeding before a discussion or the nurse-directed experience of feeding a newborn can spark client questions and make the nurse–client interaction more successful. Careful assessment of client literacy, language, and healthcare resources should always be considered when using independent study materials. The nurse should be familiar with available resources in their area of expertise and can be helpful in showing the client where those sources may be obtained (Box 12.5).

AFFECTIVE (VALUES)

Discussion

Discussion is useful for individual or group instruction in classroom, home, or community situations. Teacher and learner discussions commonly involve the exchange of information, ideas, and feelings during brief encounters, such as while preparing a patient for a diagnostic procedure or when the nurse administers medications. Nurses involved with family support groups and organizations such as stroke and ostomy clubs also frequently use this approach.

> **THINKING CRITICALLY**
> Would the learning needs of the clients in the chapter-opening case study be best met by a discussion approach or a lecture approach? Explain.

Values Clarification

Encouraging clients to explore and identify their values about health, sickness, and healthcare issues helps remove barriers to learning new or different approaches to managing health and illness. Identification of values in different aspects of a client's life might serve as a stimulus for changing behaviors in healthcare practices. Depending on the client's interests, a nurse might help a client understand the importance of routine

---

BOX 12.5 **Effective Internet Use for Patient Education**

1. Assess the client's computer access and computer literacy.
2. Explain that not all online resources are current or accurate.
3. Encourage the client/family to print/save resources and use them as a basis of discussion with the healthcare educator.
4. Counsel use of reputable internet sources prior to making informed decisions.

follow-up visits for hypertension by comparing it to routine maintenance of a classic car or the health maintenance of a pet.

Role-Playing

Acting out feelings or behaviors gives the learner a chance to experience, to relive, or to anticipate a situation. Role-playing emphasizes the cognitive and affective domains of learning. The client can experiment with different responses to a situation while the nurse offers guidance and feedback.

Play with puppets and dolls has proven effective in preparing young children for procedures and in helping them express negative feelings about hospitalization. Role-playing in a prenatal class is effective and necessary to help couples get through transition in childbirth. However, there are some disadvantages of using role-play with adults. Adults may feel uncomfortable with role-play teaching strategies due to self-consciousness, fear of failure, lack of experience, and the fear of being judged by peers or instructors. Role-play activities require individuals to step out of their comfort zones, assume unfamiliar roles, and engage in simulated scenarios, which can be daunting for many adults. Every effort should be made to help them feel safe to explore feelings, reassuring them that the exercise will be helpful in meeting their learning needs and kept confidential.

Role Modeling

Seeing a nurse who has overcome health challenges can help the client change attitudes and values associated with health issues. A nurse who has struggled with a weight issue, given up a dependency on tobacco, or overcome a learning disability may be able to share personal insights that are helpful to a client. Nurses who formerly smoked have been excellent role models for clients who are trying to quit smoking to improve their health. Nurses with children who have a learning disability can share beneficial learning strategies and successful outcomes.

Simulation

Simulation teaches and evaluates client learning. Because of its interactive nature, simulation promotes partnership in the learning process. By applying new information in different scenarios, the client experiences the subject matter while the nurse evaluates the client's learning. For example, a nurse could teach and evaluate how well Mr. James has learned dietary modifications for hypertension by providing a sample menu and asking him to order a meal that best meets sodium and fat restrictions. Computer simulations and internet resources for clients are becoming more readily available. Reinforcement by the computer program would be provided if the client chose correctly, or instruction could continue if an incorrect choice was made.

PSYCHOMOTOR (SKILL)

Demonstration/Return Demonstration

Demonstration is the ideal way of teaching procedures, techniques, exercises, and the use of special equipment. Models of body parts, medical practice models, and teaching simulators—such as resuscitation dolls, anatomical models, and injection mannequins—are available to help clients learn independent healthcare practices. Providing step-by-step instructions in short, sequential teaching sessions usually works best for complex procedures such as ostomy care or self-injection of insulin. Return demonstration by the client provides an opportunity for the nurse to evaluate and correct problems, to praise the client's learning, and to make plans for further reinforcement and follow-through, if necessary.

Guided and Independent Practice

Client practice—guided, then independent—should always be considered in conjunction with the demonstration strategy for psychomotor learning. After explaining and demonstrating a skill, sufficient time should be planned for the nurse to direct or guide the client through each step of a procedure, such as changing sterile dressings or operating a glucose monitor. Additional independent practice with and without the nurse present will help the client move to more independent functioning. Written materials, videotapes, CDs, DVDs, and podcasts should be given to the client for review.

> **THINKING CRITICALLY**
>
> In the chapter-opening case study, Mr. Martinez was having difficulty learning self-injection. Assuming that the nurse was using demonstration and practice as teaching strategies, what principle of learning needs emphasis in revising Mr. Martinez's teaching plan so he can be more successful?

STEPS IN THE TEACHING–LEARNING PROCESS

Client teaching is most effective when approached through the nursing process, as outlined in Table 12.3. Rather than think of client education as a separate and unique nursing function, nurses must integrate client education into their general approach to client care and address learning needs in every aspect of the nursing process. The nurse should be aware that all client interactions are teaching interactions. In some situations, the nurse can anticipate a series of learning needs, such as the standardized preoperative teaching topics needed by Mrs. Duncan in the chapter-opening case study, whereas other teaching situations are incidental to ongoing nursing care, such as teaching the purpose and side effects of a newly prescribed drug, as was needed by Mr. James in the chapter-opening case study before administration of the BP medication. The wise nurse teaches "on the go" and makes every contact an opportunity to teach.

TABLE 12.3 Comparison of the Nursing Process and the Teaching–Learning Process

Nursing Process	Teaching–Learning Process
Assessing	Determine learning needs.
Diagnosing	Identify learning needs. Formulate nursing diagnoses of learning needs.

Planning	Specify learning objectives.
	Select teaching method.
	   • Informal teaching
	   • Formal teaching
	   • Standardized teaching plans
	Select teaching strategies.

Implementing	Implement teaching plan, prepare materials, and structure teaching sessions. Control environment.
Evaluating	Evaluate teaching. Evaluate learning.

ASSESSMENT

The first and most essential step for effective learning, an organized and thorough assessment, keeps client care individualized and determines readiness to learn (Eskolin et al., 2023; Hogan et al., 2023). A basic educational assessment should include motivation level, comprehension ability, current knowledge level, attitudes about health, and factors that will affect teaching, such as sensory, physical, and mental abilities and language. Ideally, this information should be obtained on admission and during early periods of client contact, when the nurse interviews the client for the nursing database. In addition, the nurse should remain vigilant about obtaining information about the client's learning needs, as revealed through the client's questions and behaviors when the nurse is giving care.

The nurse can accomplish a basic educational needs assessment by using the following prompts as a guide during client interactions:

- What does the client know?
- What does the client think is happening and why?
- What does the client need to know; what is important to them?
- What worries the client most?
- What does the client want to know?
- How does the client feel about managing the situation independently?
- Is there someone that can help if needed?

Learning the answers to these questions helps Mary from the chapter-opening scenario discover why Mr. Martinez was having difficulty mastering his insulin injections and exactly what Mr. Wallis needed in order to be less afraid to take his wife home (see Box 12.6).

DIAGNOSIS

After collecting the necessary data, the nurse analyzes the information and identifies the nursing diagnosis or problem statement that most clearly describes the client's learning needs. According to the guidelines of the North American Nursing Diagnosis Association International (Herdman et al., 2024), there are two approaches to diagnosing learning needs. If the learning need is keeping the client from functioning optimally, the problem statement "lack of knowledge" (International Council of Nurses, 2019) can be used with additional clarification and etiology, as in the following examples.

EXAMPLE 12.1 Problem Statement for Mr. Wallis
Lack of knowledge of safety measure (body mechanics of getting out of bed related to inexperience and concern about home care management)

EXAMPLE 12.2 Problem Statement for Mrs. Duncan
Lack of knowledge of physical therapy (postoperative exercises) related to lack of information about postoperative care

Lack of knowledge may also be the etiology of the healthcare problem, such as impaired health maintenance, emotional problem, anxiety, risk for infection, and difficulty coping. Thus, lack of knowledge, lack of understanding, or insufficient information may be used as the etiology of the nursing diagnosis, as in the following examples.

EXAMPLE 12.3 Nursing Diagnosis for Mr. James
Impaired health maintenance related to lack of understanding about the disease process, treatment regimen, and home care management

BOX 12.6 Assessment of Clients in Chapter-Opening Case Study

Mr. Martinez—Client With Insulin-Dependent Diabetes

In preparation for Mr. Martinez's discharge, Mary visits him, arranging for a hospital interpreter to be present during the sessions. Mary concentrates on speaking to Mr. Martinez, not the interpreter. She learns that Mr. Martinez's mother is knowledgeable about diabetic diet management because she also has diabetes. His mother is also a respected curandera, or local healer. With Mr. Martinez's permission, Mary arranges for Mr. Martinez's mother to be included in the teaching and for the afternoon nurse to continue training in the evening. Mary learns that Mr. Martinez is knowledgeable about the signs and symptoms of hypoglycemia and hyperglycemia but has difficulty mixing and preparing his insulins, partly because he cannot see well. Mary contacts the local Visiting Nurses Association (VNA) for follow-up teaching at home and refers him to the walk-in clinic for vision testing for presbyopia.

Mrs. Wallis—Client Undergoing Postoperative Laminectomy

Mr. Wallis has never had to be responsible for an ill family member; Mrs. Wallis has always cared for their children when they were ill, has cared for his invalid mother for 5 years after a stroke until her death 2 years ago, and has cared for him after five major surgeries during the past year, including his colostomy care. Mr. Wallis can explain the principles, purpose, and instructions for applying his wife's brace but before Mrs. Wallis' surgery has avoided handling the brace or practicing its application. Mary asks for his assistance in applying the brace so Mrs. Wallis can get up to use the bathroom. Mr. Wallis' manipulative skill in arranging the brace for application is good, but he becomes extremely shaky and clumsy when attempting to apply the brace on his wife. Mr. Wallis expresses fear of hurting his wife or not being "a good nurse" like she was during his recovery from surgery. Mary arranges several more supervised practice sessions before discharge, inviting a physical therapist. These sessions include a lot of praise from both the nurse, the physical therapist, and Mrs. Wallis. Eventually, Mr. Wallis becomes the preferred "nurse" in managing the brace because of his consistent and tender approach. In addition, Mary consults VNA for support for Mr. and Mrs. Wallis at home.

EXAMPLE 12.4 Nursing Diagnosis for Mr. Martin

Delayed surgical recovery related to lack of knowledge of treatment regime of colostomy irrigation, peristomal skin care, and incorporation of ostomy care into activities of daily living

The nurse must choose a style of diagnosis. However, regardless of which style the nurse uses, both approaches give direction to nursing care and education interventions.

The NCLEX-RN *Might Ask* 12.3

The nurse is writing a teaching plan for a client with a lack of knowledge. Which of the following nursing diagnostic statements would be most accurate in writing a "lack of knowledge" etiology?

a. Anxiety related to upcoming surgery
b. Impaired ability to manage medication regime related to insufficient information and inexperience in mixing insulins
c. Risk for infection related to lowered immune system
d. Difficulty coping related to stress of job change

• See Appendix A for correct answer and rationale.

PLANNING

Writing an individualized teaching plan or emphasizing the teaching component of the client's general nursing care plan is an expectation for the registered nurse. When the client's learning needs are identified and presented in a diagnostic statement, the nurse, in collaboration with the client, develops a client-centered teaching plan that establishes outcomes and appropriate interventions.

Individualized Plans

Individualized teaching plans are generally a component of the client's overall nursing care plan. Educational outcome criteria and teaching interventions are included as one of three approaches (diagnostic, therapeutic, and educational) to resolve an identified human response pattern problem. This type of plan requires more composing and writing time for nurses, but this is the preferred method for ensuring that the unique needs of clients will be addressed.

Standardized Teaching Plan

Standardized teaching plans or model teaching plans have evolved in clinical settings in which teaching situations frequently recur. The standardized preoperative teaching plan is one of the most common plans. Specialty areas such as prenatal clinics, maternity centers, emergency rooms, outpatient ambulatory care centers, and client education clinics are developing other teaching plans to lessen the nurse's work and to make client education documentation easier.

Standardized teaching plans are available in books, preprinted guides, or computer models. The plans usually include checklists, blank lines, or empty spaces for the nurse to individualize outcomes and nursing interventions and to document the teaching provided. This type of plan should not be used as a guide because it does not address the client's individual needs and can cause the nurse to focus only on predictable problems and miss cues to unique client problems.

Nurses must always assess the client's knowledge level first to determine if all the information included in the model plan is needed and then individualize the plan to meet the client's specific needs. Most nursing care planning guides include teaching outcomes and interventions in a general abbreviated form, and nurses need to personalize the teaching plan in more detail for each client (see Box 12.7).

Expected Outcomes/Learning Objectives

Learning objectives are similar to the outcome statements used for nursing care plans in general. Learning objectives should be client-centered, simple, measurable statements of what the client will say or do to give evidence of learning. Using the mnemonic acronym SMART (specific, measurable, achievable, relevant, and time-bound) is helpful in developing meaningful objectives. Verbs in learning outcomes should be consistent with the three domains of learning:

- **Cognitive learning objectives** use verbs describing the results of the thinking process: "The client will state how diet intake affects his blood sugar levels."
- **Affective learning objectives** use verbs that disclose the client's feelings, attitudes, and values: "The client will express feelings about his colostomy stoma."
- **Psychomotor learning objectives** use verbs that clarify client actions and skills: "The client will demonstrate aseptic technique when self-administering an insulin injection."

The more specific the desired outcomes are, the easier it will be for the client to pursue learning and for the nurse to evaluate progress. A single general objective, such

BOX 12.7 Nursing Care Plan for Postoperative Laminectomy: Assessment for Mrs. Wallis

Before using the standardized model teaching plan, Mary carefully assessed Mr. and Mrs. Wallis's knowledge and abilities regarding positioning, activity precautions, and back brace management. In her assessment, Mary found Mrs. Wallis could independently log roll when changing position in bed and maintained proper body alignment while lying in bed, sitting, and standing with her walker. Mrs. Wallis was cooperative, showing personal responsibility in adhering to the 15-minute limitation on sitting without needing any reminders from the nursing staff. Mrs. Wallis needed assistance in applying the back brace when getting out of bed, and Mr. Wallis became extremely shaky and appeared awkward when trying to align and comfortably position the brace for Mrs. Wallis. Mr. Wallis always called for the nurses to assist Mrs. Wallis with the brace, and he left the room during his wife's dressing period.

Standardized Plan	Individualized Plan
Nursing Diagnosis	**Nursing Diagnosis**
Risk for injury related to lack of knowledge of postoperative position restrictions and log-rolling technique	Risk for injury related to lack of knowledge and skill in the use of a back brace
Expected Outcomes	**Learner Objectives**
1. The client will demonstrate correct positioning and log-rolling techniques within 4 hours. 2. Mr. Wallis will express a feeling of confidence in assisting Mrs. Wallis in donning the back brace.	1. Client will demonstrate correct application of the back brace. 2. The client will verbalize implementing necessary activity precautions by the end of this shift. 3. The client will demonstrate proper application and use of the back brace.
Interventions	**Interventions**

1. Teach client to use arms and legs to transfer weight properly when getting out of bed.
2. Encourage walking, standing, and sitting for short periods as soon as permitted after surgery.
3. Teach the client precautions to maintain proper body alignment:
  a. Log-rolling techniques
  b. Side-lying position in bed
  c. Positions to avoid
  d. Standing and weight bearing
4. Teach the proper use of a back brace, if indicated.
5. Teach client to avoid:
  a. Prolonged sitting
  b. Twisting the spine
  c. Bending at the waist
  d. Climbing stairs
  e. Automobile trips while wearing the brace
	1. Demonstrate the proper use of a back brace:
	  a. Explain the mechanism and purpose of the back brace.
	  b. Show Mr. Wallis proper positioning of brace while it is being worn by Mrs. Wallis.
	  c. Demonstrate how to secure the back brace.
	  d. Demonstrate and explain how to minimize skin irritation from wearing the brace.
	  e. Show pictures and describe skin breakdown to be assessed each time the brace is applied and removed.
	  f. Demonstrate skin care and massage after brace removal.
	2. Encourage Mr. Wallis to discuss his concerns about responsibilities in helping his wife put on the back brace.
	3. Give verbal praise each time Mr. Wallis participates or takes charge in assisting his wife to put on her back brace.

> **BOX 12.8**
>
> ### Sequenced Learning Objectives for Mr. Martin's Individualized Teaching Plan
>
> 1. Mr. Martin will empty and change the colostomy bag using supplies provided.
> 2. Mr. Martin will perform colostomy irrigation independently.
> 3. Mr. Martin will accurately assess skin area and describe the management of skin irritation if it occurs.
> 4. Mr. Martin will describe plans for resuming his preoperative lifestyle.
> 5. Mr. Martin will discuss feelings about the stoma with significant others.

as "Mr. Martin will become independent in colostomy care," may be accurate but is too general and does not provide enough direction for meeting the client's individual needs. Listing objectives in a step-by-step sequence (Box 12.8) can make the teaching plan easier to implement, gives the nursing team clearer direction, and enables the nurse to better evaluate client learning.

Interventions

When learning objectives have been identified, the nurse chooses teaching strategies appropriate for the type of content, the client's learning style, and the outcomes to be achieved. Strategies will not be effective if they are applied incorrectly; a demonstration will not facilitate a change in attitude or values if there is no opportunity to express feelings; the best-planned and best-delivered lecture will not achieve psychomotor skills if there is no opportunity to practice. In most client situations, integration of several teaching methods may be required. Each nurse must use their own creativity to develop and use teaching interventions.

IMPLEMENTATION

When the teaching plan is implemented, the nurse should stay alert and sensitive to the client's needs and responses. If the nurse or client becomes frustrated with the process, the nurse should take a step back and review the assessment, objectives, and interventions. Were they made with the client? Be prepared to adjust the teaching approach and to modify the pace or setting according to the client's progress. The client may have more discomfort or fatigue than expected, so the teaching session may need to be delayed or shortened. Learning a new skill—such as dressing changes, ostomy care, or self-injection—may be more complex for the client than anticipated, so additional practice sessions may need to be provided.

Remember that the nurse is part of a collaborative team, so the nurse may delegate some parts of the teaching plan to another healthcare professional. For example, Mr. and Mrs. Willis may be assisted with mobility by a physical therapist. Drug information for Mr. James can be obtained by the unit pharmacist. In many instances, other team members can be part of the teaching team. Dr. Lotte may have an advanced nurse practitioner that assists him in educating clients about medication. Regardless of the support personnel, it is Mary's responsibility to assess, plan, coordinate, and evaluate the teaching.

When appropriate, possible, and permitted by the client, include family members and support people in the teaching plan and instructional sessions. Their involvement will help them assist in the client's home care and can reinforce the client's learning.

EVALUATION

Evaluation of an individual teaching plan should include the achievement of desired outcomes, the adequacy and appropriateness of teaching materials/methods, and the effectiveness of the nurse as a teacher. Do not assume that learning has occurred without some type of validation. Such evaluation of learning flows logically from the learning objectives of the teaching plan if the teaching–learning process is developed systematically from the nursing process.

Learning can be evaluated in a variety of ways, including by written tests, questionnaires, oral questioning, observation, return demonstration, and home follow-up calls or visits. The method of evaluation should be consistent with the type of learning: Cognitive learning can be evaluated by questioning (written or oral), affective learning through client responses, and psychomotor learning by client return demonstrations.

To be effective, evaluation should occur throughout the teaching–learning process and at completion. The nurse should always be alert for staff frustration, client confusion, inaccurate information, or improper return demonstrations by the client. Early correction will ensure that the client does not learn inaccurate information or practice skills incorrectly.

Evaluation of learning should also include an assessment of the adequacy and appropriateness of the materials and methods used. For example, if this assessment shows that the resource library contains adult education materials English only, it is essential to obtain a variety of materials (printed, audiovisual, and computerized) that include pictures or languages appropriate to other client populations.

Just as with other nursing roles, teaching requires practice and experience. The nurse should always complete a self-evaluation to improve their approach. Some questions the nurse might ask themselves include the following:

1. Did the client achieve the learning objective?
2. How was I helpful to the client's learning? How was I not helpful, and how could I have been more helpful?
3. What factors facilitated (or blocked) the client's success?
4. How could I improve this teaching session next time?
5. Nurses should also seek client feedback about the teaching–learning experience. Much can be learned from the client's perception. An anonymous questionnaire using a standardized form could be provided to the client on discharge via paper and pencil or a computerized format.
6. Communication of the results should be shared with staff and teaching changes made accordingly.

DOCUMENTATION OF CLIENT TEACHING

Documenting client teaching is an important nursing responsibility required by the following:

- State nurse practice acts
- State home health agency licensure laws
- Medicare and Medicaid program regulations
- The ANA, which established a standard of care that includes teaching as a measure of accountability for quality of nursing care rendered, in which the latter must be demonstrated through documentation

- The Joint Commission, which requires that teaching (involving the client and their support system) must be shown by documentation for a facility to receive accreditation

Documentation of teaching and learning is set by agency policy and procedures. Each agency must determine the method of documentation and the types of clinical records that meet the agency's requirements for client teaching. Teaching may be written on a care plan, in nursing notes, or on a separate teaching record, but it must be part of the client's official record. Generally, documentation of client teaching should include the following:

- Learning needs
- Teaching interventions planned
- Teaching interventions implemented
- Client outcomes achieved or not achieved
- Revisions or changes in teaching methods used

Whatever charting format or record is used, the nurse's charting must be clear, concise, accurate, and complete. The charting entries must show what was taught and how well the client or family demonstrated learning. An example of documentation of client teaching is shown in Box 12.9.

CLINICAL APPLICATION OF THE TEACHING–LEARNING PROCESS

Now that we have reviewed important principles of teaching and learning and applicable teaching strategies for varied clinical settings, let's use the teaching–learning process to help Mary complete Mrs. Duncan's preoperative teaching (Box 12.10).

ASSESSMENT FOR MRS. DUNCAN

Before using the hospital's guidelines for preoperative teaching (standardized plan), Mary assessed Mrs. Duncan's previous experiences with surgery and hospitalizations, knowledge about the procedure to be performed, and her emotional state regarding surgery.

BOX 12.9

Focus on Charting: Documentation of Client Teaching

Problem

The client requested that the nurse change the newborn son's wet and soiled diaper after circumcision procedure. The client asked many questions about how to care for a circumcised son, including diaper change and bathing instructions.

Intervention

The nurse taught postcircumcision care with diaper changes and explained and demonstrated cleansing the circumcised penis. The nurse answered questions and will supervise the client in the next diaper change and reinforce teaching.

Evaluation

The client returned a demonstration of diaper and circumcision care as taught. The client now requests nursing support for instruction on bottle-feeding the infant.

BOX 12.10 Individualized Preoperative Teaching Plan for Mrs. Duncan

Nursing Diagnosis
Anxiety related to insufficient knowledge about current anesthesia side effects and pain control management practices

Outcomes
1. Mrs. Duncan will effectively verbalize concerns regarding surgery and anticipated recovery before surgery.
2. Before surgery, Mrs. Duncan will verbalize postoperative pain management routine with the use of patient-controlled analgesia (PCA).

Interventions
1. Provide an environment with privacy and minimal disruptions to encourage the expression of feelings and concerns.
2. Listen actively, and clarify and reflect feelings as expressed by the client.
3. Return demonstrates postoperative pain controlling activities, with emphasis on the use of PCA.

Nursing Diagnosis
Lack of knowledge (coughing and deep breathing [C&DB]) related to unfamiliarity with postoperative care activities

Goal
1. Mrs. Duncan will verbalize knowledge of perioperative activities before surgery.
2. Mrs. Duncan will demonstrate correct C&DB techniques before surgery.

Interventions
1. Explain preoperative and postoperative activities and expectations for Mrs. Duncan's procedure. Ensure that family members are included and that hospital staff will call/text to keep them informed of Mrs. Duncan's situation.
2. Demonstrate C&DB using an abdominal splinting technique. Have Mrs. Duncan's return practice and demonstrate techniques.
3. Demonstrate incentive spirometry, and have her practice and return demonstrate.
4. Show Mrs. Duncan and family a DVD on postoperative respiratory care.
5. Coordinate visit by respiratory therapy for use of mini-nebulizer treatments.

In her assessment, Mary found that Mrs. Duncan had two previous hospital experiences (appendectomy at age 14 years and childbirth at age 26 years), which she found to be satisfying and uneventful, except for postanesthesia nausea and vomiting after her appendectomy. Mrs. Duncan cannot recall what the nurses and providers expected of her after her previous surgery, but she is apprehensive about postsurgery pain management and nausea, and the postoperative length of stay (she has no sick leave accrued from her new job as a legal secretary and needs to return to work as soon as possible).

Mrs. Duncan restates her surgeon's instructions regarding her procedure and potential complications that may arise with her surgery. She expresses confidence in her provider and trust that the nurses will keep her pain and nausea free. On physical examination, Mary finds that Mrs. Duncan's lungs are clear to auscultation. She was a moderate smoker for 10 years but has not smoked in the last 2 years. Based on the nurse and client partnering efforts, they developed and implemented the individualized teaching plan outlined in Box 12.10.

CONCLUSION

To be able to teach effectively, the nurse must be a good communicator. Through the proper application of the principles of communication, teaching, and learning, the nurse gains the trust and respect of client in meeting their many self-care needs for the maintenance and promotion of health and recovery from illness or injury. Respect for the client's unique needs is necessary for a successful teaching–learning experience.

When possible, the client and the nurse must work as a team toward meeting mutually agreed on objectives, goals, and interventions. The nursing process provides an effective framework for assessing, planning, implementing, and evaluating client learning. Varied strategies involving with direct personal interactions between the nurse and the client are essential to the client's learning. Nurses as health professionals must play a major role in meeting the public's health education needs. Nurse–client interactions provide an excellent opportunity for ongoing client health education.

REFERENCES

Ballering, A. V., Olde Hartman, T. C., Verheij, R., & Rosmalen, J. G. M. (2023). Sex and gender differences in primary care help-seeking for common somatic symptoms: A longitudinal study. *Scandinavian Journal of Primary Health Care, 41*(2), 132–139. doi:10.1080/02813432.2023.2191653

Bastable, S. (2017). *Essentials of patient education* (2nd ed.). Jones and Bartlett.

Eskolin, S., Inkeroinen, S., Leino, K. H., & Virtanen, H. (2023). Instruments for measuring empowering patient education competence of nurses: Systematic review. *Journal of Advanced Nursing, 79*(7), 2414–2428. doi:10.1111/jan.15597

Herdman, T. H., Kamitsuru, S., & Lopes, C. T. (Eds.). (2024). *Nursing diagnoses: Definitions and classification 2024-2026* (13th ed.). NANDA International, Inc.

Hogan, A., Hughes, L., & Coyne, E. (2023). Understanding nursing assessment of health literacy in a hospital context: A qualitative study. *Journal of Clinical Nursing, 32*(19/20), 7495–7508. doi:10.1111/jocn.16809

Hood, L. (2021). *Leddy and Pepper's professional nursing* (10th ed.). Wolters Kluwer.

International Council of Nurses. (2019). *Nursing diagnosis and outcome statements.* https://www.icn.ch/sites/default/files/inline-files/ICNP2019-DC.pdf

Knowles, M. S., Holton, E. F., Swanson, R. A., & Robinson, P. A. (2020). *The adult learner: The definitive classic in adult education and human resource development* (9th ed.). Routledge.

Kopec, M., Quartey, N. K., Snow, M., Stechkevich, A., Giuliani, M. E., & Papadakos, J. (2023). Improving access to patient education: An audit of extant educational materials. *Journal of Cancer Education, 38*(3), 885–894. doi:10.1007/s13187-022-02202-7

Miles, J. (2017). Facilitation of learning. In S. R. Hardin & R. Kaplow (Eds.), *Synergy for clinical excellence* (2nd ed.). Jones and Bartlett Learning.

Mursa, R., Patterson, C., & Halcomb, E. (2022). Men's help-seeking and engagement with general practice: An integrative review. *Journal of Advanced Nursing, 78*, 1938–1953. doi:10.1111/jan.15240

National Center for Education Statistics. (n.d.-a). *Fast facts: Adult literacy.* U. S. Department of Education. https://nces.ed.gov/fastfacts/display.asp?id=69

National Center for Education Statistics. (n.d.-b). *Program for the international assessment of adult competencies (PIAAC).* U. S. Department of Education. https://nces.ed.gov/surveys/piaac/state-county-estimates.asp#4

National Center for Education Statistics. (n.d.-c). *U.S. skills map: State and county indicators of adult literacy and numeracy*. U. S. Department of Education. https://nces.ed.gov/surveys/piaac/skillsmap/

Ng, S. X., Wang, W., Shen, Q., Toh, Z. A., & He, H. G. (2022). Effectiveness of preoperative education interventions on improving perioperative outcomes of adult patients undergoing cardiac surgery: A systematic review and meta-analysis. *European Journal of Cardiovascular Nursing, 21*(6), 521–536. doi:10.1093/eurjcn/zvab123

Petrie, K. A., Chen, J. N., Miears, H., Grimes, J. S., & Zumwalt, M. (2022). Gender differences in seeking health care and postintervention pain outcomes in foot and ankle orthopedic patients. *Women's Health Reports, 3*(1), 500–507. doi:10.1089/whr.2021.0076

Taylor, C., Lynn, P., & Bartlett, J. L. (2023). *Fundamentals of nursing: The art and science of nursing care* (10th ed.). Wolters Kluwer.

SUGGESTED READING

Boggs, K. U. (2023). *Interpersonal relationships: Professional communication skills for nurses* (9th ed.). Elsevier.

Kozak, R. (2021, March 12). *RÁPIDO—A new Spanish acronym to raise stroke awareness*. American Heart Association. https://www.heart.org/en/news/2021/03/12/rapido-a-new-spanish-acronym-to-raise-stroke-awareness

On the WEB

Adult Education and Literacy Facts & Figures: https://www2.ed.gov/about/offices/list/ovae/pi/AdultEd/facts-figures.html

CMS Tipsheet for Meaningful Learning: https://www.cms.gov/Regulations-and-Guidance/Legislation/EHRIncentivePrograms/Downloads/Stage2Overview_Tipsheet.pdf

Health Care Education Association Tools and Resources for Patient Education: https://www.hcea-info.org/educational-tools

The Interactive Teach-back Learning Module (This is an easy-to-use toolkit to teach nurse's how to teach using the teach-back method): http://www.teachbacktraining.org/interactive-teach-back-learning-module

The Joint Commission's Speak Up Fact Sheet: https://www.jointcommission.org/resources/news-and-multimedia/fact-sheets/facts-about-speak-up/

The Learning Pyramid: https://www.educationcorner.com/the-learning-pyramid.html

Newest Vital Sign by Pfizer: https://www.pfizer.com/products/medicine-safety/health-literacy/nvs-toolkit

PART B | MANAGER OF CARE

Managing the Care of Unique Clients

CHAPTER 13

LEARNING OUTCOMES

By the end of this chapter, the student will be able to:
1. Discuss the following concepts related to diversity: culture, subculture, customs, beliefs, attitudes, values, and ethnocentrism.
2. Explain why the process of developing cultural awareness/competency/humility is ongoing, requiring continuing education and sensitivity.
3. Discuss how values, beliefs, and attitudes affect the nurse–client relationship.
4. Identify communication skills that foster open discussion between the nurse and the client.
5. Perform accurate assessments that incorporate client uniqueness.
6. Analyze how uniqueness impacts the nursing care planning process.

KEY TERMS

attitudes
beliefs
culture
cultural competence
cultural humility
cultural relativism

customs
ethnocentrism
gender identity
heritage
multicultural
sexual orientation

stereotyping
subculture
underrepresented
uniqueness
values

Case STUDY

To help staff their community hospital, Sacred Heart Hospital administrators have recruited José Cruz, LPN, from his home country of Colombia, South America. José is enjoying his orientation and is motivated to begin caring for patients. His colleagues at the hospital have welcomed José and other nurses who have been recruited from various countries. José has entered the accelerated LPN–RN program at a local community college and is talking to one of his professors.

PROFESSOR: How are you, José?

JOSÉ: I'm happy to be in America, although I miss Colombia and my family. I enjoy living here, but the pace is faster. I am having some problems communicating with the Anglo nurses and physicians. They talk so fast. Sometimes they use phrases that don't make sense to me. We don't have as many different medicines in Colombia, either. Even though we speak the same language, communication is difficult at times. Everyone here is so strict about time, too. In my country, we are much more relaxed.

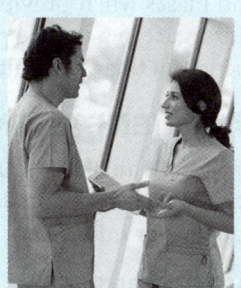

PROFESSOR: What do you think would be helpful to you?

JOSÉ: I think if people would just slow down, be more patient. Maybe if they could go to another country and work, they would see how difficult it is to think and understand in a different language. Having Juan Perez, the Hispanic nurse manager in telemetry, mentoring me has meant a lot. We've had many similar experiences.

PROFESSOR: Yes, in the United States, we tend to be pressured about time, and we need to slow down. Juan was a graduate of our program; I'm glad he's helping you. Would you be willing to share what you're experiencing in class? It would help the other students to see another cultural perspective.

JOSÉ: Sure. I want people to learn how different but similar we are.

Nurses strive to assess, plan, and intervene based on an individual's response to illness. In addition to anatomical and physiologic factors, when planning care, nurses must consider the uniqueness of the client in terms of their cultural, social, sexual, and spiritual background. Nurses incorporate diversity into the nursing process, allowing them to develop effective plans of care.

UNDERSTANDING UNIQUENESS

According to the U.S. Census Bureau (2022) American Community Survey Five-Year Estimates, 21.6% of the population speaks one or more languages other than English. These numbers reflect only previously established large cultural groups; they do not reflect the full **multicultural** nature of the U.S. population. Population statistics have increasingly become more fluid, with a growing percentage of individuals reporting they are members of **underrepresented** groups (U.S. Census Bureau, n.d.). In the United States, 81% of nurses providing patient care are White females (Huston, 2023; Smiley et al., 2023). As the population becomes increasingly diverse, sharing multicultural perspectives has the potential to improve healthcare professionals' awareness of client needs.

Communication and understanding of how diversity impacts competent and compassionate care are imperative for all nurses. Discrimination has a negative impact on population health. Health disparities are influenced by health policies, individual discriminatory actions, marginalization, and prejudice. The American Nurses Association (2018) states nurses must confront discriminatory practices, whether intentional or unintentional. Nurses must be aware and examine their own attitudes, ideals, beliefs, and biases when providing care to all clients, families, communities, and populations. Nurses are in a unique position to lessen potential misunderstandings and clarify information in their daily interactions with diverse clients.

UNIQUENESS AND CULTURE

Each individual's **uniqueness** is affected by many factors, including culture, ethnicity, gender, sexual orientation, socioeconomic status, spiritual orientation, and education. Each factor influences an individual's life journey.

DEFINITIONS
Stereotyping
Each individual must be considered an individual and be treated as such. To assign fixed characteristics to an individual based on overgeneralized or preconceived ideas is referred to as **stereotyping** (Boyle et al., 2025). When stereotyping occurs, an individual is no longer recognized as being different from a larger group. Their uniqueness as a person—including their feelings, values, and customs—is overlooked. Tools the nurse can use to assess diverse customs, beliefs, attitudes, and values are referred to at the end of this chapter.

Culture
Each human society has a body of norms governing behavior and other knowledge to which an individual is socialized, beginning at birth or at the time the individual becomes a member of the social group. **Culture** is characterized as a common set of moral principles, standards of behavior, and beliefs that provide social structure to daily activities (Taylor et al., 2023). Cultures to which an individual may belong include family unit, nationality, religion, social class, and profession. Culture is the binding agent of families, neighborhoods, and communities in a relationship of shared meaning.

Culture is learned through socialization with those who are near (Taylor et al., 2023). The socialization process comes from **heritage**, which comprises the traditions, histories, and stories that are passed down from generation to generation. An individual may or may not incorporate heritage into their life experience.

The United States is composed of many cultures with social groups (subcultures) coming together to form a larger social group (dominant culture). A **subculture** is a subset of a larger community that adheres to values, norms, standards, and beliefs that set them apart from the mainstream wider society (Boyle et al., 2025). Subcultures have special needs because individuals in subcultures may identify with the main culture, with the minor culture, with none of the cultures, or with a blend of them.

Customs
Customs are learned behaviors that are shared and practiced by some individuals who belong to a particular group. Customs are based on beliefs, attitudes, or values. The importance of a custom is related to the importance of the belief, attitude, or value on which it is based. Many customs that are important to a particular client are easily assessed because those customs can be observed or can be elicited by direct questioning. For example, an older custom in the nursing profession is to wear a pin signifying the school from which the nurse graduated.

Beliefs
Beliefs include opinions, knowledge, and faith. A belief is the acceptance of the truth or the reliability of something with or without proof. Another term for a belief is *supposition*.

Attitudes

An **attitude** is a way of feeling about or behaving toward a person, object, or idea. Attitudes comprise many beliefs. Judgments of "good" and "bad" are called binary opposites and are derived from attitudes.

Values

Values are a set of personal beliefs and attitudes about the truth, beauty, and worth of any thought, object, or behavior. Values:

- Are action oriented
- Give direction and meaning to life
- Develop from associations with people, the environment, and the self
- Are derived from life experiences

Cultural Competence and Cultural Humility

Cultural competence is an individual's lifelong endeavor to learn skills that can help with competent care (Purnell & Fenkl, 2021). However, skills are not enough to provide culturally competent care; nurses must also engage in cultural humility. **Cultural humility** is a lifelong process of self-reflection and self-critique in which nurses are encouraged to view each client's situation as if the nurse were experiencing the problem themselves. Cultural humility fosters the nurse's recognition of the impact of oppression and discrimination of individuals from underrepresented communities (Frie & Timm, 2023; Wall, 2023). When nurses are culturally humble, they become a part of the client's shared experience.

Culturally competent care occurs when healthcare professionals and institutions can successfully meet the cultural needs of their clients (Catalano, 2024). Cultural competence is the ability to work within a client's environment, including the client's family, community, cultural values, behaviors, and beliefs. Learning more about your own cultural background is the first step in understanding culturally diverse client populations. Box 13.1 provides suggestions on how a nurse can become more culturally sensitive. More information on cultural competence and developing cultural proficiency is included in Chapter 4.

Self-Assessment and Cultural Relativism

Individuals are socialized into viewing the world a certain way. They naturally believe that their way of viewing the world is the correct way. This narrow, one-sided view is called **ethnocentrism**, which is the inclination in someone to see their own group as the most important, superior to all other groups (Boyle et al., 2025). Atrocities of one group against another have been widely documented throughout history.

BOX 13.1

Suggestions to Enhance Cultural Competency

- Engage in student foreign exchange programs.
- Take a foreign language course or online language resource.
- Visit other countries on guided tours.
- Talk to nurses from other countries about their experiences.
- Read books and journals about other cultures.
- View DVDs or online programs with cultural themes.
- Enroll in courses with culturally diverse teachers/populations.

The opposite of ethnocentrism, stepping out of one's comfort zone to learn about another culture, is called **cultural relativism**. Because people live in a multicultural society and because it is impossible to know everything about all cultures, the journey toward cultural relativism is a lifelong process. For nurses, this process requires becoming culturally competent.

THINKING CRITICALLY
Make a list of the culture/subcultures to which you belong. Write down what you value most about communication, space, social organization, and time. Find a friend, another student, or a nurse and ask them to do the same; then, compare your notes. What is the same? What is different?

THINKING CRITICALLY
Watch movies about different cultures. Write down what the main characters value most about communication, space, social organization, and time. Now compare these to the values you wrote down about yourself and a friend, student, or nurse in the previous exercise. What is the same? What is different?

SENSITIVELY ASSESSING A CLIENT'S UNIQUENESS

Assessing a client's uniqueness can be a challenge for the RN. As discussed in Chapter 10, the nursing care plan must be individualized for each client. Following are some suggestions for data collection strategies for assessing each client's unique characteristics:

- **Customs:** The most easily identifiable unique behaviors are those that can be observed or elicited by questioning.
- **Beliefs:** An individual's beliefs can be ascertained in discussion.
- **Values:** Distinct values—those that form the basis for beliefs and customs—may be difficult to uncover during conversation or observation.

Note that the nurse must be sensitive to a client's customs, beliefs, and values, even if they differ from their own.

For examples of how assessments can be performed with sensitivity, read the following examples.

EXAMPLE 13.1 A 3-year-old Hmong American child is hospitalized for dehydration. As the nurse prepares to start an intravenous (IV) line, he notices an embroidered cloth bracelet on the child's wrist. The nurse wants to remove it so an IV can be started. The sterile insertion of the IV is extremely important. Before cutting the bracelet off the patient's wrist, the nurse says to the child's parent, "Tell me about this bracelet." The nurse learns that children wearing bracelets is a Hmong custom. Pursuing the discussion further, the nurse learns that this custom is based on the belief that the bracelet will protect the child from harm. The nurse is culturally humble to this belief, and they do not remove the bracelet. To respect the significance of the bracelet, the nurse chooses an insertion site where the bracelet can be easily retained and will not restrict IV access. To prevent interference with the IV insertion, the nurse secures the bracelet out of the way by wrapping it with a protective cover. After the procedure is finished, the nurse uses a transparent adhesive dressing to secure and protect the inserted IV.

EXAMPLE 13.2 A 6-month-old Mexican American infant is brought by her mother to the clinic. The admitting nurse states, "Your baby is so beautiful!" The mother responds, "Oh, this is the ugliest, naughtiest child." The nurse questions, in a genuinely curious tone, "Why do you say negative things about your baby?" By direct questioning, the nurse learns that in their culture it is a custom to say negative things about an infant. The mother believes that this will ward off the *mal de ojo* (evil eye) and explains that admiration of infants by strangers attracts this curse.

When caring for the infant, the nurse keeps this information in mind. To ensure culturally respectful care, the nurse communicates the mother's beliefs during bedside report, with the care team during interdisciplinary rounds, and by documenting it in the electronic health record.

The nurses in these examples use sensitive assessment techniques to incorporate uniqueness into the care plan. In both cases, the nurses used observational skills, and their communication was open, inquiring, accepting, and free from judgment. The nurses did not judge the worth of the stated customs.

A nurse's best source of information about the details of cultural, social, sexual, and spiritual uniqueness is the client. It is best to ask the client to help you understand their experience and then you need to listen carefully. It is also beneficial to ask another more culturally knowledgeable nurse, educator, or manager for help. Experienced nurse leaders are in a position to bring needed institutional resources into the environment if they are made aware of the challenges facing nurses in daily interactions.

THINKING CRITICALLY

The below exercises are designed to stimulate discussion about how the attitudes, beliefs, and values of the nurse may affect the caring, collaborative nurse–client relationship when the client holds different beliefs and attitudes. In groups of three, role-play three situations: One person will play the client; another, the nurse; and a third, the observer/recorder. Change roles for each situation.

Situation 1
Client: You are a 30-year-old gay individual hospitalized for leg pain. The provider has just left your room after telling you that your leg will need to be amputated. You are crying when the nurse walks into the room.
Nurse: Use therapeutic communication to allow your client to express their feelings.
Observer: Note the nonverbal techniques that are used; note any statements that are judgmental or neutral.

> **Situation 2**
> *Client:* You are a 43-year-old patient newly diagnosed with HIV. You are in the hospital receiving IV antibiotics for pneumonia. You are afraid to tell your partner about your diagnosis.
> *Nurse:* Teach the client the causes and preventive measures for infections.
> *Observer:* Note the nonverbal techniques that are used; note any statements that are judgmental or neutral.
>
> **Situation 3**
> *Client:* You are a 56-year-old client about to undergo treatment for severe anemia. You are a Jehovah's Witness and are refusing all blood products.
> *Nurse:* Discuss the impact of the client's religious preference on their treatment.
> *Observer:* Note the nonverbal techniques that are used; note any statements that are judgmental or neutral.
>
> After completion of each of the above exercises, have each member of the group answer the following questions:
> - *Client:*
>   - How did it feel to play the client character? What was difficult for you?
>   - How did the interaction affect you and your responses?
>   - Did you feel your character was supported?
> - *Nurse:*
>   - What approach did you take during the interaction?
>   - What statements or questions were easiest for you to answer?
>   - What other information did you gather?
> - *Observer:*
>   - What communication techniques were used during the interaction?
>   - Which techniques were facilitative, and which blocked the interaction?

ASPECTS OF CLIENT UNIQUENESS

This section explores four broad aspects of client uniqueness: cultural, social, sexual, and spiritual. The nurse can use assessment information related to these aspects of uniqueness to provide holistic, individualized nursing care. Keep in mind that the nurse should not make assumptions based on any of these aspects; instead, they should ask the client questions to assess their values and beliefs.

THE CLIENT AS A CULTURAL BEING
A client who is a member of a particular cultural group may identify solely with that culture or group or may adapt values and customs from another group into their lifestyle.

Verbal and Nonverbal Communication
Never assume English literacy when caring for a client; it is important to clarify meanings and avoid idioms, slang, and jargon. For example, instead of saying, "You've hit the nail on the head," a simple "That's right" or "Correct" would be best. Because of

enacted federal mandates and HIPAA regulations, institutions can no longer use a client's friends and family members as translators. If the client requires a language translator, it is important to obtain a translator, preferably one who can converse in the dialect or accent found in the region the patient is from. For example, if a client is from Colombia, they may have difficulty understanding a Spanish-speaking translator from Spain.

Language also includes nonverbal communication. In the United States, nodding the head while smiling can be interpreted as signifying an understanding. However, among some groups, these nonverbal messages are only a sign of respect.

Customs, Beliefs, and Values

Even after a thorough assessment of customs, beliefs, and values, omissions of needs or incorrect assumptions can still be made. Time, personal space, customary healing foods, and rituals for the dead are some of the issues around which inaccurate assumptions or omitted assessment data can affect patient care. To provide sensitive, culturally competent care, nurses must ask questions to investigate and integrate the customs, beliefs, and values of the client whenever possible.

THE CLIENT AS A SOCIAL BEING

The social aspects of each person include interpersonal relationships, economic status, and intrapersonal sense.

The NCLEX-RN *Might Ask* 13.1

The nurse is caring for a Hindu client. Which would be the most culturally sensitive way to approach this client?

a. Base interactions on preconceived knowledge about Hindus.
b. Assess this client for individual preferences.
c. Assign this client to a nurse who is Hindu.
d. Ask an experienced colleague if they can teach the nurse about Hinduism.

- See Appendix A for correct answer and rationale.

Interpersonal Relationships

Interpersonal relationships can include families, friends, and other people in the community. This section focuses on families.

The meaning of the word *family* may differ from person to person, but its basic definition is a unit composed of two or more persons who are joined by emotional closeness or bonds of sharing and who identify themselves as being part of a family (Boyle et al., 2025). Families may include single-caregiver households, same-sex couples, multigenerational families, and biracial families; also, families may or may not include children. It is important when working with families to know who is considered to be included and how long the family has been together.

Many families embrace the idea that individuals should be free to choose roles and responsibilities based on their abilities and preferences rather than their gender. A client may not only be the caretaker of children but also may be the caregiver of older adult parents. When planning care, the nurse needs to know what family, friend, or community support is available. It is also important to assess the beliefs and values of each individual about independence versus dependence.

> **BOX 13.2**
>
> **Ten Tips for Effectively Working With Families**
> 1. Be prepared for family chaos. Critical illness can trigger this in even stable families.
> 2. Involve significant others in a fact-finding conference with the healthcare team and all stakeholders. Reassure them that no decisions will be made at this time.
> 3. Assess the coping mechanisms used by family members.
> 4. Seek to reestablish a sense of control for family members.
> 5. Distraction may come in the form of unresolved conflicts. Redirect attention back to the client's needs.
> 6. Use an organized, simple, straightforward manner to give medical information. Provide written booklets and educational tools when needed.
> 7. Allow time to answer questions.
> 8. Encourage emotional expression.
> 9. Provide a safe zone if emotions become difficult to control.
> 10. Agree to a plan. Remind all family members that they need to step outside themselves and view any decisions in light of what the client would want.

Nurses help families manage intense interpersonal processes. Many nurses may feel unprepared to deal with these interactions, especially during decision-making. Box 13.2 provides some tips on how to respond with sensitivity when working with families and the decisions a family may have to make.

Economic Status

Each client has a unique means of financial support. When planning nursing care, nurses must identify and understand the effect of disease or illness on the client's financial support and economic status. Loss of the ability to earn money is a major concern. A prolonged illness may bankrupt even the most financially secure individual. Many households are managed by a single caregiver, whose income pays the rent and buys food and little else. Older adult clients may not be able to pay for prescribed medications or suggested nutritional supplements. An individual experiencing homelessness or an undocumented noncitizen may not know how to access available support systems for basic needs and healthcare. Socioeconomic status has an impact on health, and health has an impact on socioeconomic status (Bastable, 2017).

When assessing financial ability and economic status, the nurse can learn through thoughtful questioning and by carefully listening to the client's concerns. The nurse should not be swayed into false assumptions by material trappings; a client may be well-dressed but may be recently unemployed. It is appropriate to ask the following:

- "Do you have resources to purchase medications?"
- "What support systems do you have in place?"
- "What will you need to attend to your needs?"

These questions can help the nurse plan what institutional or community resources will be appropriate for the client.

Intrapersonal Sense

The client who feels a lack of control over a situation may not be able to participate in care, and a client who believes that their illness is deserved may be an unwilling participant in care. At particular risk are individuals in violent relationships, individuals with substance use disorder, and individuals with chronic diseases that require lifestyle changes to remain healthy. When assessing in this area, the nurse needs to listen for clues. A client may say, "I can't" or "I shouldn't" or have excuses for their inability to agree with a plan of care. This is often a sign that the individual does not have the ability to make independent healthy decisions. Psychosocial interventions in the form of counseling or therapy groups may be necessary before the client is willing to take charge of their own life.

THE CLIENT AS A SEXUAL BEING

Sex is a basic human need about which all nursing students must learn. Consensual sexual activities are a natural and healthy part of human life. An individual's attitudes and beliefs are just as important as genitalia and hormones in defining sexuality (Taylor et al., 2023). Attitudes regarding sexuality can vary widely across different cultures, societies, and individuals. These attitudes are shaped by complex factors, including cultural, religious, social, and personal beliefs. It is important for nurses to recognize that attitudes toward sexuality are diverse and can change over time. Societal shifts, increased awareness, and ongoing conversations about sexuality contribute to the evolution of attitudes and beliefs in different communities. It is especially important for nurses to consider how the client's own sexuality and the sexuality of those in the client's support system affect the client's life.

Barriers to Communicating About Sexuality

Although nurses agree that sexuality should be considered when developing the plan of care, they may struggle to construct a plan that meets an individual's sexual needs (Niemet & Rice, 2022; Yu et al., 2023). The barriers to communicating about sexual topics with the client include items listed in Box 13.3. An important component of communication is self-discovery—that is, the nurse must be aware of their own beliefs, ideals, and bias. The nurse must be accepting and open when assisting the client with sexual issues. Discussing sexual-related problems with clients requires sensitivity, empathy, and effective communication; see Box 13.4 for tips for doing so.

Variations in Sexual Openness

A person's sexuality is expressed in the context of culture. Openly discussing sexual matters may be comfortable to one person but intimidating to another. Nurses need to be

---

BOX 13.3 Barriers to the Nurse's Discussion of Sexual Issues

1. Inadequate education of the nurse
2. Embarrassment/anxiety of the nurse and/or perceived embarrassment/anxiety of the client
3. Low priority for the client in view of other physiologic needs
4. Lack of time and heavy workload
5. Inability to intervene or follow up on a client's sexual problem

BOX 13.4 Tips for Helping the Nurse Discuss Problems Related to Sexuality

Before the Discussion With the Patient
1. Seek educational offerings to enhance the nurse's competence and confidence.
2. Role-play difficult conversations with a knowledgeable advanced practice nurse, unit manager/educator, social worker, or psychiatrist.
3. Do not expect the client to bring up the subject. Clients expect the nurse to start the conversation.

During the Discussion With the Patient
1. Begin the conversation by establishing trust and emphasizing confidentiality. Assure the client that the information shared will be kept private.
2. Be mindful of using inclusive and nonjudgmental language. Avoid assumptions about the client's sexual orientation, preferences, or practices.
3. Use open-ended questions to encourage the client to share their concerns and experiences.
4. Practice active listening by giving your full attention, making eye contact, and nodding appropriately.
5. Frame the discussion in a way that normalizes sexual health as an essential aspect of overall well-being.
6. Assess the client's level of knowledge about sexual health and any specific concerns they may have.
7. Offer information about sexual health, addressing any misconceptions and providing resources for further education.
8. Use clear, simple language, avoiding medical jargon.
9. Recognize and explore the emotional aspects of sexual health. Discussing sexual concerns can be emotionally charged, so be prepared to address emotional reactions with sensitivity.
10. Provide information about available resources, such as sexual health clinics, counseling services, or support groups. Ensure that the client knows where to obtain additional help if needed.
11. Be aware of and respect cultural differences related to sexuality.
12. Maintain professional boundaries while being empathetic. Clarify the scope of your role and responsibilities in providing support.

Source: Jadoon, S. B., Nasir, S., Victor, G., & Pienaar, A. J. (2022). Knowledge attitudes and readiness of nursing students in assessing peoples' sexual health problems. *Nurse Education Today, 113*, 105371. https://doi.org/10.1016/j.nedt.2022.105371; Niemet, C. J., & Rice, K. (2022). LGBTQ & A: Development of a needs assessment to define access, needs, and barriers to health care services among LGBTQ older adults. *Journal of Prevention & Intervention in the Community, 50*(1), 1–15. https://doi.org/10.1080/10852352.2021.1915937; Yu, H., Dalmacio, D. F., Bonett, S., & Bauermeister, J. A. (2023). LGBTQ+ cultural competency training for health professionals: A systematic review. *BMC Medical Education, 23*, 1–83. https://doi.org/10.1186/s12909-023-04373-3

aware of their personal attitudes about sex before they can be comfortable with a client's ability to express sexual concerns. The first step is often to give permission to the person to discuss sexual concerns in an open way.

Variations in Sexual Orientation and Gender Identity

Sexual orientation refers to an individual's emotional or romantic attraction and preference of gender of a partner (Taylor et al., 2023). Sexual orientations include heterosexual, bisexual, asexual, or gay. **Gender identity** refers to the gender people perceive themselves as, including what they call themselves and the pronouns they use. Gender identities include cisgender, agender, and transgender; pronouns include he/him/his, she/her/hers, and they/their/theirs. Sexual orientation and gender identity are often not apparent upon observation of the client. A frequently used term that nurses must familiarize themselves with is LGBTQIA+, which stands for: lesbian, gay, bisexual, transgender, questioning or queer, intersex, and asexual; the "+" refers to members of other LGBTQIA+ communities and allies.

Recognizing and respecting a client's sexual orientation and gender identity are fundamental in providing inclusive care, impacting communication and trust between the client and the nurse. Open discussion about sexual health and behavior is important in developing an appropriate plan of care. Nurses must tailor their care and health education to address each client's specific needs and risks.

Healthcare screenings and preventive measures may be recommended based on a person's sexual orientation or gender identity. For instance, sexual health screenings, counseling on safe sex practices, and discussions about pre-exposure prophylaxis (PrEP) for HIV prevention may be more relevant for certain individuals. Nurses who are aware of a client's sexual orientation and gender identity are better equipped to offer support, resources, and referrals.

When interviewing clients, it is important for the nurse to approach the conversation with sensitivity, respect, and inclusivity. For example, appropriate questions might include:

- "With what gender do you identify?"
- "What pronouns do you use?"
- "Do you have any questions or concerns about your sexual health?"
- "Is there anything about your sexuality that is important to your care or that you want me to know?"

Social stigma, structural barriers, and lack of culturally sensitive care contribute to the health issues seen in LGBTQIA+ populations (Mukerjee et al., 2022).

The NCLEX-RN *Might Ask* 13.2

The nurse is caring for the child of a biracial couple. Recognizing that this couple's value system may differ from the nurse's is known as:
a. prejudice.
b. acculturation.
c. ethnocentrism.
d. cultural relativism.

• See Appendix A for correct answer and rationale.

THE CLIENT AS A SPIRITUAL BEING

Spirituality is an individual's journey to find the purpose of their life. Religion is often thought of as being the same as spirituality; however, religion is an organized system of beliefs about a higher power (Taylor et al., 2023). Therefore, religion falls under the umbrella of spirituality. Religious groups practice worship, prayer, meditation, or healings and may practice in a church, temple, synagogue, or mosque. Usually, there is a religious leader who plays a pivotal role in the development and guidance of religious aspects of life; this may be a priest (Catholicism), pastor (Fundamentalist Christianity), rabbi (Judaism), elder (Anabaptist Christianity [Amish]), or imam (Islam) (Purnell & Fenkl, 2021).

The nurse must be open and willing to learn about a variety of religions. The receptive and accepting nature of nursing helps foster the bonds needed when providing spiritual care. The best way to be receptive to others' ideas is to be aware of and be comfortable with your own spirituality. As nurses explore and learn more about their own beliefs, they are better able to recognize and support the client's spiritual needs and beliefs.

Religious Beliefs

Each organized religious group has its own values and beliefs. Occasionally, these affect either the client's ability to participate in their own care or the nurse's ability to give care. The challenge is to give judicious care without violating the religious beliefs of the client. Nurses must not only clarify their own values but also assist the client in clarifying theirs. It is not necessary for the nurse to agree with the client's values and beliefs, but it is necessary to respect them. One of the ways the nurse can show respect for the client's religious beliefs is to incorporate the client's spiritual leader into the plan of care.

Religious or Spiritual Symbols or Treatments

Religious or spiritual groups may use symbols, talismans, or special treatments as part of their rituals; many of these have been in use longer than organized Western medicine has been in existence. Using a crystal, candles, folk medicine, or an herbal remedy is therapeutic when doing so supports a client's personal belief system. Practices such as acupuncture and acupressure, meditation, therapeutic touch, Tai chi, and Reiki are examples of nontraditional health belief choices that a client might consider therapeutic. By incorporating these choices into the plan of care, you are showing respect for the client's belief system, which can promote their health.

INCORPORATING UNIQUENESS INTO THE NURSING CARE PROCESS

The nursing process supports diversity by recognizing uniqueness and by recognizing the needs, backgrounds, and experiences of diverse client populations. By following the stages of the nursing process, nurses are able to plan and to provide care that is equitable and inclusive.

ASSESSMENT

A thorough assessment helps nurses identify the specific needs and preferences of each client, taking into account factors related to gender, sexual orientation, socioeconomic status, spirituality, and other aspects of diversity. The ability to obtain a full assessment depends on communication skills. Asking questions in an open way allows the nurse to gain valuable information about the way each individual will achieve a state of health that is personally satisfying.

Which questions are asked and the way in which they are asked are important. Box 13.5 provides some sample questions to use in a cultural assessment.

BOX 13.5 Assessment of Cultural Uniqueness

1. What are your views on health and healthcare, and/or your present healthcare situation?
2. Tell me about your family and community relationships.
3. What language is spoken at home?
4. Do you have ties to another country or another part of this country?
5. Describe the types of foods you usually eat.
6. What are your spiritual/religious beliefs? How much of a part of your life is spirituality/religion?
7. In your family, who cares for the children?
8. Who is the decision maker at home?
9. What are your views about death, and do you follow any death rituals?

THINKING CRITICALLY

Locate the Health Research and Educational Trust (HRET) website at http://www.hretdisparities.org. Find the HRET Disparities Toolkit, which can be used to collect race, ethnicity, and primary language information from clients. Then, contact the healthcare organization that employs you and ask if they use a tool for collecting client diversity information. If they do, compare your organization's tool to the HRET tool. What are the similarities? What are the differences? What is the impact of such tools on the quality of nursing care for clients? If your organization does not use such a tool, inquire about their interest in using one.

DIAGNOSIS

Nurses must consider the impact of diversity and inclusion when determining appropriate nursing diagnoses. By recognizing how factors such as ethnicity, socioeconomic status, and access to healthcare services can influence a client's health, nurses are able to plan care that is culturally sensitive. Although International Classification for Nursing Practice nursing diagnoses (Box 13.6) and NANDA-I nursing diagnoses that address cultural, spiritual, and social variations exist, there is a continued need for diagnosis development that accommodates diverse cultural practices and religious beliefs.

The NCLEX-RN *Might Ask* 13.3

The nurse is formulating a nursing diagnosis for a client who speaks and reads only Chinese. Which of the following nursing diagnoses would be *most* appropriate?
a. Lack of knowledge related to surgical procedure
b. Communication barrier related to inability to speak and read English
c. Sensory deficit caused by inability to hear
d. Spiritual distress caused by hopelessness

• See Appendix A for correct answer and rationale.

> **BOX 13.6** **Sample International Classification for Nursing Practice Cultural/Social/Spiritual Nursing Diagnoses**
>
> Powerlessness
> Risk for spiritual distress
> Impaired sexual behavior
> Conflicting religious belief

PLANNING

The process of planning and setting goals that align with the client's values and beliefs requires collaboration between the client, their significant others, and the nurse. At the client's request, a spiritual advisor may also be part of the client's support team. Care goals should reflect the client's individual needs and preferences, include interventions to accommodate diverse cultural practices, and empower the client with the knowledge and skills needed to actively participate in their care.

IMPLEMENTATION

Uniqueness must be recognized and incorporated into the plan for client-centered care. Nurses should implement interventions that are culturally sensitive and that respect diverse traditions and practices. Standard care protocols may need to be adapted to accommodate cultural practices. Asking the client about intervention preferences might include inquiring whether there is a need for specific clothing and draping during physical examinations, whether they would like family to be involved in care discussions, and which foods are culturally acceptable. Box 13.7 offers interventional strategies that can be used by the nurse to be more culturally sensitive.

> **BOX 13.7** **Interventions for the Culturally Competent Nurse**
>
> - Be aware of how ethnocentric tendencies affect your perception.
> - Identify cultural groups within the community.
> - Ask for help from the client, family, or other healthcare workers, if needed.
> - Commit to ongoing education and self-reflection on diversity, cultural competence, and cultural humility.
> - Apologize for making mistakes; this is a learning process.
> - Be observant of client behaviors.
> - Listen closely to what the client says.
> - Speak slowly and simply; avoid medical jargon and slang.
> - Use gestures cautiously.
> - Use open-ended questions to explore the client's cultural identity.
> - Advocate for the client's cultural needs and preferences.
> - Incorporate practices/ideas from the client's healthcare beliefs.
> - Assess the role of family and community in the client's healthcare decisions.
> - Facilitate access to religious or spiritual support, if desired.
> - Respect food preferences when possible.
> - Use a clinically approved nonfamily, culturally similar interpreter.
> - Provide translated materials and signage in commonly spoken languages.
> - Ensure that educational materials are available in multiple languages.
> - Be sensitive to nonverbal cues and expressions of discomfort or agreement.

EVALUATION

Client uniqueness must be considered throughout the nursing care planning process. In the evaluation phase, nurses assess client satisfaction and the effectiveness of interventions based on diverse outcome measures. If the evaluation of the plan is unsatisfactory, the nurse should consider that unique factors might have been missed. Understanding diverse perspectives and expectations helps nurses gauge the effectiveness of care from the client's point of view. The evaluation process should include gathering feedback from clients about their satisfaction with their care, monitoring outcomes, and adjusting interventions based on cultural considerations. When goals are unmet, nurses should continue to seek education and increase the use of resources that they did not previously consider.

CONCLUSION

Cultural awareness helps nurses provide respectful, inclusive, and patient-centered care. Nurses who recognize the unique needs and backgrounds of diverse client populations provide care that is equitable, respectful, and inclusive. Cultural awareness and cultural humility contribute to understanding an individual's health needs and allow tailored healthcare interventions that promote overall well-being. The nursing process supports diversity and promotes individualized culturally competent care. By incorporating the steps of the nursing process, nurses develop plans of care that are culturally sensitive and contribute to improved health outcomes.

REFERENCES

American Nurses Association. (2018). *ANA position statement: The nurse's role in addressing discrimination: Protecting and promoting inclusive strategies in practice settings, policy, and advocacy.* https://www.nursingworld.org/~4ab207/globalassets/practiceandpolicy/nursing-excellence/ana-position-statements/social-causes-and-health-care/the-nurses-role-in-addressing-discrimination.pdf

Bastable, S. (2017). *Essentials of patient education* (2nd ed.). Jones and Bartlett.

Boyle, J. C., Collins, J. W., Ludwig-Beymer, P., & Andrews, M. M. (2025). *Transcultural concepts in nursing care* (9th ed.). Wolters Kluwer.

Catalano, J. T. (2024). *Nursing now: Today's issues, tomorrow's trends* (9th ed.). F.A. Davis.

Frie, K., & Timm, J. (2023). Developing cultural humility through an interprofessional clinical education experience. *Nurse Educator, 48*(5), E153–E157. https://doi.org/10.1097/NNE.0000000000001379

Huston, C. (2023). *Professional issues in nursing: Challenges and opportunities* (6th ed.). Wolters Kluwer.

Jadoon, S. B., Nasir, S., Victor, G., & Pienaar, A. J. (2022). Knowledge attitudes and readiness of nursing students in assessing peoples' sexual health problems. *Nurse Education Today, 113,* 105371. https://doi.org/10.1016/j.nedt.2022.105371

Mukerjee, R., Wesp, L., & Singer, R. (Eds.). (2022). *Clinicians guide to LGBTQIA+ care: Cultural safety and social justice in primary, sexual, and reproductive healthcare.* Springer Publishing.

Niemet, C. J., & Rice, K. (2022). LGBTQ & A: Development of a needs assessment to define access, needs, and barriers to health care services among LGBTQ older adults. *Journal of Prevention & Intervention in the Community, 50*(1), 1-15. https://doi.org/10.1080/10852352.2021.1915937

Purnell, L., & Fenkl, E. (Eds.). (2021). *Textbook for transcultural health care: A population approach: Cultural competence concepts in nursing care* (5th ed.). Springer Publishing.

Smiley, R. A., Allgeyer, R. L., Shobo, Y., Lyons, K. C., Letourneau, R., Zhong, E., Kaminski-Ozturk, N., & Alexander, M. (2023). The 2022 national nursing workforce survey. *Journal of Nursing Regulation, 14*(1), S1–S90. https://www.journalofnursingregulation.com/article/S2155-8256(23)00047-9/pdf

Taylor, C., Lynn, P., & Bartlett, J. L. (2023). *Fundamentals of nursing: The art and science of nursing care* (10th ed.). Wolters Kluwer.

U.S. Census Bureau. (2022, December 08). *American community survey 2017-2021 5-year data release.* https://www.census.gov/newsroom/press-kits/2022/acs-5-year.html

U.S. Census Bureau. (n.d.). *2020 Decennial census: Race and ethnicity.* https://data.census.gov/profile/United_States?g=010XX00US#race-and-ethnicity

Wall, A. (2023). Practicing cultural humility toward Black and Brown communities in the ED. *Nursing, 53*(4), 41–44. https://doi.org/10.1097/01.NURSE.0000920456.10204.1a

Yu, H., Dalmacio, D. F., Bonett, S., & Bauermeister, J. A. (2023). LGBTQ+ cultural competency training for health professionals: A systematic review. *BMC Medical Education, 23*, 1-83. https://doi.org/10.1186/s12909-023-04373-3

SUGGESTED READING

Apodaca, C., Casanova-Perez, R., Bascom, E., Mohanraj, D., Lane, C., Vidyarthi, D., Beneteau, E., Sabin, J., Pratt, W., Weibel, N., & Hartzler, A. L. (2022). Maybe they had a bad day: How LGBTQ and BIPOC patients react to bias in healthcare and struggle to speak out. *Journal of the American Medical Informatics Association, 29*(12), 2075–2082. https://doi.org/10.1093/jamia/ocac142

Kelleher, S. T., Barrett, M. J., Durnin, S., Fitzpatrick, P., Higgins, A., & Hall, D. (2023). Staff competence in caring for LGBTQ+ patients in the paediatric emergency department. *Archives of Disease in Childhood,* https://doi.org/10.1136/archdischild-2022-325151

Ličen, S., & Prosen, M. (2023). The development of cultural competences in nursing students and their significance in shaping the future work environment: A pilot study. *BMC Medical Education, 23*, 1-9. https://doi.org/10.1186/s12909-023-04800-5

Osmancevic, S., Großschädl, F., & Lohrmann, C. (2023). Cultural competence among nursing students and nurses working in acute care settings: A cross-sectional study. *BMC Health Services Research, 23*, 1-7. https://doi.org/10.1186/s12913-023-09103-5

Quallich, S. A. (2023). Treating all patients the same does not equal person-centered care. *Urologic Nursing, 43*(1), 9-9,13. https://doi.org/10.7257/2168-4626.2023.43.L9

On the WEB

American Nurses Association—Racism in nursing: https://www.nursingworld.org/practice-policy/workforce/racism-in-nursing/

EthnoMed—Information for integrating cultural information into clinical practice: https://ethnomed.org/

Every Nurse—Seven steps to become a more culturally sensitive nurse: https://everynurse.org/7-steps-culturally-sensitive-nurse/

Hartford Institute for Geriatric Nursing—Includes the ConsultGeri resources: https://hign.org/

Health Information Translations—Free, easy-to-read, shareable health education in 15+ languages: https://www.healthinfotranslations.org/

Health Professionals Advancing LGBT Equity: https://www.glma.org/

Health Research & Educational Trust (HRET): http://www.hret.org

Journal of Transcultural Nursing: http://www.tcns.org/journal

National Institutes of Health—Cultural Respect: https://www.nih.gov/institutes-nih/nih-office-director/office-communications-public-liaison/clear-communication/cultural-respect

United States Census Bureau—Useful statistics for patient uniqueness: http://www.census.gov

Decision-Making and Managing Time, Conflict, and Resources

CHAPTER 14

LEARNING OUTCOMES

By the end of this chapter, the student will be able to:
1. Summarize factors that influence time management.
2. Describe strategies to manage time more effectively.
3. Discuss various contexts in which conflict occurs.
4. Identify strategies for conflict resolution.
5. Apply the guidelines for conflict resolution to a hypothetical situation.
6. List the steps in the decision-making process.
7. Recognize the role of the nurse in cost-containment activities.
8. Analyze the role of the nurse in managing a safe environment.

KEY TERMS

accommodation
chunking
conflict
conflict management
conflict resolution
cost containment
decision-making
delegation
effectiveness
efficiency
emotional intelligence
multitasking
Pareto principle
procrastination
perfectionism
quality management (QM)
time management
unlicensed assistive personnel (UAP)
worksheet

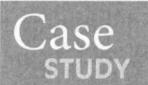
Case STUDY

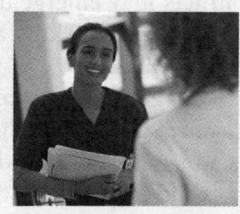

Nancy is the preceptor to Juanita, a new RN graduate who was formerly an LPN. Juanita has to "pay back" her student loan at New Berry Hospital by staying in their employment. Due to staff turnover, Juanita is orienting on the same unit where she was functioning as an LPN before graduation. Nancy is discussing her orientation with Juanita.

NANCY: You're doing well. Patients are complimentary about your care. Your assessment skills are really improving. The discharge planners are very impressed with your teamwork and early referral. If you could pinpoint an area where you need the most help, what would that be?

329

> **JUANITA:** I believe the areas I would identify are conflict management and having enough time to finish work. I seem to be irritating the other aides and LPNs that I've worked with for years. Suddenly, since I've assumed this new role, I'm "putting out fires" with people I've always gotten along with. I find myself doing things myself just to avoid conflict, which I know isn't a good use of my time. This is much more difficult for me than the actual tasks I have to do. Any words of advice?
>
> **NANCY:** I understand what you're saying. Sometimes it's better to either change units or change hospitals, especially if the institution is small and people really know each other. It's especially difficult being on the same unit because people often have difficulty adjusting to your newly expanded role. The first step is always to assess the situation. Since you have already done that, you need to assess how frequently issues occur and with whom. Keep track of the issues factually and unemotionally, if you can.
>
> I would try to identify the MOST problematic relationship and focus on working with that person in a nonthreatening way. Arrange to meet with the person when you both have time and you can openly discuss issues privately. When you approach your coworker, let them know you want to work on building a good working relationship. If you can't come to some resolution, you may need a neutral third party to discuss the issues. Hope this helps! Now about time management…

Today's healthcare system requires that RNs be prepared to assume the management of care for large, unique groups of clients. This includes completing assigned tasks in a timely manner, delegating work to others, managing conflict, making wise decisions, and maintaining a safe environment for all clients. Juanita is aware she has a time management issue. She has successfully identified that she needs to settle conflicting relationships with some coworkers in order to be a successful time management steward.

The frustration that Juanita is feeling is familiar to many nurses who have changed responsibilities and roles. Unless a nurse is in a new unit or has mentors who have taught them how to cope with other staff while transitioning into the new role, conflicts may emerge during a role shift. Coping strategies, leadership abilities, and communication skills are essential in transitioning from the LPN/LVN role to the RN role.

Managing client care requires the nurse to assess the needs of the clients; to plan, organize, and direct the implementation of care; and to evaluate care effectiveness. As a manager of care, the nurse is in the combined role of care provider, coordinator, and overseer. Managing care includes the ability to organize time effectively, establish priorities, delegate appropriately, and ensure effective and efficient client care. Conflict management and decision-making are also important components of the manager of care role.

As roles and responsibilities shift, the student must have a foundational understanding of organizational and managerial skills. This chapter includes strategies to manage time more effectively on the job, methods of conflict resolution in the work setting, how to make decisions, and strategies for managing resources.

MANAGING TIME

Although we cannot add more hours to a day, we can work toward effectively managing the time we have. Time management is useful at home, work, and school. Strategies for prioritizing, planning, and scheduling are necessary when balancing multiple responsibilities. Time management can be enhanced by using tools and strategies that increase productivity. Nurses have numerous responsibilities, and effective time management is essential. In managing client care, the task of time management becomes more complex and highly variable. Time management is similar to the nursing process; needed activities are assessed, a time for completion of tasks is identified, priorities and goals are established, and the results of the process are evaluated. Nurses can determine if they are managing time efficiently by examining how they use their time.

TIME MANAGEMENT SELF-ASSESSMENT

Because of the new responsibilities in the RN role, time management is even more important for RNs than for LPN/LVNs. Although you may already be well organized, your new role may require you to improve your skills. Take some time to assess your time management abilities and to identify methods that will help you gain even more skill in this area.

Self-assessment will help determine whether a nurse needs to adopt better time management strategies. Think back on the past workweek and answer the following questions. Have you experienced:

- An increase in the number of hours it takes to complete daily work?
- Feelings of resentment about the lack of "free time"?
- A decrease in the regularity of completing work items at home or on weekends?
- An increase in the feeling of being rushed or "out of control"?

Many nurses have had similar experiences but do not despair. Managing time more effectively is a learned skill. The first step is realizing, like Juanita, that better time management requires planning and effort.

TIME ASSESSMENT

Time management is the process of organizing and using time wisely (Albert et al., 2022). Because you are already an LPN/LVN, you recognize that managing time with respect to client care is dictated by the number of clients assigned and the role assumed for that particular clinical day. Although time is somewhat controlled by what else happens with clients or by having to wait for an instructor to supervise procedures, completing the requirements of the assignment requires appropriate planning. As an LPN/LVN, you are also familiar with caring for a larger number of clients and not having much flexibility in planning time. The shift is dictated by predetermined schedules for care and procedures; however, planning needs to be flexible in order to provide for sudden interruptions. (Just as in your role as an LPN/LVN, you have to anticipate interruptions; RNs also anticipate that interruptions will occur throughout the day.)

As you transition into the RN role, the focus of how you spend your time will change. RNs dedicate their time to assessment, identifying interventions, implementing interventions, and evaluating the results of each task. Having well-developed time management strategies usually lead to feelings of accomplishment because completing tasks goes according to plan. Even with exceptional planning, at one time or another every nurse feels overwhelmed; however, learning to develop and implement time management strategies will increase your confidence in managing care.

The Pareto Principle

One strategy to improve efficiency when managing time is the 80/20 rule identified in the **Pareto principle**. In 1906, an Italian economist named Vilfredo Pareto discovered the 80/20 rule (Pareto principle) when making observations about wealth distribution. Over time, researchers discovered that the principle could be applied to other fields, like time management. According to the principle, 80% of results come from 20% of effort (Carver, 2022). When applying the rule to time management, identifying the tasks that generate the most results will lead to the greatest productivity. In other words, when prioritizing tasks, 20% of our effort will result in 80% of the results. If we fail to plan, 80% of our effort will result in only 20% of the results.

Time Activity Log

A time activity log is a useful tool to assess how effectively you use your time. The log provides a detailed visual record of how you spend your time, helps you become more aware of your daily activities, and identifies how much time you allocate to completing tasks. You can construct time logs for any time interval increments. However, because the amount of time it takes to complete nursing tasks varies widely, using 30-minute intervals will likely work best for an initial activity assessment. An example activity log with 30-minute intervals is shown in Box 14.1. After listing your shift hours, record the start and end times for each activity you perform in the time intervals. Do not use

BOX 14.1 Time Assessment

Day 1		Day 2	
Time	Activity	Time	Activity
7:00		7:00	
7:30		7:30	
8:00		8:00	
8:30		8:30	
9:00		9:00	
9:30		9:30	
10:00		10:00	
10:30		10:30	
11:00		11:00	
11:30		11:30	
12:00		12:00	
12:30		12:30	
13:00		13:00	
13:30		13:30	
14:00		14:00	
14:30		14:30	
15:00		15:00	
15:30		15:30	
16:00		16:00	

generic terms (e.g., hygiene; meds); be specific and include details about each task. It is helpful to record activities for at least 3 days to recognize patterns, determine types of interruptions, and identify how unexpected events are handled. The goal of a time log is not just to record your activities but to gain insights that lead to improved time management and productivity. Keeping a log for several days also helps analyze how a nurse copes with interruptions, what aspects of organization the nurse needs to be improve, and where the nurse's most productive time occurs.

PLANNING

When working as a care manager, the idea of planning may be seen as unnecessary or pointless because time limits and unit policies already dictate most of the work. In the case study, Juanita failed to anticipate problems with other staff in her new role. Although Juanita was able to adjust to her new role, the other staff had difficulty recognizing how her role had changed. Managing conflict with her coworkers was more time consuming than Juanita had anticipated. The plan Juanita's preceptor suggested may help alleviate the problems she is facing and allow her to regain some poorly spent time.

In nursing care, careful planning is one of the best ways to maximize efficiency. Start by developing a time schedule, which can be done by using a **worksheet** (see Box 14.2). Take a few minutes to examine what goals need to be achieved and develop a plan to meet them. Estimating the time required to complete assigned tasks improves time management and efficiency. Next, determine which item is the highest priority, which is the next highest, and so on (Huston, 2023). If something unexpected happens, reprioritize based on the new situation. Two of the most common pitfalls in planning are failure to plan and not allowing enough time to plan. The more experience a nurse gains in priority setting in the RN role, the more accurate time requirements for the work the nurse will be able to estimate, and the easier it will become to develop a basic routine. Obviously, this daily plan cannot account for crises, but it should allow for flexibility and reorganization when those unexpected interruptions occur. Like Juanita, consult a more experienced nurse or the instructor to compare what was accomplished to how the day was planned. As you learn to manage care in the RN role, seek out timely tips

BOX 14.2 Sample Worksheet for Medical–Surgical Unit

Room	Name	Med Times	Procedures	IV Sites	IV Fluids	Adm & Hx	
Diet							

Delegate	VS	Assessment	Glucometer		
			Time	BS	TX

To Do:

TABLE 14.1 Comparison of Workday Planning and the Nursing Process

Planning Your Workday	Nursing Process
1. Assess the tasks for the day. (Make time to plan.)	1. Assessment of the client
2. Identify and prioritize tasks and determine who will complete them.	2. Diagnosis
3. Develop a daily plan and time-related challenges or constraints that may impact task completion.	3. Planning
4. Complete assigned tasks. (Pick the highest priority task and finish it.)	4. Interventions
5. Evaluate the results of the plan. Set new priorities as needed. (Reprioritize based on new data or remaining tasks.)	5. Evaluation

and advice on organizing your day, especially from experienced nurses. See Table 14.1 for a comparison of how the process of planning your workday compares to the nursing process.

Setting Priorities

When developing a daily plan, the activities that need to be accomplished should be listed in an organized and easy-to-read format. Although most electronic health records (EHRs) incorporate "to do lists" and nursing hand-off report pages, many nurses find it useful to make a worksheet, or "nursing brain," from their daily plan (Box 14.2). This worksheet lists essential information and needed tasks for each patient. It also assists in establishing priorities by determining what is essential and what is important but not critical. Needed care can be designated or color coded into "do now," "delegate," "do later," "do whenever," and "don't do" priorities. The "to do list" should be organized in terms of urgency of care, safety of care, patient's priority of care, and ongoing care (Table 14.2).

It is often beneficial to indicate what absolutely must be done by highlighting or color-coding different priorities. For example, preoperative patients take priority, so color code those patients in red. Early regular insulin and blood glucose checks are also

TABLE 14.2 Planning Priorities Hierarchy[a]

Care Priorities	Types of Care	Examples
Urgency of care	• ABCs of care (airway, breathing, circulation) • Life-threatening situations	• Blocked airway • Hypotension
Safety of care	• Change in assessment status • Protection from injury	• Avoiding medication errors • Prevention of falling • Seizures
Patient's priority of care	• Tasks to be done routinely or at client's request • Partner with the client to set priorities; remember that the patient is the champion of their own care	• Administering medications and treatments • Informed consent • Patient education
Ongoing care	• Not essential; could be put off until a later time	• Following up with psychologist on low self-esteem needs • Nutritional consult

[a]May change with the situation. For example, if a client's self-esteem needs are so low that the client is suicidal, then safety becomes the priority.

a priority but can have a bit of flexibility; color code those tasks in blue. Although this may seem simplistic, when the nurse is in a hurry, this can save time by enabling the nurse to see priorities at a glance and get back on schedule.

THINKING CRITICALLY

Planning sheets (reports) are frequently used by RNs to organize a workday. Meet with other students in the class. Compare and contrast the various types of time management sheets. Take the best of each sheet and combine them into one. Use this sheet in clinical. The following week, report back to the group what worked or what did not. Also, discuss the workflow of clinical time. Was it more or less organized?

Another aspect of developing and maintaining a worksheet is to get in the habit of writing things down. If there is a bedside computer or a workstation on wheels, save time by documenting each activity and task as you complete it. Although some nurses may be able to remember everything, most nurses find it useful to keep notes and write down key facts. The worksheet is an excellent place to write down information as you work. This information can include abnormal assessment findings, laboratory results, and PRN medications given. The worksheet is not meant to replace appropriate documentation; it is a method to assist in accuracy and continually updating the establishment of priorities for critical tasks.

A final aspect of the worksheet is to determine who is the most appropriate person for completing a task. A green color code might be used to delegate skills to be performed by the **unlicensed assistive personnel (UAP)** (such as vital signs, glucose checks, and walking a client). This documentation can also help verify that the work was completed and describe patient outcomes, both of which are essential components of managing client care in your role transition.

One of the rewarding aspects of planning or using a worksheet is checking off or crossing out tasks that have been completed. This method of tracking care will identify what tasks remain to be accomplished by the oncoming shift and will give you a sense of accomplishment from the completed tasks.

Quiet Time and "No-Interruption" Zones

Time to plan is critical in preparing for patient care. Many hospital administration groups are beginning to recognize how critical preparation and "quiet time" are to nurses; they understand that nurses need time for the complex thinking required to perform the duties and responsibilities of a nurse. Some hospitals have designated no-interruption zones or no-interruption time frames (especially during medications passes).

DELEGATION

The process of **delegation** often proves troublesome for new nurses and for those who are making the transition from LPN/LVN to RN. Some of the reasons that nurses avoid delegating tasks are as follows:

- Lack of understanding about the process of delegating
- Inability to assess what should be delegated and to whom
- Guilt about not doing as many tasks as the rest of the team members are doing

- Desire to be liked by everyone
- Inability to organize
- Distrust of others' abilities or the need to take care of everything personally
- Being caught in the trap of "we've always done it that way"

Delegation is covered in more depth in Chapter 11. Because delegation is an important function in nursing practice today, be sure to review that chapter.

> ### The NCLEX-RN *Might Ask* 14.1
>
> The RN's client assignment team includes one LPN and two UAPs for 10 clients on night shift. Before assigning tasks to perform, the RN must (Select all that apply):
>
> a. free themselves to deliver care to only the most acutely ill.
> b. assess the skills of the workers assigned.
> c. check on every task assigned to the UAP.
> d. assume that all standards of care are upheld.
> e. prioritize who needs to be seen first.
>
> • See Appendix A for correct answer and rationale.

EFFICIENT AND EFFECTIVE USE OF TIME

A comprehensive approach to managing time involves a combination of various factors beyond assessment, planning, priority setting, and delegation. Time management effectiveness and efficiency are two key aspects of optimizing how you use your time. **Efficiency** is the process of doing something right; **effectiveness** is doing the right thing right (Zerwekh & Garneau, 2023). As simplistic as this may seem, as a nurse, you have to make choices about what needs to be accomplished (the right thing) and then do it right. Table 14.2 may be helpful in planning for efficiency and priorities throughout the day.

Take Advantage of Your Energy

One of the best methods for increasing effectiveness is to be self-aware of energy levels as they relate to the time of day. Determine what time of day is the most productive for you while allowing for some variations regarding the time of year and the multiple demands on your time. It is useful to pay attention to the high-energy periods and plan to do the things that require more energy at those times. It is also helpful to recognize that efficiency may not be as great at the low-energy times, even though important tasks need to be completed. During times of low energy, the nurse may work with less speed and focus. Some methods to boost energy include providing for basic human needs, such as eating appropriately, sleeping adequately, and planning regular exercise.

Learn to Function in a Teamwork Environment

Being prudent when offering or seeking assistance is another method for increasing effectiveness. Learning to function in a teamwork environment requires careful thought and evaluation of needed tasks. To maintain effective use of time, one must not only recognize when it is best to ask for help but also when it is and is not appropriate to provide assistance to others. Knowing when it is appropriate to help others while managing your time involves finding a balance between being supportive and safeguarding your own priorities. Some considerations to help you determine when it is appropriate to assist others include urgency and importance, priorities, communication, boundaries, recurring requests, and your own expertise. By considering these factors, you can find a balance that allows you to be supportive while still protecting your time and well-being. Because effective use of time is a cause of stress and tension among coworkers, some units have developed policies such as at least every 2 hours all RNs must ask each other if they need help.

Streamline the Documentation Process

Resolving the documentation and paperwork dilemma will also increase efficiency and effectiveness. Despite the fact that computers streamline most tasks, nurses still need to minimize the quantity of papers they handle. Although nurses must fulfill the requirements of the agency for which they work, there are ways to streamline paperwork and documentation. For instance, if using paper worksheets, limit worksheets to one page to reduce shuffling through several pages. Some EHRs include computerized worksheets that eliminate the need for paper forms and improve the efficiency in managing the care for a group of clients.

Because of the many factors associated with documentation, many institutions have gone "paperless" in which standardized forms are accessible to all need-to-know professionals. This decreases the interruptions on nursing time in providing report of retrievable information such as vital signs, meal consumption, and activities of daily living. Efficient documentation will make you more effective in managing client care. Box 14.3 provides tips for personal effectiveness, and Box 14.4 provides tips for efficient documentation. By incorporating these strategies into your daily routine, you can enhance your time management skills and streamline the nursing documentation process, allowing you to provide optimal patient care.

BOX 14.3

Tips for Personal Effectiveness

- Pay attention to basic human needs (sleep, nutrition, exercise).
- Plan frequently (daily, weekly, yearly).
- Take breaks (more frequent for mental work).
- Declutter and organize any work areas.
- Find a quiet place without interruptions when doing paperwork.
- Work as a team when possible.
- Delegate appropriately.
- Handle paper only once.

BOX 14.4

Tips for Efficient Documentation

Document in Real Time

- Whenever possible, document patient care in real time.
- Documenting immediately after completing a task reduces the risk of forgetting important details and minimizes the time needed for retrospective documentation.

Use Standardized Forms

- Utilize standardized forms and templates whenever possible to streamline the documentation process.
- Standardized forms help to ensure consistency and save time by reducing the need to recreate similar documents.

(Continued)

BOX 14.4 (Continued)

Utilize Electronic Health Records
- If the healthcare facility uses EHRs, take advantage of features that automate and simplify documentation.
- Use shortcuts, templates, and copy-paste functions within the EHR system to speed up data entry.

Minimize Interruptions
- Find a quiet and focused environment for documentation to minimize interruptions.

Use Approved Abbreviations and Acronyms
- Only document using standardized abbreviations and acronyms.
- Ensure that you follow guidelines for safe abbreviations.

Stay Organized
- Develop a consistent system for organizing patient information for documentation.
- Utilize a "nursing brain."

Continuous Training
- Stay updated on the latest features and improvements in your facility's EHR system.
- Attend training sessions to enhance your proficiency and efficiency in using documentation tools.

Quality Over Quantity
- Focus on the quality of your documentation rather than the quantity.
- Ensure that your documentation is accurate, concise, and reflects the patient's condition and care accurately.

Seek Feedback and Improvement
- Regularly seek feedback on your documentation practices.
- Look for opportunities to improve efficiency and effectiveness based on input from colleagues or supervisors.

MINIMIZING TIME WASTERS

The last aspect of managing time is to identify and minimize tasks that waste time or decrease the ability to be efficient and effective. Some of these items are personal time wasters, and others are outside factors. The following subsections highlight some of these issues and provide suggestions on how to control or minimize them (see also Box 14.5).

Interruptions

Interruptions, where nurses are stopped in the middle of one activity to give attention to another, frequently occur during patient care. Although some interruptions are necessary and essential to the well-being of a client or to the general management of a group of clients, other interruptions are less urgent and should be limited for greater efficiency. The task for the nurse is to determine which interruptions

> **BOX 14.5 Common Time Wasters**
> - Interruptions
> - Socialization/personal cell phone calls or texts
> - Poor communication (lack of information or feedback)
> - Personal disorganization
> - Procrastination
> - Perfectionism
> - Meetings
> - Paperwork

are necessary. Many interruptions cannot be avoided and are part of the job. For example, if a patient call light is on, it is necessary to answer the call, just as it is necessary to answer the telephone to speak with a client's family members or their provider.

Mobile phones allow the nurse to manage phone calls while performing other tasks and decreases travel time to a stationary phone. However, because mobile phones interrupt the nurse in the process of completing tasks, the nurse must rearrange tasks once the call is answered. Personal phone calls that are nonurgent are negative interruptions and should be conducted during breaks to prevent interference with patient care duties. When interruptions occur, nurses must determine how to manage their time to decrease any negative impact on required duties. Following an interruption, the nurse must try to refocus as much as possible on finishing the first task before continuing to another task. Unfortunately, if there are frequent interruptions, nurses may begin numerous tasks but never finish them.

Multitasking is the ability to handle many tasks simultaneously. A nurse rarely has the chance to finish one task prior to starting another. For example, it is not unusual for a nurse to balance teaching a patient with diabetes, preparing a preoperative patient, administering medications, and performing colostomy care all in one shift. Having a to-do list helps to keep nurses organized so they will avoid missing tasks they need to perform.

Socializing

Socializing in nursing is not always negative; in fact, it often contributes positively to the work environment. Although socializing can have both positive and negative aspects, its impact largely depends on the context, setting, and the extent to which it interferes with professional responsibilities. Some positive aspects of socializing include team building, stress relief, enhanced communication, and professional development. Unfortunately, there are negative consequences to inappropriate socializing. Excessive socializing during work hours can interfere with productivity and time management. It is important to strike a balance between social interactions and fulfilling professional responsibilities. In some instances, socializing can lead to the formation of cliques, which result in exclusionary dynamics within a team that may negatively affect teamwork and collaboration. Too much socializing, especially during busy periods, can be distracting and may compromise patient care.

THINKING CRITICALLY

Review the cell phone policy implemented by staff of the Association of periOperative Registered Nurses that is described in the article "A Plan for Cell Phones in the OR" at https://www.aorn.org/article/2019-10-22-Phones-in-the-OR and discuss the advantages and disadvantages of this type of policy. Compare this policy with current cell phone practices in your clinical setting or place of employment and suggest what could be done differently.

Poor Communication

Even when a nurse has thoughtfully planned out their day, circumstances can change, and a task that was previously low on the list of priorities may become urgent. Poor communication or lack of information that helps in decision-making can contribute to a disruption. Nurses should always ask clarifying questions about important details before beginning any task. The use of standardized charting forms or report sheets enables proactive planning to reduce the potential lack of communication of crucial information. The nursing care plan is an excellent tool to communicate what patient care has been accomplished, evaluation of completed tasks, and any further client needs. Remember that nursing care is frequently "around the clock." Because the nurse may not always be able to complete everything during their shift, it is important to communicate to the following nurse what remains to be done and its priority (Huston, 2023).

Nurses should also routinely seek feedback on their communication and performance, especially if assuming a new task or role. Feedback provides information about what is completed well (strengths), where improvements can be made (weaknesses), and helps nurses adapt to unexpected changes in care requirements or situations. Feedback can provide insight into what adjustments are needed to keep work on track and prevents the need to redo work when requirements may not be fulfilled.

Personal Disorganization

Personal disorganization wastes time. Personal organization is often reflected in how a nurse organizes work. The use of a worksheet, daily or weekly planners, or calendars assists in being more organized.

Also, save time and energy by gathering the supplies that you will need and grouping them in the same area, if possible, before engaging in an activity (Huston, 2023). Going back and forth from a client room to the supply room for needed items wastes time and energy. Many hospitals have implemented strategies to minimize the added time for gathering supplies by storing commonly used items in the client's room. Careful planning can also alleviate wasted steps. Review procedures and needed care, then make a list of items that will be required to accomplish those tasks. Gather the needed supplies before proceeding to the client room.

Improve your personal organization by making wise use of downtime. Everyone has spent time waiting in various situations for various reasons. When you encounter a long wait time, boost productivity by working on brief items, reading research articles, catching up on correspondence, and completing small segments of larger time-consuming projects. Have a note pad and pen handy to jot down ideas before bed. When on the go, use the cell phone dictation features to save ideas. Creativity can help you find a few extra minutes each day that will add up.

Procrastination

Procrastination, which is delaying a project or item without a cause, is high on the list of time wasters (Huston, 2023). Procrastination usually occurs when a person has a high-priority task that is viewed as difficult, large, or unpleasant. For example, no one enjoys preparing their income tax returns. Even though the prepared forms can be submitted any time from January to mid-April, an individual may wait until a day or two before the deadline because the task is unpleasant to complete. To make the task less daunting, the needed data and calculations could be spread out from January to mid-April, so only a small amount of time would need to be invested each month.

If there is a particular procedure to be done during your nursing shift, it is beneficial to complete the task as soon as you have time because unforeseen circumstances may sometimes prevent you from finishing it at all. Waiting to complete a task will usually have negative consequences. For example, waiting until shift change to complete a procedure could result in handing over an incomplete task to the next shift, potentially compromising patient care continuity and causing unnecessary stress for the incoming nursing staff. Delaying the completion of continuing education modules until the last minute may result in rushed completion and limited retention of material. In addition, waiting until the due date leaves no time to work out technical issues or unexpected obstacles that could prevent timely submission, risking noncompliance with licensure requirements or employer policies.

To avoid procrastination, follow these steps:

1. Recognize and admit that procrastination is occurring.
2. Identify the consequences of the delay (e.g., I won't get my promotion, the job won't get done, I will look inefficient, I will feel bad about not completing the task).
3. Consider if the task could be most efficiently delegated to someone else.
4. If you decide not to delegate the task, develop an action plan. Start by breaking the task into small steps that seem more manageable (sometimes called "**chunking**"). Keep in mind that perfection is not always necessary as long as standards are maintained.
5. Assign a reward for accomplishing the dreaded chore (Box 14.6). A reward is important. The positive reinforcement for self-initiated actions creates an expectation for future rewards. Over time, the anticipation of a reward leads to an increase in task completion (Michaelsen & Esch, 2023).

BOX 14.6

Tips to Prevent Procrastination

- Recognize that procrastination is occurring and determine why.
- Analyze what is being avoided.
- Determine the cost of putting off the task.
- Start the task with planning.
- Divide tasks into small pieces over a period of time (chunking).
- Don't take past failures personally.
- Don't dwell on the past; move on to the next project.

Perfectionism

Perfectionism in nursing comes with both advantages and disadvantages. In school, student nurses are educated to practice until skills are performed without error. Standards for demonstrating skills are set high for several reasons, with the most critical reason being to prevent harm to the client. Although performing clinical procedures requires 100% accuracy, there are other tasks required of nurses for which perfection is not the expectation. In practice, it is essential to recognize that perfectionism exists on a spectrum; moderate levels may be beneficial, whereas extreme perfectionism can be detrimental.

Extreme perfectionism can result in rigid thinking, making it difficult for nurses to adapt to changing circumstances or to accept constructive feedback. Striving for perfection may result in spending excessive time on tasks, which can lead to challenges with time management. This can be particularly problematic in a fast-paced healthcare environment in which efficiency is crucial.

For instance, the nurse searching for the perfect teaching tool may not complete adequate client teaching required for discharge. A student striving for the perfect paper may miss assignment submission deadlines. In dynamic and complex environments like healthcare, there may be instances in which perfection is unattainable. Rather than setting unrealistic expectations to perform some tasks to perfection, strive to meet the standards of care.

LEARNING TO SAY "NO"

It is common for nurses to attempt to please everyone. In the process, nurses frequently attempt to do too much and take on unachievable tasks. Overcommitting, or taking on tasks beyond the nurse's capacity, can jeopardize client safety. For nurses, saying "no" is an important skill that can contribute to their well-being, effective client care, and maintaining professional boundaries. By saying "no" to additional responsibilities when appropriate, nurses can focus on their core duties, reducing the risk of errors or oversights that may affect client care.

Although a nurse cannot say "no" to assist a client in pain or to follow up with a UAP who has abnormal findings, nurses must express their limitations, concerns, or needs clearly to colleagues, supervisors, and other team members. Saying "no" does not mean a nurse is avoiding responsibilities. Rather, the nurse must make informed decisions to prioritize and balance the various demands on their time and energy. It may be necessary for the nurse to opt out of committee work or other activities when those responsibilities might compromise client care. Saying "no" to additional tasks or responsibilities that exceed the nurse's capacity helps prioritize essential duties and prevents spreading oneself too thin.

Just as it is crucial for the nurse to say "no" to certain tasks, it is equally important for the nurse to communicate when extra activities can be undertaken. Helping other nurses who may be overwhelmed strengthens teamwork and collaboration and contributes to a positive work environment.

The NCLEX-RN *Might Ask* 14.2

The RN should be efficient and effective in delivering client care. Common time wasters a nurse should avoid are (Select all that apply):

a. socialization.
b. handling a paper once.
c. organizing supplies ahead of time.
d. calling providers to report changes in a client's assessed condition.
e. procrastination.

- See Appendix A for correct answer and rationale.

MANAGING CONFLICT

Because no two people think or behave exactly the same, there is the possibility of **conflict**. Conflicts can arise between individuals, groups of individuals, and organizations. Although it may be thought of as detrimental to relationships in the workplace, conflict is not necessarily a negative phenomenon. Conflict is often a catalyst in building stronger bonds with others and in promoting organizational change (Albert et al., 2022). Examples of positive outcomes of conflict include exchange of ideas and a greater understanding of another person's feelings that leads to innovative change.

Conflict is common in the high-stress environment of healthcare. When managing client care, various conflicts may arise, either in interactions with clients and their families or with other members of the healthcare team. Conflict may lead to antagonism and incompatibility among individuals or groups and can be disruptive.

Conflict can be uncomfortable for some individuals. The tension produced during conflict may lead to unusual or uncharacteristic behavior. **Conflict resolution** skills are essential for maintaining a positive work atmosphere. The RN must be able to manage conflict and disagreements professionally, promote effective communication, and find collaborative solutions.

TYPES AND CAUSES OF CONFLICT

There are many reasons that conflicts may arise in nursing, and the form conflicts take can vary. Some typical types of conflict include those related to role, communication, goals, personality, and ethics or values (Zerwekh & Garneau, 2023).

Role Conflict

Conflict can occur when people share similar responsibilities but boundaries are not well defined. For example, shift-to-shift conflict about who is responsible for particular procedures during certain hours is common. Nurses may experience conflict when trying to balance direct client care responsibilities with administrative or managerial tasks. For instance, a nurse in a leadership role may find it challenging to allocate time between administrative duties and hands-on client care. Because nurses work closely with providers, therapists, and other healthcare professionals, collaboration is essential. Role conflict can arise when there are disagreements or different approaches to patient care among team members.

Communication Conflict

Communication conflicts can arise in various situations and relationships due to misunderstandings, differences in communication styles, or conflicting expectations. The most common communication conflicts are the result of misinformation and misinterpretation (Boggs, 2023). Misinterpretation can occur when words or phrases are interpreted differently by different people. A breakdown in communication can occur when information is not communicated because it was forgotten or overlooked (e.g., provision of incomplete information during handoff report). Other communication conflicts can occur because of poor listening skills, assuming intent, mixed nonverbal signals, differences in communication styles, and inappropriate tone. Whatever the reason, because communication is critical in healthcare, a breakdown in the process may lead to conflict.

Goal Conflict

In some situations, an individual's goals may not align with the goals and objectives of the client, group, or organization. A client's goals must be taken into consideration in formulating nursing goals; otherwise, the goals will not be achieved. In addition, conflicts can occur when client preferences or needs clash with established protocols or organizational policies. Nurses working for an organization need to be keenly aware of the organization's mission, goals, and values, both the written and the understood culture (Catalano, 2024). Choosing a goal that is in direct violation of those values can result in negative consequences.

Personality Conflict

A personality conflict refers to a situation in which individuals experience disagreement, stress, or tension due to differences in personalities, behavioral styles, or temperaments. Personality conflicts often arise from contrasting communication styles, values, attitudes, or approaches to problem solving. Certain personality traits, such as impulsivity or a tendency toward aggression, can predispose individuals to lashing out in stressful situations. When individuals perceive others as a threat to their beliefs, values, or self-esteem, they may respond defensively.

In the healthcare environment, if families feel the care of their loved ones is inadequate, they may direct their anger toward nursing staff. Staff may lash out at others during conflict because of poor coping mechanisms.

Ethical or Value Conflict

Ethical or value conflict can pose a significant dilemma. For example, disagreement about the code status of a client or the type of treatment to be implemented for a terminally ill client can be a source of conflict. Chapter 17 examines ethics that are relevant to nursing practice, providing students with the opportunity to analyze potential conflicts between ethics and values.

CONFLICT RESOLUTION

Effective conflict resolution involves open communication, active listening, empathy, and a willingness to find mutually acceptable solutions. Resolving conflict contributes to a healthier and more productive environment, whether in professional or personal settings. Encouraging a positive and respectful dialogue can help individuals navigate conflict productively.

Due to the dynamic nature and high pressure within healthcare environments, resolving conflict can be challenging. Because conflicts can arise among colleagues, with other healthcare professionals, or even with clients and their families, conflict resolution skills are crucial for RNs. In some instances, the nurse may feel like withdrawing from the issue rather than facing the conflict; however, the ability to resolve conflict is necessary to promote patient safety, to foster a positive work environment, and to support effective teamwork. Some methods for resolving conflict include accommodation, avoidance, competition, compromise, and collaboration. The method chosen is determined by the situation, the comfort level, and personal reaction to the conflict. Conflict resolution styles are listed in Box 14.7.

BOX 14.7 Conflict Resolution Strategies

- Accommodating: "A little bit of sugar goes a long way."
- Avoidance: "Leave it alone … it will go away."
- Competition: "I win… You lose."
- Compromise: "One for you, one for me. Two for you, two for me."
- Collaboration: "The more heads, the better!" "None of us is as smart as all of us."

CHAPTER 14 • Decision-Making and Managing Time, Conflict, and Resources

The NCLEX-RN *Might Ask* 14.3

An RN delegates obtaining vital signs to the UAP. When the RN reviews the vital sign results before giving medications, the RN observes that vital signs were obtained on only four of the six clients. When the RN alerts the UAP of the missing vital signs, the UAP states, "I thought I only had to take vital signs on these four." This type of potential conflict is known as a _____ conflict.

a. role
b. communication
c. goal
d. personality

• See Appendix A for correct answer and rationale.

Accommodation

Accommodation is a conflict resolution strategy in which one person willingly yields or adjusts their position to meet the needs or preferences of the other person. Concessions or compromises are made to maintain harmony and to facilitate a resolution. Accommodation is usually characterized by a conciliatory attitude, with the goal of preserving relationships and promoting a positive working environment. Accommodation can be a useful strategy when an issue is more important to one person than another or when maintaining a relationship is a priority (Yoder-Wise & Sportsman, 2023).

A nurse may accommodate in a conflict for several reasons:

- There is a short-term decrease of the potential for conflict to escalate.
- The issue may not be a high priority for the nurse; other issues may be of greater concern.
- If there is a significant power gap between the nurse and the other person (such as if the other person is a cardiothoracic surgeon).

The nurse may want more time to plan a solution to the conflict. Although accommodation can be a beneficial strategy in certain situations, it is important to be mindful of the potential drawbacks. Over time, the accommodating person may harbor resentment because their needs and concerns may be consistently overlooked or downplayed in favor of the other person's preferences. Unresolved anger on the part of the accommodating nurse may be misplaced to someone who has no stake in the issue, such as a client or other staff under the nurse's supervision. Accommodating may lead to a temporary solution; however, the strategy does not address the root cause of the conflict. Eventually, the unresolved issue may resurface. Excessive accommodation can reinforce negative behaviors such as dependency, entitlement, manipulation, and avoidance of responsibility in those who consistently benefit from the accommodation.

Avoidance

Using the avoidance strategy, individuals choose to ignore or evade the conflict rather than addressing or resolving it directly. For example, if a nurse refuses to engage in discussion related to the conflict, that limits the development of effective solutions. Nurses who are uncomfortable with conflict may avoid addressing issues or may try to remain neutral.

There are times when avoiding conflict is preferable, such as when insufficient information is available or when the particular problem is low priority. However, in most instances, avoiding conflict is not a positive way to deal with issues (Yoder-Wise &

Sportsman, 2023). Many of the same negative results encountered with accommodating can also arise when avoiding conflict. Although avoidance may provide temporary relief from tension or stress, it does not lead to a resolution of the issue and can allow underlying problems to persist. In some instances, nurses have gone as far as quitting their jobs rather than having to deal with interpersonal work conflicts, which in turn may lead to regret and guilt.

Competition

Competitive conflict resolution is a strategy in which one person advances their own interests and goals with disregard of the other person. With this strategy, the focus is on winning and gaining an advantage by using aggressive behaviors such as outtalking, outshouting, and possibly threatening the opponents. Competitive conflict resolution is characterized as a win-lose situation in which one person's success comes at the expense of the other person. A possible advantage of this strategy is that it may be beneficial if the conflict warrants moving beyond a deadlock. Competitive resolution is sometimes used when one person is more knowledgeable than the other person (Yoder-Wise & Sportsman, 2023).

Competitive conflict resolution can strain relationships and may not lead to mutually beneficial or sustainable solutions. The obvious disadvantage to this approach is that someone always loses. Negative feelings may last longer than the original conflict.

Compromise

Compromise is a conflict resolution strategy that requires all participants to make concessions in reaching solutions that are agreeable to all involved. Compromise requires effective communication, a willingness to understand the other person's perspective, and the ability to find common ground that addresses the core issues of the conflict. Issues are directly discussed so that all participants are aware of what is transpiring and the resolution process (Yoder-Wise & Sportsman, 2023).

There are several advantages for using compromise to resolve conflict. Because compromise requires active participation, everyone has a voice in negotiations. Compromise maintains positive relationships by fostering cooperation and collaboration. Individuals work together toward a solution that accommodates everyone's needs. Although everyone may not get everything they want, compromise ensures that everyone derives some level of satisfaction from the resolution.

For compromise to be effective, there must be open communication, including active listening and the articulation of needs and concerns. Face-to-face interaction and dialogue can be time consuming and intimidating. A third-party negotiator, such as a union representative, may be needed if solutions cannot be achieved. Because confrontation can be uncomfortable, many nurses prefer to use avoidance or accommodation to resolve conflict rather than compromise.

Collaboration

Collaboration is the preferred conflict resolution method endorsed by the AACN (2016). During collaboration, individuals work together cooperatively to find a mutually beneficial solution to an issue. This strategy requires open communication, active participation, and a shared commitment to understanding and addressing each person's concerns. Collaboration fosters a win-win outcome that builds on compromise to create a solution that all participants feel good about and can support (Yoder-Wise & Sportsman, 2023).

The steps necessary in constructing a solution are identifying each person's concerns, clarifying assumptions, communicating honestly to identify the underlying issue, and working cooperatively to find a solution that satisfies everyone (Boggs, 2023). The collaborative method requires a high level of trust, empathy, and a willingness to explore creative solutions that address the root causes of the conflict. Collaboration requires respect for each contributor's expertise and abilities. Although this strategy requires a lot of work and effort, collaboration is strongly advantageous because it has long-reaching benefits, builds teamwork, encourages joint problem solving, and results in sustainable and positive outcomes.

THINKING CRITICALLY
Recall a recent conflict. Develop possible methods of resolving the conflict using accommodation, avoidance, competition, compromise, and collaboration. Compare and contrast the advantages and disadvantages of each method for resolving the conflict.

GUIDELINES FOR DEALING WITH CONFLICT

Remember that conflict is a natural part of human interaction. The goal is not to eliminate conflict but to manage it constructively to achieve positive outcomes. Resolving conflict when managing client care may seem overwhelming; however, resolving conflicts is essential for creating and maintaining healthy relationships, promoting productivity, and fostering positive environments that support positive client outcomes.

Successfully navigating conflicts contributes to personal and professional growth by developing problem-solving, communication, and interpersonal skills. In your experience as an LPN/LVN, you likely have seen conflict and may have used some of the discussed strategies to resolve problems. Although each situation is unique, there are some basic guidelines to help defuse tempers and emotions (see Chapter 11: Blocks in Communication). As discussed in the following subsections, you can apply the nursing process to guide development of conflict resolution strategies (see also Table 14.3).

Assessment
Assess the situation and identify the problem. Ask questions to clarify any misunderstandings, identify the scope of the problem, and identify the source. Practice active listening skills, and take the time to hear the concerns of clients, families, staff,

TABLE 14.3 Comparison of Conflict Resolution and the Nursing Process

Conflict Resolution	Nursing Process
1. Identify the conflict and gather information.	1. Assessment
2. Analyze the root cause and clearly define what the conflict is about.	2. Diagnosis
3. Establish goals and define a successful resolution.	3. Planning
4. Communicate and facilitate open and honest dialogue.	4. Implementation
5. Assess the outcome and determine if the resolution interventions were successful.	5. Evaluation

providers, and administrators. Pay close attention to the concerns and perspectives of others. Demonstrate empathy and understanding to promote effective communication. Ask questions to gain a deeper understanding of the other person's viewpoint. Maintain composure and avoid reacting impulsively. Take a moment to collect your thoughts before responding. It may be beneficial to review the therapeutic communication skills outlined in Chapter 11.

Diagnosis

Analyzing the root cause of a conflict and identifying the underlying issues that contribute to the conflict is necessary to develop targeted interventions to resolve the conflict and to restore working relationships. Clearly define the conflict and its effects on everyone involved. Various factors such as misunderstandings or ineffective communication, differing priorities, and personality clashes may amplify conflicts.

Planning

Once the problem or issue is clearly identified, plan for a successful outcome. Emphasize the desire to find a win-win, or collaborative, resolution. Identify shared goals or interests to build a foundation for collaboration. Collaborate to find mutually acceptable goals. Whenever possible, create a positive environment conducive to clear, private, and calm interaction by:

- Selecting a neutral location
- Establishing a quiet environment
- Minimizing distractions and interruptions
- Ensuring the privacy of all involved

Implementation

Now comes the real work of conflict resolution. Clearly express your thoughts and feelings. Use "I" statements to convey your perspective without blaming others. To foster a positive atmosphere, focus on areas of agreement. Brainstorm, and be open to creative alternatives that address the root cause of the conflict. Be flexible and open to finding middle ground that meets the needs of everyone involved. It may be helpful to focus on consequences. For instance, what will happen if conflict continues?

Avoid inflammatory or accusatory language. Frame statements to promote understanding and resolution rather than to escalate tension. Keep the discussion focused on the specific issue at hand rather than making personal attacks. To maintain respect, separate the problem from the person. Consider your own actions or behaviors that may have contributed to the conflict, and be willing to take responsibility for them. Clearly define acceptable behaviors and expectations moving forward. Establishing boundaries can help prevent future conflicts.

To avoid getting caught up in the emotions of the moment, develop **emotional intelligence**, which is the ability to recognize, understand, manage, and effectively use one's own emotions; the term also encompasses the ability to notice, analyze, and respond to other people's emotions. Skills such as self-awareness, self-regulation, and empathy enhance communication and facilitate cooperation. Emotional intelligence influences how individuals navigate relationships, make decisions, and handle challenging situations (Goleman, 1998). Box 14.8 summarizes the interventions to implement during conflict resolution.

Encourage collaboration by identifying shared goals and working together to find mutually acceptable solutions. Emphasize teamwork and a collaborative approach to

BOX 14.8 Conflict Management Strategies

- Stress consequences of unresolved behaviors on the team/patient care.
- Focus on the issues, not on the personalities.
- Take responsibility for your part in the conflict.
- Don't assign blame.
- Communicate openly.
- Listen carefully.
- Seek to understand first and then to be understood.
- Move to a neutral, private area.
- If aggressive behaviors occur, use assertiveness strategies.
- Let intelligence and not emotion rule.
- Seek possible solutions.

problem solving. Demonstrate empathy by trying to understand the emotions and viewpoints of others and by acknowledging and validating their feelings, even if you don't agree with their position.

When appropriate, document the details of the conflict resolution process. Documentation can be valuable for future reference and may be necessary for organizational records. Summarize accomplishments and achievements.

Evaluation

Determine whether the conflict resolution interventions were successful in achieving the established goals. Although not all conflicts will have a positive resolution, view conflicts as opportunities for learning and professional growth. Reflect on the conflict resolution process, and identify areas for improvement. After a resolution is reached, follow-up to ensure that the agreed-upon solutions are implemented. Monitor the situation over time to assess the effectiveness of the resolution. In some instances, an impartial third party such as a nurse manager, legal counsel, or ethics committee may be needed to provide resources and to assist in navigating complex situations.

Conflict management is not an easy task. Nurses should participate in conflict resolution training or workshops to enhance their skills in managing and resolving conflicts effectively. Maintaining communication and trust, together with the nurse's commitment to conflict resolution, are necessary for positive client outcomes.

MAKING DECISIONS

As you transition from LPN/LVN to RN, an important element in your new role will be the ability to make client care decisions based on information that has been reported or observed. Deciding what action to take is a process that uses complex cognitive skills (Huston, 2023). When making decisions, you will rely on clinical judgments that can positively or negatively affect client care. Problem solving, clinical judgment, and critical thinking are components of the clinical reasoning process (see Chapter 9).

Although the terms decision-making and problem solving are sometimes used interchangeably, they have different meanings. *Problem solving* entails selecting various alternatives that will solve an issue. In contrast, **decision-making** focuses on selecting the best course of action from various alternatives to achieve a specific goal or outcome.

TABLE 14.4 Comparison of Decision-Making and the Nursing Process

Decision-Making Steps	Nursing Process
1. Identify the problem and gather data.	1. Assessment
2. Analyze the data.	2. Diagnosis
3. Establish goals, outcomes, and plans of action.	3. Planning
4. Implement the plan.	4. Implementation
5. Evaluate the results.	5. Evaluation

Note that making a decision does not necessarily solve a problem, and it is not necessarily the result of a problem. In fact, nurses who are good decision makers may fail to solve long-term problems.

Factors that influence decision-making include values, life experiences, perceptions of the issue, possible risks involved, and personal approaches to making decisions. Decision-making combines personal ability and learned skills. As the healthcare system becomes more focused on cost containment and client outcomes, the need to be a competent decision maker will become increasingly crucial.

Similar to the nursing process, the process of making a decision consists of five steps (Table 14.4). Nurses don't always have time to carry out this formal process for many of the decisions they must make; quick judgments must be made on a number of issues, and many decisions must be made within seconds. However, it is beneficial to follow the decision-making process as much as possible when learning to make decisions because as more experience is gained, the process enables the nurse to make more efficient and effective decisions.

ASSESSMENT

The first step is to identify the problem and gather data. Based on the nurse's assessment, the problem must be clearly defined, and the problem's priority and context must be determined. Once the problem has been identified, relevant information must be collected. This step is similar to the assessment step of the nursing process; the quality and comprehensiveness of information can significantly impact the decision-making process.

DIAGNOSIS

After data are gathered, the nurse will *analyze the information*. Using analysis, the nurse can compare and contrast different options to solve the problem. This step involves considering and exploring the implications of possible decisions, weighing advantages and disadvantages, and assessing potential outcomes.

PLANNING

The third step is to *establish goals*. In developing goals, the nurse determines what is realistic and what actions will result in an improvement or positive change. This step involves choosing the best course of action or selecting the most suitable option. The nurse must consider values, preferences, and goals. It is important to note that not all decisions will have a single best option, and alternatives may need to be considered. Seeking alternatives ensures all sides of the issue are addressed. Analysis of each goal and possible outcome will help determine whether a decision is beneficial and cost-effective, and whether there are resources available. The selection of a strategy will be based on the methods of implementation available, time involved, and resources.

IMPLEMENTATION

The next step is to *implement*. Once a decision is made, it needs to be put into action. This step involves developing and executing a plan. The nurse must clearly communicate the decision and the reason for the decision. Implementation may be initiated by the nurse or be delegated to others; however, the nurse remains accountable for overseeing implementation and must establish a system for monitoring the implementation progress.

EVALUATION

The final step of the process is *evaluation*. As with any evaluation, the nurse compares the results of the implementation with the goals. Evaluating a decision is not a one-time event; it requires ongoing monitoring. Nurses should assess the impact of the decision and allow for adjustments and refinements as needed.

Making knowledgeable decisions is the basis of managing client care. The quality of decisions influences the quality of client care. Another area of client care management is resource management.

THINKING CRITICALLY

You are a new nurse in a long-term care facility; the oncoming charge nurse tells you that you are spending too much time giving report. Although your feelings are hurt, you must face the need to shorten reports and pass along information that you feel to be essential. Using the five steps of the decision-making process, develop a plan to resolve the problem.

MANAGING RESOURCES

Resources are the things that are necessary to do a job. Resources include work space, supplies, equipment, budgeted funds, and services. In today's health-conscious world, attention to resource management has greatly increased. The expectation is that high-quality care will be delivered to a large number of clients by fewer people (particularly professional people) with a cost-conscious use of resources. In addition, the environment will be conducive to maintaining high standards of quality and client safety. This is an enormous challenge for nurses and other healthcare members.

DEVELOPING COST AWARENESS

One of the first steps in managing resources is to develop cost awareness, which is the understanding and consciousness of the financial implications associated with various activities, decisions, or resources within an organization including budgetary constraints related to salaries and resources. It is important for nurses to recognize the costs involved in client care and to be mindful of how these costs impact the overall budget and financial health of the organization.

Cost awareness is often promoted as part of a broader strategy to enhance financial responsibility and accountability. Nurses are sometimes involved in decision-making related to the allocation of resources, such as medical supplies, equipment, and staffing. Being cost-aware helps nurses make informed choices that optimize the use of resources, ensuring efficient and effective client care.

CONTAINING COSTS

A second step in managing resources is **cost containment**. Organizations implemented this strategy to control or reduce expenses and to prevent unnecessary spending while maintaining or improving the quality of products or services. In healthcare, cost containment refers to developing a more businesslike approach to managing client care with efforts made to reduce rising healthcare costs.

The primary goal of cost containment is to decrease the ineffective use of resources and time while finding more efficient and cost-effective methods to deliver care. Many healthcare agencies have initiated strategies to deliver client care with an emphasis on conserving supplies and equipment. When monitoring client supplies, nurses oversee and manage the availability, usage, and replenishment of supplies necessary for safe and effective client care. Monitoring ensures that the necessary supplies are readily available, reducing the risk of errors, delays, or compromise in the delivery of needed care.

MANAGING QUALITY

Quality management is a systematic method that involves processes, standards, and continuous improvement initiatives to enhance efficiency and effectiveness (Roux & Halstead, 2018). Important elements of quality management include setting quality standards, monitoring and measuring performance, implementing corrective actions, and fostering a culture of continuous improvement throughout an organization. In healthcare, the goal is to provide high-quality client care while containing costs.

Although some cost containment measures are beyond the nurse's control, at the bedside, nurses have had an impact on preventing incidents such as falls, pressure injuries, and the use of restraints (see web source "Institute for Health Improvement" at the end of this chapter). Many hospitals reference The National Database of Nursing Quality Indicators (NDNQI) to measure and benchmark nursing-sensitive quality indicators. Developed by the American Nurses Association, The NDNQI is a comprehensive database that collects and analyzes nursing-sensitive performance indicators to assess and improve the quality of nursing care in healthcare facilities.

As an LPN/LVN, you may have participated in the interventions related to quality indicators. In your new role as an RN, you will design care that has a significant impact on cost containment, quality, and client safety.

Financial concerns will always have an impact on the delivery of healthcare. In your role as an RN, you will combine the need to provide high-quality, safe, and responsible care to clients with the necessity of being cost conscious and efficient. Cost-aware nurses advocate for their clients by considering the financial implications of care options that maintain standards of care without compromising quality and safety.

CONCLUSION

In today's healthcare system, the RN collaborates with other healthcare professionals to ensure care coordination, applies critical thinking to identify problems and make decisions, effectively organizes and manages time, and participates in improving the quality of care within their healthcare setting. The RN's role as manager of client care is vital in resolving conflict, making decisions, containing costs, promoting positive patient outcomes, and maintaining standards of excellence in nursing practice.

STUDENT Exercises

Exercise 14.1

Consider the following scenario:

Diane, a new ADN graduate, is working on a 30-bed adult surgical unit where she had previously been employed as an LPN. After she completed her orientation, she began working three evenings a week. When Diane arrives one evening, she is assigned as the nurse for half of the unit, which currently has 12 clients. Her team consists of one LPN and several UAPs. During report, she learns that there are five new postoperative clients, all of whom are having problems with nausea. Two clients are scheduled for surgery in 1 hour. The postoperative client from yesterday who had a colon tumor removed just tore off his colostomy bag and is screaming that the nurses are trying to kill him. Four of the clients are older adults who require assistance with activities of daily living. The client in Room 4 has just fallen out of bed. The unit secretary for the floor has called in sick, and the float unit secretary will not be in for 1 hour. Diane tells the charge nurse that she is concerned she will not be able to attend to everything. The charge nurse says he "cannot be too available" because he is orienting a new nurse. The charge nurse thinks that Diane's experience on the unit as an LPN will help her manage care for the day and that she will not need any more help.

  a. What does Diane need to do to get organized?
  b. What should the work plan or worksheet include?
  c. Prioritize Diane's client care assignments.
  d. What does Diane need to know about the people assigned to her team?
  e. Does Diane need additional personnel? If yes, what skill level is required?
  f. What is Diane's role in this situation? What responsibilities should Diane perform without delegating?
  g. What advice would you give to Diane?
  h. What might you discuss with the charge nurse if you were in this situation?

Exercise 14.2

Consider the scenario with Juanita and Nancy in the chapter-opening case study. Imagine you are in the same situation.

  a. If you were Juanita, how would you enhance your relationship with coworkers who are no longer your peers?
  b. How could the situation lead to inefficient utilization of resources?
  c. What strategies for conflict resolution would offer some solutions to this situation?
  d. When would managers or directors need to intervene, and what could they do to help the transition?

REFERENCES

Albert, N. M., Pappas, S. H., Porter-O'Grady, T., & Malloch, K. (2022). *Quantum leadership: Creating sustainable value in health care* (6th ed.). Jones & Bartlett Learning.

Boggs, K. U. (2023). *Interpersonal relationships: Professional communication skills for nurses* (9th ed.). Elsevier.

Carver, J. (2022). *Pareto principle: Unleash the true power of the Pareto Principle (the secret strategy to optimizing every area of your life)*. Zoe Lawson Publisher.

Catalano, J. T. (2024). *Nursing now: Today's issues tomorrows trends* (9th ed.). F. A. Davis.

Goleman, D. (1998). *Working with emotional intelligence*. Bantam Books.

Huston, C. J. (2023). *Leadership role and management functions in nursing: Theory and application* (11th ed.). Wolters Kluwer.

Michaelsen, M. M., & Esch, T. (2023). Understanding health behavior change by motivation and reward mechanisms: A review of the literature. *Frontiers in Behavioral Neuroscience, 17*, 1151918. https://doi.org/10.3389/fnbeh.2023.1151918

Roux, G., & Halstead, J. (2018). *Issues and trends in nursing: Practice, policy, and leadership* (2nd ed.). Jones & Bartlett Learning.

The American Association of Critical-Care Nurses. (2016). *AACN standards for establishing and sustaining healthy work environments: A journey to excellence* (2nd ed.).

Yoder-Wise, P. S., & Sportsman, S. (2023). *Leading and managing in nursing* (8th ed.). Elsevier.

Zerwekh, J., & Garneau, A. Z. (2023). *Nursing today: Transitions and trends* (11th ed.). Elsevier.

SUGGESTED READING

Cherry, B., & Jacob, S. R. (2022). *Contemporary nursing: Issues, trends, and management* (9th ed.). Elsevier.

Covey, S. (1989). *The seven habits of highly effective people*. Simon & Schuster.

Dryden, W. (2022). *Overcoming procrastination* (2nd ed.). Sheldon Press.

Estelle, M., & Nicolas, M. (2022). When emotional intelligence predicts team performance: Further validation of the short version of the Workgroup Emotional Intelligence Profile: Research and reviews. *Current Psychology, 41*(3), 1323–1336. https://doi.org/10.1007/s12144-020-00659-7

Kapadwala, S., & Joseph, S. (2022). Emotional intelligence in the IT industry: A study on emotional intelligence among IT professionals. *Cardiometry, 25*, 756–763. https://doi.org/10.18137/cardiometry.2022.25.756763

Matilda, O. K., Anthony Kwarteng, A.-A., & Kuranchie, A. (2022). Do emotional intelligence, cognitive intelligence and social intelligence modulate leadership qualities? *International Journal of Social Sciences & Educational Studies, 9*(4), 98–110. https://doi.org/10.23918/ijsses.v9i4p98

On the WEB

The Consortium for Research on Emotional Intelligence in Organizations: http://www.eiconsortium.org

Institute for Health Improvement—free downloadable tools to support your work to improve healthcare quality and safety: http://www.ihi.org/resources/Pages/Tools/TCAB.aspx

PART C | MEMBER OF THE DISCIPLINE OF NURSING

Professional Responsibilities

CHAPTER 15

LEARNING OUTCOMES

By the end of this chapter, the student will be able to:
1. Recall the five professional responsibilities of RNs, as set out by the ANA's *Code of Ethics*.
2. Examine how verbal statements and behaviors impact nursing's image.
3. Describe areas of professional growth of the RN as a member of the profession.
4. Develop a professional plan for growth in response to societal changes.
5. Describe ways in which the RN promotes and maintains standards of nursing practice.
6. Explore the role of the RN in research and evidence-based practice.
7. Describe the RN's role in professional stewardship and the advancement of nursing.

KEY TERMS

accountability
advocacy
evidence-based research
healthy workplace
magnet hospital designation
mentee
mentor
nursing informatics
patient advocacy
peer review
professional stewardship
professional values
referrals
self-regulation

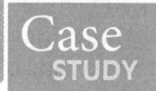

Case STUDY   Jennifer and Courtney have been friends since LPN school 5 years ago. They have kept in contact via Facebook and e-mail despite distance and time factors. Jennifer is in her second semester of RN school as an advanced placement student, and Courtney is considering returning to school. This is a transcript of their e-mail conversation.

COURTNEY: It's discouraging sometimes in nursing. The work is hard, the hours are difficult, some new graduates are making more money than the experienced staff, and you hit a ceiling where you can't advance if you stay at the bedside. Would it be a waste of time, effort, and money for me to go back to school?

JENNIFER: You're raising some serious and important questions. Despite the very real challenges you bring up, it's never been a better time to become an RN! RNs continue to be one of the professions the public respects most. We need to take our professional responsibilities seriously to keep it that way. School is impressing upon me our contract to the public—our Code of Ethics.

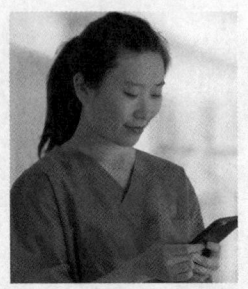

What the two of us have been doing for years is networking. Now, thanks to school and the internet, I have other LVNs—mentors, colleagues, teachers, and professors—who are networking with me. School is also teaching me more about advocacy, responsibility, and duty to myself along with the many professional advancement organizations that help nurses. I feel a renewed sense of spirit. Yes, going back to school to become an RN is time-consuming, hard work, and expensive, but school has truly been an eye-opening, positive experience.

COURTNEY: You sound so excited and full of energy. Will it rub off on me? I need to be injected with something!

JENNIFER: Well, let's keep in touch. I can also help you by sending you some websites and podcasts to help you get excited and energized. These show the RN's professional role functions in much more detail. I'm attaching them now. I'll text you later this weekend to see what you think about them.

COURTNEY: Thanks, Jen. You've really made my day, and now I want to go back to school to become an RN. I'm going to fill out that application to nursing school now and send it in. I'll text you later about how things work out.

The conversation Jennifer and Courtney are having is common between nursing friends. It might have been one you had with a fellow nurse before applying to nursing school. What are an RN's professional responsibilities? In what ways, and how, will an RN candidate assume a more expanded role with greater advocacy and accountability within the profession? What role will professional advancement and organizations play within the profession? Both LPN and RN graduates practice within their respective scopes and adhere to legal and ethical standards. Both are client advocates and engage in continuous learning and professional growth. The concept Jennifer is learning more about as an associate degree nursing student is how to be proactive in governance, self-regulation, and advancement of the profession. Some of the documents Jennifer is sending Courtney may help Courtney understand these expanded roles. However, until the LPN/LVN actually assumes the RN role, the RN's level of professional responsibilities may not be clear.

This chapter presents the responsibilities of an RN as a member of the profession and provides guiding principles that all members of the profession accept. You may want

> **BOX 15.1**
>
> **Professional Responsibilities According to the Ethical Code for Nurses**
>
> Advocacy
> Accountability to self, colleagues
> Professional growth
> Professional advancement
> Professional organizations

Source: American Nurses Association. (2015). *Code of ethics for nurses with interpretive statements* (2nd ed.).

to review the characteristics of a professional, which were covered in Chapter 2, before reading this chapter. Professional responsibilities set out by the *Code of Ethics for Nurses* (2015) are revised periodically; the current ones are set out in Box 15.1.

ADVOCACY

The RN's accountability for client advocacy has remained an essential responsibility since the inception of nursing (Potter et al., 2023). **Advocacy** is the upholding and defending of another's rights and interests (Taylor et al., 2023). **Patient advocacy** means speaking on the client's behalf or representing the client's point of view and promoting the client's dignity and worth (see Chapter 13 on caring for unique clients). Advocacy may involve translating or articulating the client's intent or original thinking when it is not being heard, perceived, or understood accurately or consistently. As an LPN/LVN, you advocate for clients by ensuring their basic needs are met, providing emotional support, and communicating their concerns to the RN and healthcare team. However, as an RN, you will have the ultimate accountability in advocating for the client and in ensuring that the client's desires are understood and the patient's rights (and freedom of choice) are protected.

> **The NCLEX-RN *Might Ask* 15.1**
>
> The nurse is interceding for a client who has refused radiation treatment for a slow-growing malignant tumor. In this role, the nurse is acting as (Select all that apply):
> a. teacher.
> b. benefactor.
> c. advocate.
> d. proxy.
> e. spokesperson.
>
> • See Appendix A for correct answer and rationale.

SUPPORTING THE CLIENT

At times, the client may need help communicating their desires. Respiratory devices, lowered states of consciousness, or other physical impairments may impede or limit the client's ability for self-expression. Language or cultural barriers may be present. The client may be mentally disabled or illiterate, or they may be unable to read, comprehend, or communicate adequately. The client may simply not grasp the information being explained. Your educational preparation in communication and assessment skills as an RN will assist you in ascertaining the client's needs and in serving as a spokesperson and client advocate.

HELPING THE CLIENT MAKE INFORMED DECISIONS

It is the RN's responsibility and commitment to ensure clients are well informed to make choices and decisions about their care. Information and instructions should not be provided in a hurry or rushed, and they should always be given both verbally and in writing. By using knowledge and application of effective communication skills, the nurse must ensure that the client has been provided with and comprehends the information. A common method to ensure understanding is the "teach back" method; the client should be able to describe the procedure or treatment and explain its positive and negative consequences. When there are alternatives, the nurse must describe each option and ensure comprehension of all material. The nurse must communicate in a nonjudgmental and unbiased manner; when the client exhibits signs of uncertainty, the nurse should assist them in gathering additional information, getting a second opinion, or taking other steps to alleviate their concerns. Informed consent and the nurse's role related to advance directives (e.g., living wills) are discussed in Chapter 16. To assist the client in making decisions, review the techniques for decision-making discussed in Chapter 14.

RNs empower and advocate for clients to make informed decisions about their health by accessing accurate and reliable information online. Today's healthcare consumer is internet savvy. Because there is an abundance of false information on the internet, nurses have a responsibility to educate consumers about reputable websites and how to find reliable, accurate information. The nurse should offer clients a list of reputable websites and online resources that have been vetted by healthcare professionals; teach clients how to evaluate the credibility of health information online; explain common red flags that may indicate unreliable health information, such as exaggerated claims, lack of references, or websites promoting unproven treatments; and if available, suggest that clients use online client portals provided by healthcare organizations. These portals often contain accurate and personalized health information, including test results, treatment plans, and educational materials.

MAKING REFERRALS

In addition to assisting the client in gaining more information, the RN also advocates for the client by making referrals. RNs may make referrals in various situations to ensure comprehensive and specialized care for their clients. **Referrals** are indicated when the client needs information or intervention outside the scope of RN practice or when an intervention will occur under another nurse's care (e.g., in the transfer from acute to ambulatory care).

Referrals are generally within the healthcare environment and include specialty care by cardiologists, endocrinologists, neurologists, or other specialists. Other services for which the RN may refer the client are diagnostic tests or imaging studies, such as magnetic resonance imaging, computed tomography scan, or a biopsy; mental health services such as care by a psychologist or a psychiatrist; rehabilitation services such as physical therapy, occupational therapy, or speech therapy; home health services; community resources; educational programs; and legal or social services.

PROTECTING CLIENT RIGHTS

The RN actively supports and safeguards each client's rights, ensuring that they are protected when receiving healthcare services. This advocacy guarantees that clients are treated with dignity, respect, and autonomy. Nurses uphold principles such as informed consent, privacy, confidentiality, and the right to make decisions about one's own healthcare. Ensuring client rights includes protecting medical records, conversations, and any other personal health information; ensures that clients are not discriminated against based on race, ethnicity, gender, religion, sexual orientation, or any other protected characteristic; acknowledges and respects a client's right to refuse treatment, even if the nurse disagrees with the decision; and ensures a safe and secure environment by implementing interventions to prevent harm and to protect clients from abuse, neglect, or any form of mistreatment. Client rights are usually outlined in healthcare organizations' policies and are supported by ethical principles and legal frameworks. By incorporating these principles into their practice, RNs ensure that clients receive high-quality, client-centered care that maintains their autonomy and dignity.

ACCOUNTABILITY

Accountability means being answerable for one's conduct and taking ownership of the consequences, whether positive or negative, that result from those actions (Potter et al., 2023). **Accountability** extends beyond the responsibility of ensuring high standards of nursing care and includes evaluating implemented care to ensure consistency with written standards and consulting with healthcare providers, colleagues, and other professionals as needed. (Accountability in the legal context is discussed in more depth in Chapter 16.) Because registered nurses continue to gain more responsibility in the delivery of client care and the execution of their professional duties, accountability and professionalism have become critically important. By embracing increased accountability, nurses are less likely to be governed by non-nursing organizations and have greater influence over the future of the profession.

In addition to being accountable to the profession, nurses are also accountable to themselves and to their colleagues.

ACCOUNTABILITY TO SELF

The Code of Ethics for Nurses (ANA, 2015) provides the guiding principles of professional practice for all nurses. One of the provisions in *The Code* is that the nurse is accountable to self. This means that nurses are responsible to keep themselves healthy, safe, and whole. Nurses cannot provide quality care to others without personal well-being that ensures they are physically, emotionally, and mentally healthy and prepared. Mental preparedness—the psychological readiness, focus, and resilience to handle a task or challenge effectively—fosters wholeness of character. Wholeness of character is supported in the provision by giving nurses the right to consciously object if they feel that an aspect of client care violates the standards of care (Lackman et al., 2015).

Nurses are accountable to themselves and build resilience by committing to continuous self-care, self-improvement, maintaining personal and professional integrity, and taking proactive steps to ensure their well-being. Resilience is more than learning to cope with stressors. Resilience enables nurses to adapt, to navigate challenges, and to sustain a fulfilling and successful career. Nurses can foster their resilience by engaging in reflection and mindfulness, by seeking support from colleagues and support groups, by embracing continuous learning, by setting clear boundaries, and by acknowledging and celebrating personal and professional achievements (Faraco et al., 2022; Tsui, & Adam, 2023).

Modeling Professional Values of Nursing

Self-care, professionalism, and modeling are interconnected. Self-care is essential for maintaining the energy and resilience required to meet professional standards. When nurses prioritize their well-being, they are better equipped to deliver high-quality and compassionate care. **Professional values** are the foundational principles that guide nursing practice and contribute to the delivery of high-quality care. Nurses model professional values through their actions, behaviors, and interactions within the healthcare setting.

The self-care practices of nurses also impact the public image of the profession. A positive public image is vital for gaining the confidence of clients, the community, and peers. Demonstrating qualities such as competence, accountability, empathy, and ethical conduct enhances public trust. It is imperative for nurses to lead by example in everything they do. Nurses who prioritize their well-being are more likely to be perceived as competent, caring, and dedicated; if nurses are visibly stressed, overworked, or experiencing burnout, it may negatively affect the public's perception of the nursing profession (Peng, 2022).

When nurses embrace a culture of self-care and emphasize professionalism, doing so helps change outdated perceptions of nursing as a high-stress and burnout-prone profession. This cultural shift can positively influence how the public views nursing and how nurses view their own careers and profession. Prioritizing self-care enhances professionalism, which, in turn, positively influences how nurses view the nursing profession. Nurses must continue to believe that what they do is essential and important—that is, nurses must value nursing. This holistic approach is essential for maintaining a vibrant, respected, and sustainable nursing workforce.

Historically, nurses have received little reward for what they do (Gordon, 1997). The collaborative nature of the profession may sometimes result in nurses' individual contributions being overlooked or absorbed within the healthcare team. In addition to hands-on client care, nurses work behind the scenes providing essential support. Although doctors and other healthcare professionals may be more visible, nurses are frequently the ones managing day-to-day patient care, making critical decisions, and ensuring the smooth operation of healthcare facilities (Huércanos-Esparza et al., 2021). Many of these duties may go unnoticed or underappreciated by the general public, creating the phenomenon of "the invisible nurse" described by Gordon (2005), which can still be observed today:

> [W]hen a nurse makes a contribution into patient care ... the system often gives credit for [their] actions and contribution to the physician. This means that the nurse is stuck in the most pernicious Catch 22 of all: Whatever the nurse does confers credit on the physician (p. 48).

One way nurses can increase their visibility is to enhance their professional influence and power through a combination of strategies that focus on education, advocacy, leadership development, and collaboration. Working within their institution, nurses can create an environment that empowers nurses. Nurses can increase their visibility and power by seeking leadership opportunities within healthcare organizations, by participating in hospital committees, and by actively participating in interdisciplinary collaborations to demonstrate the value of nursing contributions to client care and positive outcomes.

The magnet hospital concept capitalizes on the strength and power of nursing. The American Nurses Credentialing Center and the American Nurses Association (ANA) designed the **magnet hospital designation**, which recognizes organizations that provide nursing excellence. The program also provides a vehicle for disseminating successful nursing practices and strategies. Requirements for designation as a magnet hospital are stringent; many standards must be met. Magnet workplaces recognize that nurses need to be supported and valued. Because magnet facilities place a high value on nursing contributions and recognize that nurse satisfaction and patient safety and outcomes are intertwined, they have a low nurse turnover and a high rate of client satisfaction. Box 15.2 provides ideas to increase the visibility and value of nursing.

THINKING CRITICALLY
What is your response when someone asks you what a nurse does and how you like being a nurse? How do you model and value what you do? What do you do to help promote moral resiliency? Share your thoughts with others in your group who are LPNs/LVNs. Next, share them with an RN, and compare the differences/similarities.

BOX 15.2 Daily Ways to Display Modeling and Valuing Nursing

1. When you introduce yourself in client interactions, state that you are the RN.
2. Volunteer to be on committees at your institution that promote the professionalism of nursing, including those trying to achieve magnet status.
3. Emphasize the positive impact you make by reducing costs, complications, and deaths.
4. Get involved with community service activities.
5. Inspire interest in nursing in children and others in the community; appear as a guest speaker for Brownies or Cub Scouts or at the local schools, community centers, or places of worship.
6. Lead by example and demonstrate professionalism, empathy, and dedication in your interactions with patients, families, and other healthcare team members.
7. Use nursing research to add power to your image.
8. Support ongoing education and skill enhancement for nurses through training programs, workshops, and access to resources.
9. Refer to the nursing shortage as an opportunity.
10. Join and participate in local, regional, and national nursing organizations that are promoting nursing politically.
11. Acknowledge and celebrate the accomplishments of nurses, whether through formal recognition programs and verbal praise, or by small gestures of appreciation.
12. Donate money, supplies, or support to a nursing student in another country.

ACCOUNTABILITY TO COLLEAGUES

Nurses are accountable to their colleagues through various mechanisms that promote professional responsibility, ethical behavior, and collaboration within the healthcare team. Accountability to colleagues is crucial for maintaining a high standard of patient care and fostering a positive work environment. Nurses are accountable to adhere to established professional standards and codes of ethics. This includes guidelines set by nursing organizations and regulatory bodies. The nurse demonstrates accountability by promoting these standards and ensuring that all nurses uphold them in their practice.

As a member of the discipline of nursing at the RN level, the nurse maintains accountability for the standards of practice. In *Nursing's Social Policy Statement*, the ANA (2010) notes that nursing as a profession gains its authority from the social contract it holds with society. Under its terms, society grants the nursing profession authority over functions vital to itself and permits considerable autonomy in the conduct of the nursing profession's own affairs. In return, the nursing profession is expected to act responsibly, always mindful of the public trust. Self-regulation to ensure quality in performance is at the heart of this relationship. **Self-regulation** is one of the hallmarks of a profession; it is how a profession ensures that standards of practice within the profession are met (Taylor et al., 2023). The major vehicle for the profession's self-regulation is its professional organizations. Through activities and forums of professional organizations, nurses are able to establish and maintain standards for nursing practice. This is discussed later in this chapter.

RNs have a number of opportunities and responsibilities to engage in peer review to support the standards of nursing practice. One of the self-regulation methods within professional practice, **peer review** occurs when a member of a profession reviews the work of another member of the profession. Peer review processes are implemented to evaluate and ensure the competence and performance of nurses. Some examples of the peer review process include shared governance, peer nurse employee evaluation processes, nursing peer review panels, record audits, quality councils, quality assurance procedures, staffing ratio committees, and ethics committees. Through self-regulation and peer review, it is every nurse's responsibility to take the initiative to report behaviors or actions performed by nurse colleagues that are inconsistent with standards of nursing practice.

PROFESSIONAL GROWTH

As a member of the discipline of nursing, the RN makes a commitment to ongoing professional growth and lifelong learning. According to the NLN (2012), graduates of ADN programs must be able to make decisions for safe care based on the application of nursing science. Nurses are accountable for their own professional development and education. This includes continuous professional development to stay informed about advancements in healthcare, attending relevant training, and sharing knowledge with peers. Attending conferences, workshops, and seminars is beneficial to expand your network and knowledge base. You may decide to pursue higher education, such as advanced degrees (master's or doctorate) or certifications in specialized areas. Specializing in a particular field or becoming an expert in a specific nursing area can increase your knowledge and authority. Encouraging and supporting each other's ongoing education contributes to a culture of accountability.

When transitioning into the professional RN role, the graduating nurse assumes a leadership role in the profession, which includes a broader scope of responsibility and

> **BOX 15.3**
>
> **Areas for RN Professional Growth**
>
> The RN continually strives:
> - To maintain a current knowledge base
> - To remain technologically current
> - To apply current research to practice
> - To respond to societal changes

accountability, and will be making a commitment to professional growth at the RN level (Box 15.3). The nurse continually strives to maintain an updated knowledge base, to remain technologically current, to apply the latest research to practice, and to respond to societal trends.

MAINTAINING A CURRENT KNOWLEDGE BASE

Although maintaining a current knowledge base is an ongoing challenge, RN, it is a critical responsibility as a member of the profession of nursing. You may have heard a nurse say, "I've been a nurse for 20 years, so I know what I'm doing!" However, longevity, seniority, and the passage of time do not necessarily equal expertise. Nurses need current information to provide safe and effective client care. Outdated knowledge may lead to errors in assessment, diagnosis, medication administration, and treatment planning, which jeopardizes client safety.

Continuous learning is a hallmark of the nursing profession. Nurses who do not prioritize ongoing education may become stagnant in their professional growth, hindering their ability to adapt to changing healthcare environments and evolving patient needs. On what areas should the nurse focus when seeking to update their knowledge base? Chapter 8 discusses competencies of the RN as a member of the professional discipline. Each nurse must acquire and utilize new information in the biologic, physical, behavioral, social, and nursing sciences.

Maintaining a current knowledge base can be accomplished in several ways. In-service programs are available in most health networks; however, the nurse should not limit themselves to only network-based educational opportunities. If health networks do not provide adequate educational opportunities, the RN must take the initiative to find various other learning programs.

Local, state, regional, national, and international conferences are held regularly in nursing and in disciplines that support and inform nursing. Schools of nursing often offer courses, clinical updates, refresher programs, and independent study options with an advisor, mentor, or preceptor. In addition, numerous nursing journals feature articles and case studies to maximize dissemination of new knowledge in nursing, and most journals offer online continuing education that can be accessed within the work or home setting. Nurses can also access information online from reputable and reliable sources and government agencies. Nurses committed to lifelong learning have positive attitudes toward—and even embrace—change. They understand that actively seeking change can positively boost their growth experiences.

Nurses are accountable for their own professional development and education, including sharing knowledge with peers. Encouraging and supporting each other's ongoing education contributes to a culture of accountability. As you advance in your expertise, you may want to act as a mentor to junior nurses and nursing students.

Offering educational sessions within your organization or community and sharing your expertise will contribute to the professional development of your peers. Sharing your experiences and knowledge will empower others in the profession.

THINKING CRITICALLY

A plan for designing learning lies squarely on the shoulders of each nurse. As a student enrolling in a program, you had to plan carefully how, where, and when to further your nursing education. But do you have a yearly plan, or a 5-, 10-, or 20-year plan? Have you ever thought of what you want to accomplish or a legacy you want to leave prior to retirement? What educational requirements would you need to complete these plans? Share your plans with the members of your class either during a discussion or in an online chat room or student café. As President Dwight D. Eisenhower famously once said, "Plans are nothing, but planning is everything." Although you should always plan ahead, be prepared to make adjustments because of unexpected events.

REMAINING TECHNOLOGICALLY CURRENT

Equally important for professional growth is the nurse's need to be technologically current to practice competently in the care provider and manager roles. New technology continues to emerge, including cardiorespiratory diagnostic and supportive devices, pharmacotherapeutics, computer-based treatment devices, and client documentation systems. In-services are often provided as new technology is introduced in healthcare agencies, and schools of nursing may provide workshops or courses for technology upgrades.

Nursing informatics "is the specialty that transforms data into needed information and leverages technologies to improve health and health care equity, safety, quality, and outcomes" (American Nurses Association, 2022, p. 3). Nursing informatics encompasses the design, implementation, and evaluation of information systems and technologies within the nursing profession. There is a growing demand for nurses with advanced training in the application of informatics in this rapidly expanding nursing specialty. The link between nursing informatics and evidence-based practice (EBP) needs to be valued and strengthened (Ramage, 2023).

At the bedside, nurses need to be familiar with new tools, devices, and electronic health record (EHR) systems. Knowledge of the latest technology enhances the nurse's ability to adapt to evolving healthcare practices and to contribute to healthcare innovation. Lack of familiarity with current technologies can hinder efficient and accurate documentation, communication, and patient monitoring. Nurses often use technology to educate patients about their conditions, treatment plans, and self-management strategies. Medical equipment such as infusion pumps, ventilators, and diagnostic tools often involves digital interfaces and connectivity. Nurses must understand how to operate and troubleshoot these devices to ensure patient safety (Box 15.4).

Examples of technologies the nurse must be familiar with include EHRs, which nurses use to document care, to track patient histories, and to improve communication and collaboration among healthcare team members. Computer-assisted medication

> **BOX 15.4**
>
> ### Competencies for the Technologically Current Nurse
> The RN should be familiar with the following technologies and topics:
> - Mobile phones, cell phones, and voice-activated devices
> - iPad applications
> - Electronic medical administration record and medication administration via bar coding/automated systems
> - Use of point-of-care technology
> - Telecommunications
> - Internet and intranet
> - Electronic health record (EHR) and clinical information systems

administration in the form of bar coding and automatic dispensing systems enhance client safety. Nurses can conduct virtual consultations, monitor patients remotely, and provide education and support through digital platforms. Mobile applications and devices support patient engagement and self-management, and nurses may recommend health apps for tracking vital signs, medication adherence, and lifestyle modifications.

Although technology allows nurses and clients to immediately access data, the value of such devices depends on the proficiency of the user. Nurses unfamiliar with using various digital equipment may feel apprehensive about learning to use it. The first step in overcoming the fear is to recognize and acknowledge that feeling afraid or anxious about learning new technology is normal. Begin by learning the basics and gradually build your knowledge. Trying to understand everything at once can be overwhelming. Focus on mastering one aspect of the technology before moving on to more advanced features. For an optimal learning experience, do not hesitate to communicate with educators, IT support, and colleagues, asking questions, seeking clarification, or requesting additional training if needed.

To prepare technology-savvy nurses and the digital aspects of healthcare, schools of nursing integrate technology into their programs. You are most likely already familiar with online learning platforms and learning management systems that are frequently used for online courses, assignments, and resources. Your school may also incorporate simulation labs, EHRs, virtual reality experiences, e-books, webinars, and adaptive learning systems. For more information and guidelines on technology, refer to the ANA's *Nursing Informatics: Scope and Standards of Practice* (2022), which is now in its third edition.

Applying web-based technology as well as the use of Web 2.0 technologies can help you sort through the wealth of information now available, which can be completely overwhelming in its volume. Definitions and examples of Web 2.0 resources are available in Box 15.5.

APPLYING EVIDENCE-BASED RESEARCH

Along with maintaining a current knowledge base and staying current with technology, nurses also need to apply evidence from research to their practice. **Evidence-based research** is defined as clinical decisions based upon a patient's preferences, life experience, and values, bridged with the best available current evidence and the practitioner's clinical expertise (Masters, 2023). Nurses systematically evaluate current research, clinical guidelines, and reputable reliable sources to guide their practice. EBP (discussed

BOX 15.5 Web 2.0 Resources

Resource	Definition	Example
Blog*	Short for "web log"; usually a diary, journal, or bulletin board that is updated frequently with general comments that can be added by the public	http://www.mediblogopathy.blogspot.com
Wiki*	Online site that allows compilation of posting and editing	http://www.wikipedia.com
Social website*	Allows photographs, commentary, and access to websites by others	http://www.facebook.com
Collaborative editing website	Texts, documents, and spreadsheets may be shared between two or more participants	http://www.docs.google.com
Survey data compilation	Participants of a study or a group, such as nursing students, can be surveyed about their opinions	https://forms.office.com/Pages/DesignPageV2.aspx

*Information obtained may not be reputable. Authors of sites must be vetted before application of resource information.

in Chapters 9 and 10) ensures that interventions and decisions are based on the best available evidence, improving the likelihood of positive patient outcomes. Since the 1990s, research findings have led the nursing profession to alter some long-standing practices. Evidence-based research has been proven to improve the quality and safety of healthcare, to enhance positive client outcomes, to decrease variations in delivery of care, and to reduce costs. The steps in applying EBP are described in Box 15.6 (Melnyk & Fineout-Overholt, 2023).

BOX 15.6 Steps in Applying Evidence-Based Practice

1. **Ask:** Formulate a clear and focused clinical question based on a specific client scenario or clinical issue.
2. **Acquire:** Search for the best available evidence from research articles, systematic reviews, and clinical guidelines.
3. **Appraise:** Critically evaluate the quality and relevance of the evidence. Assess the validity, reliability, and applicability of research findings.
4. **Apply:** To make informed and individualized decisions about client care, integrate the evidence with clinical expertise and consider client preferences.
5. **Assess:** Continuously monitor and evaluate the outcomes of interventions to determine their effectiveness, and adjust the plan of care as needed.

Source: Melnyk, B., & Fineout-Overholt, E. (2023). *Evidence-based practice in nursing and healthcare: A guide to best practice* (5th ed.). Wolters Kluwer.

RESPONDING TO SOCIETAL CHANGES

The professional growth of the RN includes identifying and responding to societal changes to meet the evolving needs of clients and communities. Several societal trends influence nursing and have professional growth implications for nurses in clinical practice, including changing demographics, healthcare reform, the emerging global community, and advances that are increasing the amount, cost, and complexity of technology.

Changing Demographics

Demographic changes in healthcare clients are influenced by various factors including population aging, a rise in chronic diseases, and increased cultural diversity. Nurses must adapt their care strategies to meet the diverse needs of clients. By recognizing and proactively adapting to demographic changes, nurses can provide more effective and patient-centered care that meets the unique needs of the diverse populations they serve.

Older Adults

By the year 2050, the client population of those older than 65 years will dramatically increase by an estimated 47% due to longer life expectancy and improved management of chronic disease (Mather & Scommegna, 2024; U.S. Census Bureau, 2023). In caring for the older adult population, nurses must focus on preventive measures, manage chronic conditions, and address the unique healthcare needs that promote independence, fall prevention, and facilitating end-of-life discussions. Some considerations to keep in mind as the client population ages include the following (Dassel et al., 2022):

- When caring for older adults, the nurse must gain additional knowledge on the differing care needs of well, frail, and ill individuals.
- What new evidence-based research is available in geriatric nursing and the field of gerontology?
- What nursing intervention is needed for a client who is nearing 100 years of age?
- What safety and preventive measures are required to maintain health in frail individuals?
- What new information is available in the behavioral sciences to support nursing of older adults?

Chronic Conditions

The prevalence of chronic diseases such as diabetes and cardiovascular conditions for adults aged 50 years and older is estimated to increase from 61.11% in 2020 to 99.5% by 2050 (Administration for Community Living, 2021; Ansah & Chiu, 2023). Nurses can support clients in chronic disease management through client education, lifestyle counseling, and medication management. The rise in chronic conditions also requires that nurses and other healthcare professionals collaborate to develop comprehensive care plans that address the physical, emotional, and social aspects of living with chronic conditions.

Cultural Diversity

In light of changing demographics, nursing practice requires a dedication to cultural sensitivity and ongoing education. See Chapters 4 and 13 for more on managing the care of unique clients, including practicing cultural humility and sensitivity.

Healthcare Reform

A hotly debated concern in the United States is healthcare reform, which refers to the process of making changes and improvements to the healthcare system with the goal of enhancing efficiency, accessibility, affordability, and overall quality of care. Healthcare reform initiatives can take place at various levels, including local, regional, and national, and they often involve changes to healthcare policies, regulations, and delivery models. Healthcare reform is a complex and ongoing process, and its success depends on collaboration among policymakers, healthcare providers, payers, patients, and other stakeholders. Reforms are influenced by current or ongoing health problems, technological advancements, and shifts in population health patterns.

Because nurses spend a great amount of time advocating for clients and working in communities, they should actively engage in healthcare reform. Some ways nurses can be involved in shaping the future of healthcare include the following:

- Being informed about healthcare policies and actively participating in discussions about reforms at local, regional, and national levels
- Maintaining membership in nursing organizations that advocate for healthcare reform
- Providing education to the public about healthcare issues, preventive care, and the importance of health insurance coverage
- Advocating for policies that address healthcare disparities and promote equitable access to care, especially for vulnerable populations
- Developing programs that enhance health literacy to help individuals better understand healthcare options and make informed decisions
- Participating in initiatives that focus on client safety, quality improvement, and EBPs

Nurses are uniquely positioned to influence public health and to advance professional nursing. Nurses can actively voice their ideas for healthcare reform through various channels and platforms such as professional organizations, advocacy groups, legislative advocacy, social media and online platforms, letters to editors, op-eds, professional conferences, community outreach, and research publication.

Global Communities

Global communities form around topics such as culture, environment, health, human rights, and more. Global communities bring together people from different regions to work collectively to address common problems or to pursue shared goals. Because of advances in technology and communication, the nursing profession has a presence online as a global health community. Nurses in this global community work together to address global health challenges, to share resources, and to contribute to the development of healthcare policies and practices that transcend international borders. This international collaboration encompasses the exchange of knowledge, expertise, and best practices among nurses and healthcare professionals worldwide to improve health outcomes, to promote cultural competence, and to enhance the overall quality of nursing care on a global level (Lal, 2023; Naz, 2023).

Advances in distance communication provide opportunities for nurses to participate in professional development activities with colleagues across the United States and internationally, creating exciting professional growth opportunities for RNs around the world. Nursing education programs that incorporate global health perspectives give students opportunities for international clinical experiences, exchange programs, or collaborations with healthcare institutions in other countries.

Understanding and navigating the complexities of global healthcare and nursing practice is essential for modern nurses. Nurses contribute to global health initiatives aimed at addressing widespread health challenges such as infectious diseases, maternal and child health, and noncommunicable diseases. This work often involves collaborating with international organizations and governments to implement and support healthcare programs. Nurses may volunteer or be part of international teams providing healthcare services in the aftermath of natural disasters, conflicts, or public health emergencies.

Organizations such as the International Council of Nurses provide a platform for nurses worldwide to address common issues, to share insights, and to advocate for nursing at a global level.

Advances in Technology

The rapidly increasing amount, cost, and complexity of technology advancement in healthcare can be overwhelming for both the nurse (discussed earlier) and the client. Advances in technology have significantly impacted the field of nursing, transforming the way healthcare is delivered and enhancing client outcomes.

In providing care, the RN must strike a balance between "high tech" and "high touch" in their role as care manager. Clients need to feel that the RN values them, is accessible, and pays attention to their needs. The nurse must find ways to strike a balance between high tech and high touch as flowers and personal possessions are removed to provide space for equipment, and as loved ones struggle to get close enough to touch, hug, and provide emotional support.

> **The NCLEX-RN *Might Ask* 15.2**
>
> Two nurses are developing a nursing plan of care for a community experiencing an outbreak of Zika virus. The nurses are using evidence-based research to update the community on the latest methods to help prevent spread of the virus. These nurses are using which of the following qualities of professional behaviors? (Select all that apply.)
> a. Tradition
> b. Evidence-based research
> c. Autonomy
> d. Current knowledge base
> e. Accountability
>
> • See Appendix A for correct answer and rationale.

ADVANCING NURSING AS A PROFESSION

Nurses have a responsibility to advance nursing as a profession—that is, to elevate the overall standing of nursing in the healthcare system. Advancing the profession is a dynamic and ongoing process that requires collaboration, innovation, and a commitment to continuous improvement within the nursing community; it includes maintaining and promoting the high standards of nursing practice, adding to the body of nursing research and knowledge, and recruiting and mentoring new nurses.

STANDARDS OF NURSING PRACTICE

Contributing to the establishment of high nursing standards and ensuring adherence to them is every nurse's responsibility. In Chapter 8, you learned about the standards of practice, which are different from regulations and policies in organizations. Participation in professional organizations helps practicing RNs generate standards that are comprehensive and based on daily nurse–client interactions in the clinical area.

Professional nursing organizations develop standards of practice through a collaborative and systematic process that recognizes input from nursing professionals, educators, regulatory bodies, and healthcare organizations. The goal is to establish guidelines that ensure safe, effective, and ethical nursing care. Nurses promote high standards by contributing to the continuous development of nursing problem statements, nursing diagnoses, and relevant nursing outcomes through EBP. Standards of practice are developed from evidence-based research. The profession integrates the latest research findings, clinical evidence, and best practices into their standards to ensure that care is based on the most current and effective methods.

Standards of practice are not static; they require regular review and updates to reflect advancements in healthcare, changes in technology, and evolving client needs. Routine review of standards of practice, guidelines, and regulations set by national and international nursing organizations, regulatory bodies, and professional associations identifies gaps in knowledge or areas that need to be updated. Ensuring that standards reflect the needs and experiences of frontline nurses is critical.

Through EBP, nurses improve standards of care by critiquing existing diagnoses to ensure their applicability to clients with diverse socioeconomic, religious, cultural, and ethnic needs. RNs promote autonomous nursing practice by identifying appropriate outcomes, developing and revising nursing interventions, and evaluating client outcomes. In addition, nurses need to uphold high standards of care; stay up-to-date on clinical research about therapeutic, preventative, and rehabilitative intervention strategies; and incorporate this information into nursing care plans.

NURSING RESEARCH

The ANA (2015) states, "nurses must participate in the advancement of the profession through knowledge development, evaluation, dissemination, and application to practice" (p. 27). Although this statement does not mean that all nurses are required to *conduct* research, the ANA emphasizes that nurses must apply research to their individual practice to provide safe and efficient patient care. Research builds the scientific knowledge base for nursing practice. The knowledge gained from science, research, and clinical knowledge results in improved patient outcomes. Professional nurses apply research information in practice by developing protocols, leading change in policy and procedure, and implementing evidence-based interventions. Research that leads to EBP provides nurses with opportunities to improve clinical judgment and strengthens the profession.

Research conducted by nurses is necessary for the continued growth of the nursing profession, the improvement of patient care, and the advancement of healthcare as a whole. Those nurses who actively engage in research contribute to EBP, enhance their own professional development, and play an important role in shaping the future of healthcare. In nursing research, nurses working in the clinical setting have the following important roles:

- They are best suited to come up with study questions (Adams, 2022).
- They might participate in clinical research projects that improve health promotion and client care.
- They are responsible for implementing research findings to aid clients in regaining, maintaining, and improving health.

RECRUITING AND MENTORING NEW NURSES
Recruiting
Nursing recruitment is crucial for maintaining a strong and resilient healthcare workforce. Many regions face nursing shortages, experienced nurses are reaching retirement age, and workforce turnover is on the rise. As the U.S. population grows and ages, the demand for healthcare services has increased. Effective recruitment is crucial to address these gaps in the healthcare workforce; recruiting new nurses helps ensure that healthcare facilities have an adequate number of professionals to meet client needs (American Association of Colleges of Nursing [AACN], 2022).

Attracting and retaining talented nurses fosters long-term stability. Adequate staffing contributes to a positive work environment in which nurses are more likely to experience job satisfaction and higher morale. Recruitment efforts that focus on diversity help ensure that the nursing staff reflects the diverse backgrounds and needs of the client population. Diversity in the nursing workforce is vital for providing culturally sensitive care.

Nursing recruitment is not only about increasing the number of nurses; it is also about finding qualified nurses for specialized roles within the healthcare system. This includes nurses with expertise in various fields such as critical care, oncology, pediatrics, and mental health. Effective recruitment promotes nursing as a dynamic and rewarding career choice. Highlighting career advancement opportunities, specialized roles, and the ability to make a meaningful impact on patient lives encourages individuals to pursue and remain in the nursing profession.

Nurses play a vital part in shaping the future of the nursing profession and in ensuring a skilled and supportive healthcare workforce. Practicing nurses act as ambassadors for the nursing profession by showcasing rewards and opportunities, sharing their experiences and passion for patient care, and describing the diverse career paths available in nursing.

Participation in recruitment events such as career fairs and educational programs gives nurses the opportunity to engage with individuals interested in nursing careers. Nurses should offer information and guidance to prospective nursing students by providing insights into educational pathways, licensure requirements, and the various specialties within nursing. By demonstrating professionalism, compassion, and dedication to patient care, experienced nurses inspire others to enter into and excel in the nursing field.

Mentoring
Experienced nurses play a key role in orienting and onboarding new nursing staff by helping newcomers become familiar with the healthcare facility, policies, procedures, and the culture of the organization. Nurse mentoring is essential for professional growth, improving patient care, fostering a supportive community, addressing burnout, promoting leadership development, encouraging lifelong learning, and contributing to diversity and inclusion within the nursing profession. A **mentor** is a more experienced nurse who takes an active interest in the professional development of a less experienced nurse, who is referred to as the "**mentee**" (Masters, 2023).

Mentors offer emotional support to new nurses as they navigate the challenges of starting their careers. Experienced nurses emphasize the importance of maintaining a healthy work-life balance. They provide guidance on self-care practices, stress

BOX 15.7 Positive Effects of a Mentor on Professionalism

A nursing mentor may have the following effects:
- Increase the mentee's preparedness for career success and advancement
- Increase the mentee's personal and professional satisfaction
- Increase the mentee's self-confidence and self-esteem
- Increase the mentee's preparedness for leadership positions
- Strengthen the profession

management, coping strategies, building resilience, and developing strategies for maintaining well-being in the demanding healthcare environment.

Building a mentorship relationship involves proactive communication and expressing a genuine interest in learning and professional growth. New nurses should seek guidance and take the initiative to seek a mentor by inquiring with human resources or nursing leadership, utilizing orientation programs for new nurses, connecting with experienced nurses within the workplace or professional organizations, and exploring social media groups, forums, or professional networking platforms where nurses often share experiences and may offer mentorship. The bond between mentor and mentee improves career satisfaction and strengthens the profession (Box 15.7). This is especially true in areas with an expanded scope of practice, such as the manager of care role and aspects of the care provider role (e.g., client education and referrals).

THINKING CRITICALLY

Reflect on your own practice in nursing and the competencies you anticipate acquiring as you transition to the RN level. In what areas are you experienced and can offer to mentor others? In what areas might you seek a mentor to assist you? What qualities would you look for in a mentor that are consistent with your philosophy of education?

PROFESSIONAL STEWARDSHIP

Professional stewardship is a voluntary commitment to serve in various capacities to further the professional goals of nursing. Nurses serve as stewards by upholding the highest standards of ethical conduct and professionalism. Through their daily practice, nurses not only provide compassionate and evidence-based care but also serve as role models for aspiring nurses, embodying the values of integrity and accountability that define the nursing profession.

By contributing to the development of the nursing workforce, nurses foster a culture of continuous learning and elevate the overall competence and resilience of the profession. Nurse educators have a significant impact on the strength and vitality of the nursing profession, playing a critical role in inspiring the next generation of nurses. Nurse educators shape the future of nursing by instilling professionalism, advocating for excellence, and contributing to the ongoing development and improvement of nursing education.

Nurses play a vital role in shaping the future of healthcare by embracing leadership positions, participating in quality improvement initiatives, and advocating for policies that support nursing excellence. Through involvement in interdisciplinary collaborations and advocacy efforts, nurses influence positive changes within healthcare. As stewards of the nursing profession, nurses navigate challenges, champion patient-centered care, and work toward creating environments that empower colleagues to thrive and provide the best possible care for individuals and communities. Two aspects of professional stewardship are shared governance and decision-making, and leading by participation in professional organizations.

SHARED GOVERNANCE AND DECISION-MAKING

Nurses are strongly encouraged to participate in collaborative decision-making processes that shape policies, practices, and healthcare units or organizations by engaging in shared governance. In shared governance models, nurses contribute their expertise, insights, and experiences with committees, councils, and workgroups, where they collaborate with administrators and other healthcare professionals. Through shared governance committees, nurses have a voice in decision-making related to patient care, staffing models, quality improvement initiatives, and the implementation of EBPs. This shared approach empowers nurses to take ownership of their practice, fostering a sense of autonomy, accountability, and investment in the outcomes of patient care. Speaking out for effective change engages and empowers nurses (Epstein et al., 2023).

Participation in shared governance also includes the continuous improvement of the work environment and professional development opportunities. Nurses engage in ongoing dialogue about issues affecting their practice, advocating for resources, training, and policies that support their well-being and professional growth. By actively participating in shared governance structures, nurses not only enhance the quality of patient care but also contribute to a culture of a healthy work environment. According to the American Association of Critical-Care Nurses (2016), a **healthy workplace** includes the following components:

- Skilled communication
- True collaboration
- Effective decision-making
- Authentic leadership
- Meaningful recognition
- Appropriate staffing

At the unit level, staff nurses have increased their involvement in shared governance through scheduling, staffing, and other decision-making processes that were traditionally done by the nurse manager. Staff nurses may assume a greater role in hiring practices, peer review processes, committees for policy making, creating healthy work environments for nurses, and the development of standards of practice.

LEADING BY PARTICIPATION IN PROFESSIONAL ORGANIZATIONS

RNs provide leadership through membership and participation in professional organizations at the local, state, or national level. Participation in professional organizations provides a platform for ongoing education, networking, and collaboration within the healthcare community. Nursing organizations offer access to the latest advancements in nursing practice, research, and technology, enabling nurses to stay abreast of industry trends and best practices. Involvement in professional groups fosters a sense of community and support, allowing nurses to exchange ideas, share experiences, and seek guidance from peers. Through active participation, nurses can contribute to shaping healthcare policies, advocating for their profession, and enhancing their leadership skills, ultimately promoting their own professional development, and elevating the overall quality of patient care.

Your nursing faculty may encourage participation in activities via the National Student Nurses' Association (NSNA). Established in 1953, the NSNA is an organization managed, financed, and facilitated by students. The goals of the NSNA (n.d.) are to promote high-quality care and to provide educational programs to promote development of the whole person. Involvement in local, regional, and national workshops can help students grow and develop in the professional nursing role. Websites of both the NSNA and a similar group, the Canadian Nursing Students' Association, are included at the end of the chapter.

THINKING CRITICALLY
Visit one of the student nurse organization websites provided at the end of this chapter. How might you actively participate in one of these organizations to provide leadership for the nursing profession at your school?

Participation in professional organizations fosters collaboration between professionals, such as nurses, providers, social workers, and allied health professionals, by facilitating the exchange of knowledge, expertise, and best practices of each discipline. Through shared resources and collaborative initiatives, interdisciplinary teams are informed about advancements in each respective field, gain a deeper understanding of each other's roles, and develop a cohesive approach to patient care.

CONCLUSION

The RN has multiple professional responsibilities including autonomy, accountability, duty to self, professional advancement, and participation in professional organizations. Professional role development—which enhances skills, competencies, and knowledge—is instrumental in fostering leadership qualities, promoting advanced practice, and cultivating specialized expertise. Professional advancement, which fosters career satisfaction and fulfillment, empowers nurses to take on leadership roles, to pursue specialized areas of interest, and to contribute meaningfully to the profession's growth and innovation. Participation in professional organizations, which provide a platform for collaboration and advocacy, amplifies the voice of nurses in influencing healthcare policies and supports them by offering information about industry trends, resources for continuing education, networking with peers and experts in the field, and promotion of workforce diversity. By embracing continuous professional growth, nurses continually evolve to meet the dynamic and complex needs of diverse client populations, elevate their individual careers, and collectively strengthen the nursing profession.

STUDENT Exercises

Exercise 15.1
For several hours, observe a practicing RN in the clinical setting.
1. Cite statements made by the nurse or behaviors displayed by the nurse that tell you the degree to which the nurse values (or does not value) nursing as a profession.
2. Who was present at the time of these statements or behaviors (e.g., patients, visitors, students, other healthcare workers)? How might these observers' perceptions of nursing be influenced (positively or negatively) by what they observed?
3. How might these perceptions contribute to the evolving image of nursing and affect the advancement of the profession?

Exercise 15.2
Imagine you have just completed the ADN program and are beginning your career as an RN. Design a professional growth plan for yourself by identifying your strategies for maintaining competence in each of the following areas during your first few years of nursing practice.
1. Maintaining a current knowledge base
2. Remaining technologically current
3. Applying current research to practice
4. Participating in professional organizations
5. Responding to societal changes and needs

Exercise 15.3
Reflect on who might be your mentor as you transition to the RN role. List individuals and describe why you have selected them. How do they operationalize the strategies for professional growth discussed in this chapter?

REFERENCES

Adams, S. (2022). Identifying research questions. In N. A. Schmidt & J. M. Brown (Eds.). *Evidence-based practice for nurses: Appraisal and application for nurses* (5th ed., pp. 87–112). Jones & Bartlett Learning.

Administration for Community Living. (2021, May). *2020 Profile of older Americans*. U.S. Department of Health and Human Services. https://acl.gov/sites/default/files/aging%20and%20Disability%20In%20America/2020Profileolderamericans.final_.pdf

American Association of Colleges of Nursing. (2022, October). *Fact sheet: Nursing shortage*. https://www.aacnnursing.org/Portals/0/PDFs/Fact-Sheets/Nursing-Shortage-Factsheet.pdf

American Association of Critical-Care Nurses. (2016). *Creating a healthy work environment* (2nd ed.). https://www.aacn.org/WD/HWE/Docs/HWEStandards.pdf

American Nurses Association. (2010). *Nursing's social policy statement: The essence of the profession* (3rd ed.).

American Nurses Association. (2015). *Code of ethics for nurses with interpretive statements* (2nd ed.).

American Nurses Association. (2022). *Nursing informatics: Scope and standards of practice* (3rd ed.).

Ansah, J. P., & Chiu, C. T. (2023). Projecting the chronic disease burden among the adult population in the United States using a multi-state population model. *Frontiers in Public Health, 10*, 1082183. https://doi.org/10.3389/fpubh.2022.1082183

Dassel, K. B., Edelman, L. S., Moye, J., Catlin, C., & Farrell, T. W. (2022). "I worry about this patient EVERY day": Geriatrics clinicians' challenges in caring for unrepresented older adults. *Journal of Applied Gerontology*, *41*(4), 1167–1174. https://doi.org/10.1177/07334648211041261

Epstein, E. G., Shah, R., & Marshall, M. F. (2023). Effect of a moral distress consultation service on moral distress, empowerment, and a healthy work environment. *HEC Forum*, *35*(1), 21–35. https://doi.org/10.1007/s10730-021-09449-5

Faraco, M. M., Gelbcke, F. L., de Farias Brehmer, L. C., Ramos, F. R. S., Schneider, D. G., & Silveira, L. R. (2022). Moral distress and moral resilience of nurse managers. *Nursing Ethics*, *29*(5), 1253–1265. https://doi.org/10.1177/09697330221085770

Gordon, S. (1997). *Life support: Three nurses on the front lines*. Little, Brown and Company.

Gordon, S. (2005). *Nursing against the odds: How health care cost cutting, media stereotypes, and medical hubris undermine nurses and patient care*. Cornell University Press.

Huércanos-Esparza, I., Antón-Solanas, I., Orkaizagirre-Gómara, A., Ramón-Arbués, E., Germán-Bes, C., & Jiménez-Navascués, L. (2021). Measuring invisible nursing interventions: Development and validation of Perception of Invisible Nursing Care-Hospitalisation questionnaire (PINC–H) in cancer patients. *European Journal of Oncology Nursing*, *50*. https://doi.org/10.1016/j.ejon.2020.101888

Lackman, V., Swanson, E., & Winland-Brown, J. (2015). The new "Code of Ethics for Nurses with Interpretive Statements" (2015): Practical clinical application. Part 2. *Medsurg Nursing*, *24*(5), 363–366. 368.

Lal, M. M. (2023). Learning from our global community of nurses. *JONA: The Journal of Nursing Administration*, *53*(10), 493–494. https://doi.org/10.1097/NNA.0000000000001333

Masters, K. (2023). *Role development in professional nursing practice* (6th ed.). Jones and Bartlett Learning.

Mather, M., & Scommegna, P. (2024, January 9). *Fact sheet: Aging in the United States*. Population Reference Bureau. https://www.prb.org/resources/fact-sheet-aging-in-the-united-states/

Melnyk, B., & Fineout-Overholt, E. (2023). *Evidence-based practice in nursing and healthcare: A guide to best practice* (5th ed.). Wolters Kluwer.

National League for Nursing. (2012). *Outcomes and competencies for graduates of practical vocational, diploma, associate degree, baccalaureate, master's, practice doctorate, and research doctorate programs in nursing*.

National Student Nurses' Association. (n.d.). *About us*. https://www.nsna.org/about-nsna.html

Naz, A. (2023). Linkages between different types of globalization and socio-economic variables: Panel data analysis for 129 countries. *Journal of Economic Structures*, *12*(1), 7. https://doi.org/10.1186/s40008-023-00301-2

Peng, M. T. (2022). From invisible to visible—Validating media presence: Forging a new image of nursing in the post-pandemic era. *Journal of Nursing*, *69*(6), 84–92. https://doi.org/10.6224/JN.202212_69(6).11

Potter, P., Perry, A., Stockert, P., & Hall, A. (2023). *Fundamentals of nursing* (11th ed.). Elsevier.

Ramage, B. (2023). Evidence-based practice in perioperative nursing: Barriers and facilitators to compliance. *Journal of Perioperative Nursing*, *36*(2), e-37–e-41. https://doi.org/10.26550/2209-1092.1265

Taylor, C., Lynn, P., & Bartlett, J. L. (2023). *Fundamentals of nursing: The art and science of nursing care* (10th ed.). Wolters Kluwer.

Tsui, J., & Adam, S. (2023). Resilience in nursing education: An evolutionary concept analysis. *International Journal of Nursing Education Scholarship*, *20*(1), 1–12. https://doi.org/10.1515/ijnes-2022-0121

U.S. Census Bureau. (2023, October 31). *2023 National population projections tables: Main series*. https://www.census.gov/data/tables/2023/demo/popproj/2023-summary-tables.html

SUGGESTED READING

Blau, A., Sela, Y., & Grinberg, K. (2023). Public perceptions and attitudes on the image of nursing in the wake of COVID-19. *International Journal of Environmental Research and Public Health*, *20*(6), 4717. https://doi.org/10.3390/ijerph20064717

Delengowski, A. (2022). Bringing nursing research to the bedside: Supporting staff through the process...47th Annual Oncology Nursing Society Congress, April 27-May 1, 2022, Anaheim, CA. *Oncology Nursing Forum*, *49*(2), E72. https://doi.org/10.1188/22.ONF.E2

Dodson, T. M. (2023). Use of expert modeling videos in undergraduate nursing education: A systematic review. *Journal of Nursing Education*, *62*(2), 89–96. https://doi.org/10.3928/01484834-20221213-04

Evans, N. (2022). How to find tailored CPD opportunities for mental health nurses: Mental health-focused education and training can be difficult to access, but we have tips on finding continuing professional development to meet your needs—And how your employer can help. *Mental Health Practice*, *25*(5), 6–8. https://doi.org/10.7748/mhp.25.5.6.s2

Peykar, S., Vahedparast, H., Gharibi, T., & Bagherzadeh, R. (2023). Examining the impact of time management and resilience training on work-family conflict among Iranian female nurses: A randomized controlled trial. *BMC Nursing*, *22*(1), 1–15. https://doi.org/10.1186/s12912-023-01634-w

Topçu, N., Akbolat, M., & Amarat, M. (2023). The mediating role of empathy in the impact of compassion fatigue on burnout among nurses. *Journal of Research in Nursing*, *28*(6/7), 485–495. https://doi.org/10.1177/17449871231177164

Winland-Brown, J., Lachman, V., & Swanson, E. (2015). The new "Code of Ethics for Nurses with Interpretive Statements" (2015): Practical clinical application, Part I. *Medsurg Nursing*, *24*(4), 268–271.

On the WEB

The Canadian Nursing Students' Association: http://www.cnsa.ca/

Evidence-Based Nursing: http://www.ebn.bmj.com/

National Student Nurses' Organization: http://www.nsna.org

Nursing Organizations Alliance—an alliance created for nursing organizations to create a strong voice for nurses: http://www.nursing-alliance.org

CHAPTER 16

Legal Accountability

LEARNING OUTCOMES

By the end of this chapter, the student will be able to:
1. Compare and contrast sources of U.S. law.
2. Compare and contrast public, private, and nursing law.
3. Identify the components of accountability and their impact on nursing practice.
4. Describe how liability, negligence, and malpractice affect nursing practice.
5. Discuss methods to improve client safety and to avoid litigation.
6. Identify legal issues affecting nursing practice.
7. Differentiate the legal responsibilities of the RN versus the LPN/LVN.

KEY TERMS

accountability
administrative law
advance directive
against medical advice (AMA)
civil law
common law
constitutional law
contract law
criminal law
defamation of character
defendant
durable power of attorney (DPA)
expert witness
felony
Health Insurance Portability and Accountability Act (HIPAA)
informed consent
law
legal precedents
liability
libel
living wills
malpractice
misdemeanor
negligence
occurrence report
plaintiff
professional boundaries
risk management
slander
sentinel event
standards of care
standards of practice
statutory law
tort law

Case STUDY

Cal Thomas is in his second rotation as an RN student at City Community College. He also works per diem as an LPN at busy Willow Glen Medical Center. Cal is talking to his nurse manager, Joann Francheski. Joann has been a practicing nurse for more than 20 years; she, too, started out as an LPN.

CAL: I never really gave much thought to the differences in legal responsibilities between LPNs and RNs until recently. Now that I'm in clinical at school, I see there is a big difference. Although I have legal obligations as an LPN, I feel a bit anxious about the greater legal responsibility as an RN. Do you have any advice or insights you could share?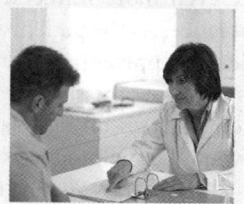

JOANN: It's completely normal to feel that way as you gain more responsibility in your nursing career. The role of an RN does come with increased legal responsibilities, but it also opens up new opportunities for growth. Let's talk about the role conflict you are experiencing. I have lots of success stories to help you understand what you are experiencing now.

CAL: I have to remember that here at work I'm an LPN. It's tempting to practice those advanced RN skills and delegation while I'm here, but I would be stepping out of my legal bounds of practice. In clinical I have a broader scope of practice, including more complex aspects of patient care, such as developing and implementing care plans, making critical decisions, and overseeing a team of healthcare professionals.

JOANN: Yes, it sounds as if you are feeling a bit of role tension now. I understand your concerns. It's a good thing that you realize the difference between roles and that you stay in the role of an LPN while here but in the role of a student while in clinicals. The role transition from LPN to RN can be tough. It's also a challenge for the staff to adjust to that new role as delegator and manager of care. However challenging, it's a rewarding step in your growth as a professional.

CAL: I'm worried about making critical decisions and being held accountable for them. As an LPN, I have a more defined scope of practice, and the thought of having more autonomy is both exciting and scary. Once I'm an RN and I'm in a more advanced role, I may face more legal consequences if something goes wrong.

JOANN: With greater autonomy comes increased responsibility, but it also means you'll have the chance to make more significant contributions to patient care. It's crucial to stay updated on regulations and guidelines, and never hesitate to consult with your colleagues or superiors when needed. Confidence comes with experience and continuous learning. Embrace the opportunities to enhance your skills, and don't shy away from learning from both successes and challenges. Remember, you're not alone in this journey—the healthcare team is here to support each other.

CAL: Thanks; I appreciate your guidance. I guess they key is to find a balance between confidence and caution. I'll make sure to approach this transition with a positive mindset and a commitment to ongoing learning.

The healthcare delivery system is extremely complex. Health maintenance and healthcare provision are the primary functions of the healthcare delivery system. Laws and standards have been developed to protect society by maintaining and promoting accountability for safe practice in the healthcare system. In the case study, Cal is grappling with the change in this role function as an LPN/LVN, as well as the increased responsibility and accountability he has in fulfilling his new role. In this role, Cal will be even more immersed in legal and ethical decisions that affect his clients and his practice. As the patient advocate, the nurse is frequently the client or family's final line of defense, preventing irreversible harm. The best defense a nurse has in preventing harm is to follow the standards of care, acting wisely and in a prudent manner. This chapter concentrates on how laws affect nursing and how to help protect your license in the event of a malpractice suit.

A **law** is a standard or rule of conduct established and enforced by the government that is intended chiefly to protect the rights of the public (Taylor et al., 2023). Laws are binding for all citizens. They are developed by people of that society and are enforced by a particular authority. U.S. laws and most Canadian laws are based on English common law. Within the United States, laws are created by local, state, and national governments. They are enforced by officers and agencies of the government and courts.

The law influences many decisions made by nurses. An RN's increased independence in function corresponds to increased accountability for decisions and actions. Many situations faced by nurses today involve concerns about protecting client rights, carrying out accepted modes of treatment, and maintaining practice standards. Issues related to confidentiality, competence, safety, and optimal care can pose challenging dilemmas for nurses, especially in a fiscally strapped economy. The legal aspects of healthcare are closely aligned with ethical concerns (Chapter 17). Frequently, conflicts in the law can arise from an ethical problem.

In this chapter, general concepts of law are introduced. There are opportunities to consider legal implications for nursing practice. Like Cal, students will develop a greater understanding of the concepts of law, a better appreciation of these principles to the practice of an RN, and an increased appreciation for how role transition affects legal responsibilities.

The expanded work role of the RN necessitates that each nurse remains informed of current laws and regulations that affect the healthcare system. Registered nurses must know and understand healthcare law to ensure ethical patient care, navigate legal complexities, and mitigate liability risks. This knowledge is essential for advocating patients' rights, making informed decisions, maintaining accurate documentation, upholding professional standards, and fostering effective interdisciplinary collaboration.

This chapter will introduce you to the origins and classifications of law in the United States. An examination of legal issues and public policies that affect nursing practice, along with issues related to accountability, contracts, negligence, malpractice, and liability, will give you the opportunity to consider the impact of legal issues on your practice.

SOURCES OF LAW

The healthcare system is affected by several sources of law. In the United States, there are four sources: constitutional, statutory, common, and administrative laws.

CONSTITUTIONAL LAW

The U.S. Constitution guarantees particular fundamental freedoms to all people in the United States; this is called **constitutional law**. Constitutional law affects nurses by protecting their basic rights. For example, freedom of speech and the right to bear arms are rights that patients and nurses have as U.S. citizens. There are controversies in constitutional laws that can affect healthcare workers. For example, the following rights affect nurses and patient care: the constitutional right for individuals to bear arms in an increasingly violent world and the fact that there is not a constitutional right of all citizens to have health insurance.

STATUTORY LAW

Statutory laws, also known as statutes, are laws enacted by a legislative body, such as a federal, state, or local legislature (Potter et al., 2023). These laws are written and codified to regulate various aspects of society, including individual behavior, businesses, and government operations. Statutory laws cover a wide range of subjects, from criminal offenses and civil matters to administrative procedures and regulatory frameworks. Statutory laws are a fundamental part of the legal system; they provide a clear and established set of rules that individuals and organizations must follow. Violations of statutory laws can result in legal consequences, including fines, penalties, or other forms of legal action.

Statutory laws can be amended, repealed, or replaced by subsequent legislative action. This process typically involves introducing a bill, debating its provisions, and voting on whether to pass it into law. If the bill is approved, it becomes part of the statutory law. Legislators may revisit and modify existing laws in response to changing societal needs, legal interpretations, or public policy considerations. Changes to laws may lead to challenges for healthcare practitioners, healthcare agencies, and individuals.

For example, the Affordable Care Act, passed in 2010, introduced several key provisions, such as expanding Medicaid eligibility, establishing health insurance marketplaces, and implementing consumer protections. These changes aimed to increase access to healthcare, to protect individuals with preexisting conditions, and to make healthcare coverage more affordable. Changes to healthcare statutes can influence healthcare costs, the availability of certain services, and the overall structure of the healthcare system, which can directly impact individuals' access to, and quality of, healthcare (Shearer & Bundorf, 2023). The Nurse Practice Acts of State Boards of Nursing are examples of statutory law. Other federal statutes that fall under statutory law are shown in Box 16.1. The Good Samaritan laws enacted in most states and the Oregon Death with Dignity Act of 1994 (which legalizes provider-assisted suicide with some restrictions) are other types of state statutory laws.

COMMON LAW

Common law, or case law, is based on precedent and judicial decisions, rulings, and interpretations in individual cases over time rather than statutory laws enacted by legislatures (Taylor et al., 2023). Common law principles are developed through the application of **legal precedents**, in which decisions in similar cases are considered binding for future cases. Common law principles emphasize the importance of consistency

---

BOX 16.1

Examples of Federal Statutes

- **Emergency Medical Treatment and Active Labor Law (EMTLA):** This law prevents hospitals from transferring those who are unable to pay to other hospitals.
- **Health Insurance Portability and Accountability Act of 1996 (HIPAA):** This federal law was enacted to prevent the release of health information without the patient's authorization.
- **Patient Self-Determination Act of 1990 and Omnibus Budget Reconciliation Act of 1990:** This law was enacted to allow clients to make decisions regarding their end-of-life care and to require medical personnel to inquire if patients have a living will or healthcare proxy. It is in effect for all federally funded hospitals.

and fairness in judicial decisions, allowing for the adaptation of legal rules to changing circumstances. New rules will be made if the precedent is no longer applicable or is outdated. Examples of violations of common law include patient abandonment, failure to obtain informed consent, and failure to accept a client's right to refuse treatment.

ADMINISTRATIVE LAW

Administrative law, sometimes called regulatory law, is a branch of law that governs the activities and operations of administrative agencies of the government. These laws are enacted by administrative agencies under the direction of the executive branch of government to relieve the courts and government of the burden of trying specific cases. Administrative law provides and outlines the legal principles and procedures that these agencies must follow in their decision-making processes and covers issues such as rulemaking, adjudication, enforcement of regulations, and the rights and obligations of individuals and businesses in their interactions with government agencies. For example, the nurse practice acts are formed by state statutory law, but the authority to regulate these acts is given to an administrative agency, the State Board(s) of Nursing, as overseen by a state's governor (Westrick, 2024).

Administrative law aims to ensure fairness, transparency, and accountability in the actions of administrative bodies, providing a framework for citizens to challenge agency decisions through administrative appeals or judicial review, if necessary. Some examples of violations of administrative laws include practicing nursing with an expired license, failure to report unethical nursing conduct, and falsifying a nursing license application. These can lead to suspension and possible revocation of a nursing license and may sometimes lead to criminal convictions. Examples of violations of the nurse practice act involve practicing without a current license, using drugs and alcohol, engaging in abusive behavior, and exhibiting incompetence (Westrick, 2024).

CLASSIFICATIONS OF LAW

Three types of laws have direct implications for nursing practice: civil, criminal, and contract.

CIVIL LAW

Civil law is the protection of individual rights and the governance of conduct between individuals and private organizations (Huston, 2023). Civil law covers a broad range of issues, including contracts, property, family law, torts, and more. The primary goal of civil law is to provide a legal framework for individuals to resolve disputes and to seek remedies for any harm or injury suffered (Potter et al., 2023). Malpractice, negligence, assault, and battery cases fall within civil law. **Tort law** creates guidelines for socially acceptable behavior and holds those who commit wrongdoings accountable for their inappropriate behavior (Mahlmeister, 2023).

Intentional torts occur when an individual deliberately engages in conduct that results in harm to another person or their property. The key element is the intent to commit the act that causes harm. The person must either desire the consequences of their actions or know that harm is substantially certain to occur. Unintentional torts, often referred to as negligence, occur when an individual's failure to exercise reasonable care results in harm to others. Unlike intentional torts, there is no requirement for the person to have intended to cause harm. Instead, the focus is on the failure to exercise the standard of care that a reasonable person would exercise under similar circumstances.

> **BOX 16.2**
>
> ## Intentional and Unintentional Torts Leading to Potential Liability
>
> **Intentional Torts**
> - Fraud
> - Assault and battery
> - Defamation of character
> - Invasion of privacy
>
> **Unintentional Torts**
> - Omitting important assessment data
> - Failure to establish priorities of care
> - Teaching not documented and a client occurrence happened
> - Client falls out of bed or is burned from intervention
> - Wrong medication given to wrong client

Source: Maher, V., & Cwiek, M. (2022). Criminal liability for nursing and medical harm. *Hospital topics*, 1–8. Advance online publication. https://doi.org/10.1080/00185868.2022.2101571

Box 16.2 provides examples of intentional and unintentional torts that involve nurses. The result of a guilty verdict in a civil law case means that the **defendant** (person accused of wrongdoing) must pay damages to the **plaintiff** (person suing). In a civil court, the plaintiff has the burden of proof, whereas in a criminal court, the state must prove the defendant guilty beyond a reasonable doubt.

CRIMINAL LAW

Criminal law involves crimes an individual commits against society or the public's general welfare. These crimes involve a willful intentional act of disregard for the safety, well-being, or life of another. Nurses, like other healthcare professionals, can potentially face criminal charges in certain situations. The decision to bring criminal charges against a nurse is typically based on specific circumstances, and not all mistakes or errors result in criminal prosecution. Box 16.3 provides examples situations in which a nurse may be charged with a criminal act. Many instances of unintentional errors or lapses in judgment are addressed through internal hospital processes, professional disciplinary actions, or civil litigation. Criminal charges are generally reserved for more severe cases involving intentional harm, recklessness, or criminal conduct. However, if an unintentional act on the part of a nurse has dire consequences, the nurse could still be tried in criminal court for felonies known as reckless endangerment or criminal carelessness (Maher & Cwiek, 2022).

There are two types of criminal charges that can be levied against a nurse: misdemeanors and felonies. The classifications for each are based on the severity of the offense and the associated potential punishment. The specific charges will depend on the nature and severity of the alleged actions. The decision to classify an offense as a **misdemeanor** or **felony** is usually based on statutory laws and can vary by jurisdiction (Maher & Cwiek, 2022). Misdemeanors are less serious offenses compared to felonies and can include traffic violations, driving under the influence of alcohol, or misuse of a controlled substance. The latter two are more common than other types of violations for nurses and can result in action by the state board of nursing (DeBrew, 2022;

> **BOX 16.3** **Situations in Which a Nurse May be Charged With a Criminal Act**
> - **Intentional harm or wrongdoing:** If a nurse intentionally causes harm to a patient or engages in criminal activities such as theft, assault, or fraud
> - **Reckless or grossly negligent conduct:** If a nurse's actions are characterized by extreme recklessness or gross negligence, resulting in serious harm or death to a patient; this goes beyond ordinary negligence and involves a higher level of culpability
> - **Drug diversion or theft:** If a nurse is involved in the diversion or theft of controlled substances, including prescription medications
> - **Forgery or fraudulent activities:** If a nurse engages in forgery, fraud, or other deceptive practices, such as altering medical records or falsifying documents
> - **Violations of healthcare regulations:** If the nurse disregards established standards, regulations, or laws, or engages in illegal practices, especially if they do so knowingly and willfully
> - **Sexual misconduct:** If a nurse engages in instances of sexual misconduct or assault; can also lead to potential professional disciplinary actions
>
> Source: Maher, V., & Cwiek, M. (2022). Criminal liability for nursing and medical harm. *Hospital topics*, 1–8. Advance online publication. https://doi.org/10.1080/00185868.2022.2101571

Mahlmeister, 2023). Punishments for misdemeanors typically include fines, probation, community service, or a short-term jail sentence of less than 1 year.

A felony is a major type of criminal law violation. Felonies in nursing may involve actions that pose significant harm to patients, violate ethical standards, or breach the trust placed in healthcare professionals. Examples of nursing-related felonies may include intentional harm to patients, drug diversion, fraudulently obtaining controlled substances, or other criminal activities that compromise patient safety and the integrity of healthcare practices. Being convicted of a felony can have severe consequences for a nurse, including potential imprisonment, fines, and the loss of professional licensure. The healthcare industry places a high value on maintaining ethical standards and ensuring patient well-being, and nurses found guilty of felonies may face both legal and professional repercussions. The majority of nurses uphold ethical standards and provide exemplary care to their patients. Felony charges in nursing are relatively rare, but when they occur, they are taken seriously by law enforcement and can result in significant consequences for the individual nurse involved Maher and Cwiek (2022).

Contrasting Two Criminal Cases

Let us look at two cases of nurses who were criminally charged with crimes: RaDonda Vaught and Charles Cullen. Although both were charged with criminal acts in the healthcare field, their cases involve different circumstances, motivations, and legal outcomes. In 2017, RaDonda Vaught, a former nurse at Vanderbilt University Medical Center, administered a paralyzing agent, vecuronium, instead of the intended sedative, resulting in the patient's death. The incident was attributed to a medication error, and Vaught faced criminal charges, including reckless homicide. The case highlighted issues related to medication administration protocols and the importance of preventing such errors in healthcare settings. Vaught's actions were characterized as a tragic mistake rather than intentional harm (Harrington, 2023; "The Case", 2022).

Charles Cullen is a former nurse who became known as one of the most prolific serial killers in the history of healthcare in the United States. Over his nursing career from

1988 to 2003 and spanning multiple hospitals in different states, Cullen was responsible for numerous patient deaths by administering lethal doses of medications. His actions were intentional, driven by a desire to end the lives of patients. Cullen's case raised concerns about the monitoring of healthcare professionals and the need for improved safeguards against serial misconduct in the healthcare system. He was convicted of multiple counts of murder and is serving a life sentence in prison (Graber, 2013).

Vaught's actions were unintentional and the result of a medical error, whereas Cullen's actions were intentional and part of a pattern of serial killings. Vaught faced criminal charges related to reckless homicide. In March 2022, Vaught was found guilty of the two lesser charges of criminally negligent homicide and abuse of an impaired adult. The legal consequences for Vaught included being fired, the loss of her professional license, and being sentenced to 3 years of probation. Cullen faced multiple counts of murder, and in March 2006, he was sentenced to 18 consecutive life terms. These cases underscore the importance of patient safety, the need for vigilant oversight in healthcare settings, and the legal distinctions between unintentional errors and intentional harm in the criminal justice system.

In Cullen's case, in which he intentionally caused harm to numerous patients over an extended period, there may have been a widespread acknowledgment of the need for legal accountability. Public support for criminal charges in such cases is often driven by a desire for justice, protection of society, and deterrence of similar actions in the future (Maher & Cwiek, 2022). The case against Vaught was quickly scrutinized by healthcare professional and the public. Public perception and understanding of medical errors can influence the response to criminal charges. Criminal charges against healthcare professionals could set a legal precedent, influencing how similar cases are handled in the future. This raises questions about the potential chilling effect on healthcare professionals' willingness to report mistakes and whether the trend to bring criminal charges will discourage a culture of openness and learning (Evans et al., 2022).

Striking a balance between accountability and recognizing the challenges inherent in healthcare delivery is essential for patient safety and to maintain public trust. There is ongoing debate about the appropriate mechanisms for addressing medical mistakes to ensure fairness, accountability, and continuous improvement in healthcare.

The NCLEX-RN *Might Ask* 16.1

A nurse accidentally administers an incorrect dose of morphine sulfate to a client. Which type of law best addresses this situation?
a. Civil law
b. Criminal law
c. Common law
d. Administrative law

• See Appendix A for correct answer and rationale.

CONTRACT LAW

Contract law is a legal framework that governs the creation, enforcement, and interpretation of contracts. A contract is an agreement between two parties in which there is a duty or an obligation (Taylor et al., 2023). Contracts are a regular part of daily life, from business transactions and employment relationships to the purchase of goods and services. In a contractual relationship, an offer is made by one party, and upon acceptance by another party, a legally binding agreement is formed. For a contract to be valid, the parties must have the legal capacity to enter into an agreement, and the purpose of the contract must be legal. Contract law provides a means for parties to enforce their rights and to seek remedies in the event of a breach, offering a structured framework for resolving disputes and upholding the integrity of agreements in both personal and business contexts.

Contracts can take various forms depending on the nature of the agreement and the preferences of the parties involved. Traditional written contracts, documented on paper or in electronic format, are common for complex agreements because they provide a clear record of terms and conditions. Oral contracts, formed through spoken communication, are also valid in many situations, although enforcing them may be more challenging. Implied contracts, arising from the conduct of the parties, and express contracts, where terms are explicitly communicated, offer flexibility in agreement formation. Unilateral contracts involve one party making a promise in exchange for the performance of another party. With the advent of technology, electronic contracts (e-contracts) have become prevalent, utilizing online platforms, e-mails, or electronic signatures to formalize agreements (Johnson, 2022).

In the United States, labor relations are governed by legislation, such as the National Labor Relations Act or similar acts at the state level. The labor relations act serves as the legal framework that outlines the rights and responsibilities of both employers and employees in matters related to collective bargaining and labor practices. Nurses generally become involved with contract law if they decide to take part in collective bargaining agreements. The labor relations act establishes the legal parameters for labor–management relations, while collective bargaining is the process through which employees and employers negotiate the terms of employment. The acts ensure fair and orderly processes, protect the rights of both parties, and contribute to the overall stability of labor relations in the workplace. The collective bargaining process is complex. To make an informed decision regarding workplace agreements, nurses working within a collective bargain unit should seek information from collective bargaining representatives (Wilson, 2023).

ACCOUNTABILITY

Accountability means that the nurse accepts responsibility for actions or behaviors. According to the American Nurses Association ([ANA], 2021) standards and the state nurse practice acts, nurses are responsible for demonstrating competence, sound judgment, and critical thinking in their role as caregivers. In order to guarantee safe care, the RN supervising LPN/LVN and unlicensed assistive personnel (UAP) must delegate appropriately and evaluate the outcomes of the delegated care (Box 16.4). A nurse can delegate tasks, but they cannot delegate professional judgment or decisions concerning a client's needs. If the nurse delegates a task that a UAP is not competent to perform, the nurse may be held accountable if the client is harmed. However, if the UAP performs a task without consulting the nurse and the work is beyond the UAP's scope of training, the UAP, not the nurse, will be held accountable for the action.

As a student nurse, you are accountable for the care you provide (see Chapter 15). The standard of care to which you are held is that of a professional nurse, not a student and not an LPN/LVN. You should perform only skills you are competent to perform, and you should never attempt an invasive procedure without the direction/presence of

> **BOX 16.4** **The 5 Rights of Delegating to Other Healthcare Personnel**
>
> 1. **Right Task:** Select the appropriate task to delegate based on the complexity of the task, the stability of the patient, and the competency of the delegate.
> 2. **Right Circumstances:** Consider the patient's condition. Is the patient stable, and is the environment conducive to safe delegation?
> 3. **Right Person:** Consider the delegatee's competence, skills, education, and experience. Delegation should only be assigned to individuals who are qualified and capable of performing the task safely.
> 4. **Right Direction/Communication:** Clear communication is essential in delegation. The nurse must provide clear and concise instructions to the delegatee, including the objectives, expectations, and any specific considerations.
> 5. **Right Supervision/Evaluation:** Delegation is not a relinquishment of responsibility and requires ongoing supervision and evaluation. The nurse retains responsibility for the overall care of the client, and regular follow-up is required to evaluate the delegatee's performance, to provide feedback, and to address any concerns or difficulties that may occur during the delegated duty.

Source: Potter, P., Perry, A., Stockert, P., & Hall, A. (2023). Managing patient care. In *Fundamentals of nursing* (11th ed., pp. 303–315). Elsevier.

your instructor or preceptor. You must always consult your clinical supervisor first if you are unclear about how to perform a skill or a procedure. Client safety is the most important issue, superseding your need to learn.

DOCUMENTATION

A major factor in ensuring accountability is accurate, complete, and comprehensive documentation (Taylor et al., 2023). Documentation in nursing is vital for maintaining accountability, supporting legal practices, ensuring patient safety, and meeting regulatory requirements. Accurate and comprehensive documentation ensures the continuity of patient care and allows healthcare providers to track and to understand a patient's medical history, treatment plans, medications, and responses to interventions. Documentation is also essential for meeting regulatory and accreditation standards in healthcare. Various regulatory bodies, such as health departments and accrediting agencies, require healthcare institutions to maintain accurate and complete patient records.

Thorough and accurate documentation provides legal protection for nurses and healthcare institutions. In the event of legal disputes or malpractice claims, well-documented records serve as evidence of the care provided and can be valuable as part of the nurse's defense. The old axiom, "If it's not documented, it wasn't done," holds true for legal issues. Generally, nurses are responsible for a major portion of the client record and must ensure that all appropriate information regarding provided care is included in the client health record. Documentation can demonstrate that healthcare professionals adhered to standards of practice, followed protocols, and acted in the best interest of the patient.

To reduce omissions and to cut down on the time required to document, many healthcare agencies provide point-of-care electronic charting that includes the standards of care and flow sheets. Point-of-care access allows nurses to document care activities in real time, ensuring that the patient's record is up-to-date. The National

BOX 16.5 Tips for Preventing Legal Problems With Documentation

1. **Be Accurate and Complete:** Ensure that documentation is accurate, thorough, and reflects the actual care provided. Avoid making assumptions or recording information that was not observed or performed.
2. **Use Clear and Concise Language:** Use clear and concise language to convey information. Avoid vague or ambiguous terms. Be specific about observations, interventions, and patient responses.
3. **Timely Documentation:** Document care in a timely manner. Delayed or retroactive documentation can be perceived as untrustworthy and may raise questions about the accuracy of the record.
4. **Follow Facility Policies and Standards:** Adhere to the documentation policies and standards of the healthcare facility. Familiarize yourself with any specific guidelines related to charting and documentation practices.
5. **Record Objective Data:** Focus on recording objective data rather than subjective interpretations. Describe what was observed, measured, or assessed, rather than personal opinions or assumptions.
6. **Document Changes in Patient Condition:** Clearly document any changes in the patient's condition, interventions provided, and the response to those interventions.
7. **Avoid Abbreviations and Jargon:** Minimize the use of abbreviations and healthcare jargon, because these can be misunderstood or misinterpreted. Stick to commonly accepted abbreviations, and ensure that they are used consistently.
8. **Document Patient Education:** Record patient education provided, including topics covered, the patient's understanding, and any educational materials provided.

Source: Potter, P., Perry, A., Stockert, P., & Hall, A. (2023). Managing patient care. In *Fundamentals of nursing* (11th ed., pp. 389–407). Elsevier.

Patient Safety Goals of 2024 challenge nurses to prevent errors and to strengthen documentation efforts to improve accuracy of patient identification, to improve safety of medications, and to reduce the risk of healthcare-associated infections (The Joint Commission, 2024). Having immediate access to accurate and timely patient information allows nurses to quickly review a patient's medical history, medications, allergies, and other relevant data to provide safe and effective care. The documentation of efforts to improve care in these areas not only will help with client safety but also will decrease liability (Mahlmeister, 2023).

Regardless of the setting in which the nurse works, clear, objective, and timely documentation protects everyone. For tips on how to avoid legal problems with documentation, see Box 16.5.

STANDARDS OF PRACTICE

Standards of practice, also called **standards of care**, are crucial in ensuring accountability within the nursing profession by defining the expectations and guidelines for each practitioner's role. The ANA's standards of nursing practice, service, and education outline the principles and expectations for delivering safe, competent, and ethical care. Adherence to these standards provides a clear framework for assessing nurse competency as well as the quality and appropriateness of healthcare services. In general, standards of practice follow the "common reasonable person" rule. This rule assumes that the expected action of a nurse would be the same as that of another nurse with similar education and experience (Catalano, 2024). As a result, during a trial, a nurse **expert witness** may be called on to verify that standard of practice (Potter et al., 2023) and to answer questions about that standard's application.

LIABILITY, NEGLIGENCE, AND MALPRACTICE

With the increasing complexity of medical treatments, technological advancements, and a growing emphasis on patient rights, nurses are held to high standards of care and accountability. To avoid negligence, nurses are expected to stay current on evolving medical practices, to adhere to established protocols, and to exercise sound clinical judgment. Strict legal regulations governing healthcare hold nurses accountable for their actions and decisions. Instances of malpractice or negligence may result in legal consequences, underscoring the necessity for nurses to practice diligence and a dedication to patient safety. Box 16.6 provides definitions of the terms liability, negligence, and malpractice.

LIABILITY

Liability refers to the legal responsibility and accountability of a nurse for their actions, decisions, and the quality of care provided to patients (Mahlmeister, 2023). Nurses have a duty to deliver care that meets established standards consistent with their professional training and scope of practice. If a nurse fails to fulfill this duty and their actions result in harm to a patient or a breach of legal standards, they may be held liable for the consequences. Liability can arise from various situations, including negligence, errors in documentation, failure to follow protocols, or inadequate communication. For example, the nurse is expected to administer the right medication, in the right dose, using the right route, to the right patient, at the right time. If any part of the process of administering that medication is incorrect and the client is harmed as a result, the nurse is liable.

NEGLIGENCE

Negligence refers to the failure to exercise the degree of care that a reasonable person would exercise in similar circumstances (Huston, 2023). Negligence is a breach of a duty of care owed to another person that results in harm or damage. In a negligence claim, the injured party typically needs to establish four key elements: duty, breach of duty, causation, and damages. Negligence can occur in various contexts, not limited to professional settings and can be applied to individuals in their everyday lives. For instance, a charge of negligence can be levied against a parent or caregiver if they failed to exercise safe care of their child by leaving the child unattended in a hot car.

BOX 16.6 Definitions of Liability, Negligence, and Malpractice

Liability: Legal responsibility for actions that do not reflect the standard of care and cause harm, or a failure to act to prevent harm

Negligence: An unreasonable or careless act, or the failure to act in a reasonable and prudent manner, that results in harm

Malpractice: Professional negligence; an act or failure to act by a professional in a reasonable and prudent manner in conducting professional duties as defined by members of the profession

Source: Westrick, S. (2024). *Essentials of nursing law and ethics* (3rd ed.). Jones & Bartlett Learning.

In the realm of healthcare, negligence might involve a healthcare professional failing to provide a standard of care that a reasonable and prudent professional would have provided, leading to harm. UAPs can be tried for negligence if they failed to lower a bed after care and the client falls, sustaining an injury. However, that UAP cannot be tried for malpractice because they are not considered professionals (Finkelman, 2021).

MALPRACTICE

Malpractice is a specific form of professional negligence in which a professional fails to follow a standard of care recognized by their profession, resulting in injury to a client (Guido, 2020). Compared to negligence, which is a broader concept that can apply to any person in various situations, malpractice specifically pertains to professionals, including doctors, nurses, lawyers, and other licensed practitioners. Medical malpractice claims typically require demonstrating the professional's actions or omissions deviated from the standard of care within their field, resulting in harm to the patient.

Examples of nursing malpractice allegations include medication errors, failure to accurately assess and monitor a patient's condition, inadequate communication with other healthcare providers, and violations of professional standards or protocols. To decrease the risk of malpractice charges, nurses must adhere to established standards of practice, engage in continuous education to stay current with developments in healthcare, communicate effectively with patients and the healthcare team, and document care accurately and comprehensively. To minimize the risk of malpractice claims, nurses are encouraged to seek guidance from their healthcare institution and to follow established protocols (Maher & Cwiek, 2022; Westrick, 2024).

In cases of medical malpractice or professional negligence, the "Four Ds" provide a framework for evaluating whether a legal claim is viable. To succeed in a lawsuit, the plaintiff typically needs to establish all four elements—duty, dereliction, direct cause, and damages—to demonstrate that the healthcare professional is liable for the harm suffered by the patient (Westrick, 2024). Box 16.7 provides brief definitions of the "Four Ds."

BOX 16.7

The Four Ds of a Successful Lawsuit

Duty: This refers to the duty of care owed by the nurse to the patient. It establishes that the healthcare professional has an obligation to provide care in a manner consistent with accepted standards and practices.

Dereliction of Duty: Dereliction occurs when there is a breach of the duty of care. It involves the failure of the nurse to meet the standard of care expected in a given situation. This breach can be a result of negligence, errors, or failure to follow established protocols.

Direct Cause: This element establishes a direct cause-and-effect relationship between the breach of duty and the harm suffered by the patient. It requires demonstrating that the nurse's actions or omissions directly led to the injury or adverse outcome.

Damages: Damages refer to the harm or injuries suffered by the patient as a result of the breach of duty. In a lawsuit, the plaintiff (patient or their representative) must demonstrate that measurable harm or damages occurred, which may include physical injuries, emotional distress, financial losses, or other adverse effects.

Source: Westrick, S. (2024). *Essentials of nursing law and ethics* (3rd ed.). Jones & Bartlett Learning.

The NCLEX-RN *Might Ask* 16.2

The scope of nursing practice is legally defined by:
a. state nurse practice acts.
b. professional nursing organizations.
c. hospital policy and procedure manuals.
d. providers in the employing institutions.

• See Appendix A for correct answer and rationale.

RISK MANAGEMENT

Risk management is a systematic process designed to identify, assess, and mitigate potential risks and adverse events in healthcare settings (Potter et al., 2023). The goal of risk management is to enhance patient safety, to improve the quality of care, and to minimize the likelihood of adverse outcomes. Nurses, along with other healthcare professionals, play a crucial role in the risk management process by actively participating in risk identification, assessment, and mitigation strategies. Ongoing evaluations of the healthcare environment, patient care processes, and staff practices identify areas where risks may arise. Risk management practices are integrated into nursing practice through occurrence reporting, process analysis, and continuous quality improvement initiatives.

Taking on the RN role will require you to be more involved in risk management, which involves identifying problems and developing solutions to eliminate or to reduce the incidence of particular situations. Because RNs are at the point of care, they are heavily involved in quality assurance or improvement programs. The steps of risk management share similarities with the nursing process. Nurses use the nursing process as a systematic framework to integrate risk management into their practice, ensuring a comprehensive approach to patient safety:

- In the *assessment* phase, nurses identify potential risks by thoroughly assessing the patient's health status, considering individual factors, and recognizing any environmental or system-related risks.
- Following assessment, nurses *diagnose* risks and prioritize areas that require attention, using critical thinking skills to categorize risks based on severity and likelihood.
- In the *planning* phase, nurses develop strategies and interventions to mitigate identified risks, incorporating evidence-based practices and established protocols. This may involve collaboration with the healthcare team and adherence to organizational policies.
- During *implementation*, nurses execute the planned interventions, ensuring proper communication, documentation, and adherence to safety measures.
- The *evaluation* phase allows nurses to assess the effectiveness of risk mitigation strategies, to make adjustments as needed, and to contribute to continuous improvement efforts.

OCCURRENCE REPORTS

Occurrence reports, also known as incident reports, play a crucial role in risk management for nurses and the healthcare team. Occurrence reports are important tools for nurses because they identify risks, support root cause analysis, drive quality improvement initiatives, serve as legal documentation, enhance communication and collaboration, and inform risk mitigation strategies. These reports are completed when an error is discovered or something extraordinary occurs that results in harm or potential harm (Guido, 2020). By actively participating in the reporting and analysis of incidents, nurses help to create a safer healthcare environment.

Reporting on incidents and occurrences also includes near misses (i.e., when an adverse event nearly happens). Occurrence reports explain the circumstances, the parties involved, and the actions done to address the issue. The purpose of the occurrence report is to analyze an issue or set of problems and to take preventative action rather than to punish employees. When completing an occurrence report, information should be factual and as complete as possible; subjective information or justifications for actions or behaviors should not be included. For example, if the nurse enters a room and discovers the patient lying on the floor at the foot of the bed, the nurse should avoid documenting, "Patient fell out of bed and found on floor." The idea that the patient fell out of bed is an assumption. Rather, the nurse should document, "Entered room. Patient found lying prone at the foot of the bed. Upper and lower side rails of bed were raised" (Mahlmeister, 2023).

The facts regarding an incident and the actions of healthcare workers should be documented in the client's medical records. However, the incident report itself is not included in the client's medical record. The Joint Commission mandates occurrence reports because they serve to alert institutions to risk management and quality assurance issues. Because incident reports are considered internal documentation, they cannot be discovered (seen) by the injured party or the lawyers acting on their behalf (The Joint Commission, 2024).

SENTINEL EVENTS

Occurrences that result in patient death or serious injury are considered **sentinel events** and require immediate attention, thorough investigation, and appropriate actions. Examples of sentinel events may include wrong-site surgery, medication errors resulting in serious harm, patient abduction, or unintended retention of a foreign object during surgery. The Joint Commission has established standards for addressing sentinel events (Box 16.8). These standards are outlined in their Sentinel Event Policy and are designed to guide healthcare organizations in responding to and learning from serious and unexpected adverse events (The Joint Commission, n.d.). Although The Joint Commission provides guidelines and standards for responding to sentinel events, how organizations implement the standards may vary.

BOX 16.8

The Joint Commission Sentinel Event Policy

1. Sentinel event occurs.
2. Respond immediately to the occurrence.
3. Conduct a root cause analysis.
4. Develop an action plan.
5. Report the event to The Joint Commission.
6. Monitor the effectiveness of the actions taken in response to the sentinel event.

Source: The Joint Commission. (n.d.). *Sentinel event policy and procedures.* https://www.jointcommission.org/resources/sentinel-event/sentinel-event-policy-and-procedures/#:~:text=The%20Sentinel%20Event%20Policy&text=A%20sentinel%20event%20is%20a,intervention%20required%20to%20sustain%20life

> **THINKING CRITICALLY**
> You have been assigned by your nurse manager to do an in-service for LPNs and UAPs regarding an update on legal implications of documentation and the 2024 National Patient Safety Goals. In your role as an RN, what would you include in this in-service? What is essential to include? What might you use to assist you in illustrating the key points?

LEGALLY SENSITIVE AREAS THAT AFFECT NURSING PRACTICE

A variety of issues within healthcare today may impact nurses. The legal implications for nurses have grown as a result of medical technology advancements and consumer education. This section addresses some of the legal issues and patient rights that may impact nursing practice.

ADVANCE DIRECTIVES

Advance directives are legal documents that allow individuals to express their preferences regarding medical treatment and healthcare decisions in the event they become unable to communicate or to make decisions for themselves (Potter et al., 2023). These directives are created when individuals are of sound mind and can include various documents such as living wills, **durable power of attorney (DPA)** for healthcare, and do-not-resuscitate orders. A **living will** outlines specific medical treatments or interventions an individual wishes to receive or avoid under certain circumstances, providing guidance to healthcare providers and family members. A DPA for healthcare designates a trusted person, often referred to as a healthcare proxy or agent, to make medical decisions on behalf of the individual if they are unable to do so (Mahlmeister, 2023). This person ensures that the individual's preferences and values are honored. Hospitals and support groups such as Compassion in Dying and Partners in Caring (https://www.compassionandchoices.org/) offer examples of advance directives for interested individuals and families.

Advance directives play a crucial role in respecting an individual's autonomy and ensuring that their healthcare wishes are followed, even if they cannot communicate or advocate for themselves due to illness or incapacitation. Advance directive documents are legally binding and must be honored by healthcare providers, emphasizing the importance of open communication between individuals, their healthcare proxies, and the medical team. Nurses have responsibilities in regard to advance directives. RNs must be knowledgeable about federal and agency rules governing advance directives, particularly the Patient Self-Determination Act of 1990. For example, federally reimbursed agencies require nurses to ask clients or their families about advance directives as part of the admissions process. It is also the nurse's responsibility to inform providers about client wishes regarding a living will or to alert the family about the wishes expressed in the client's DPA document (Mahlmeister, 2023).

Implementing advance directives or DPAs can be difficult if family members are unaware of or disagree with the patient's wishes. Nurses can encourage patients to make their family members aware of advance directives. Issues can also arise when individuals have life partners outside of marriage. In some scenarios, the partner may need to obtain legal counsel to help make judgments, especially in life-threatening or severe emergency situations (Guido, 2020). Advance directives promote patient-centered care and help healthcare professionals align medical interventions with the values and preferences of the individual, fostering a more personalized and dignified approach to end-of-life care.

INFORMED CONSENT

Informed consent is a legal and ethical principle that requires healthcare providers to obtain voluntary and comprehensible agreement, either orally or in written format, from a patient before conducting any medical treatment, procedure, or intervention. The process of informed consent involves providing the patient with clear and understandable information about the nature of the proposed healthcare intervention, including its potential risks, benefits, alternatives, and any potential consequences.

Informed consent empowers the patient, enabling them to make a voluntary autonomous and informed decision about their healthcare. It is important that consent be given freely without any form of coercion and that the client retains the right to withdraw their consent at any point if they change their mind (Mahlmeister, 2023). Clients also have the right to refuse a specific treatment; however, there have been instances in which legal authorities, such as courts, have intervened and overruled the wishes of a parent or legal guardian. In cases in which a client perceives that proper procedures for obtaining informed consent were not followed, there is a potential legal recourse wherein the client may pursue legal action, such as suing for assault and battery (see Box 16.9 for the definitions of assault and battery).

The NCLEX-RN *Might Ask* 16.3

The provider approaches the parents of an infant for permission to perform open heart surgery on their child. For the parents to give informed consent (select all that apply):

a. the nurse must leave the room.
b. the parents must realize that any information gained from the procedure may be used for research.
c. the parents must be informed about the benefits of the procedure, as well as alternatives to the procedure.
d. the parents may withdraw consent at any time before the surgery.
e. the parents have a right to know about the risks of the surgery.

- See Appendix A for correct answer and rationale.

BOX 16.9 Definitions of Assault and Battery

Assault: An intentional act of one person that causes another person to fear that they will be injured or touched in an offensive way; touching does not actually need to occur.

Battery: If the act of touching or injuring actually takes place, the act is called battery. Medical treatments and procedures done without prior consent may be considered assault and battery, with exceptions made for emergency treatment.

Source: Mahlmeister, L. R. (2023). Legal issues in nursing and health care. In B. Cherry & S. R. Jacob (Eds.). *Contemporary nursing: Issues, trends, & management* (9th ed., pp. 124–165). Elsevier.

Although the primary responsibility for discussing the risks, benefits, and alternatives lies with the healthcare provider, such as a physician or nurse practitioner, the nurse plays a crucial role in reinforcing the information provided by the healthcare provider, answering any immediate questions, and directing further inquiries or concerns back to the provider (Mahlmeister, 2023). The nurse also verifies the client's consent by witnessing their signing of the form, and they document the client's comprehension of the procedure as articulated by the client. In instances in which the client demonstrates difficulty understanding or accepting the information, the nurse is accountable for notifying the healthcare provider promptly. To ensure adherence to regulations, it is important for nurses to know their state's laws governing informed consent and to stay current on agency-specific policies. An exception to the informed consent doctrine is emergency situations. In emergent instances in which the patient is unconscious, incompetent, or otherwise unable to give consent, the institution will do what a reasonably prudent person would do, which is treat the patient (Catalano, 2024).

AGAINST MEDICAL ADVICE

Leaving **against medical advice (AMA)** refers to a situation in which a patient decides to discharge themselves from a healthcare facility or to discontinue medical treatment against the advice and recommendations of their healthcare providers. When a patient leaves AMA, they are choosing to leave before the healthcare team has deemed it medically appropriate for them to do so. This decision can apply to various healthcare settings, including hospitals, clinics, and other treatment facilities. Healthcare providers, including nurses, have a responsibility to ensure that patients fully understand the potential risks and consequences of leaving AMA. The nurse's primary role is to engage in open and honest communication with the patient, providing clear and thorough information about the risks and potential consequences of leaving AMA.

The patient may be asked to sign a form indicating their decision, acknowledging that they are leaving AMA. Despite a patient's decision to leave AMA, healthcare providers continue to prioritize the patient's safety by providing information on the potential risks associated with their decision. It is important for healthcare providers to document the patient's decision, the information provided, and any discussions held regarding the risks and benefits of continued treatment. Additionally, efforts should be made to address the patient's concerns, to provide appropriate education, and to encourage the patient to reconsider the decision, emphasizing the importance of their health and well-being (Mahlmeister, 2023).

CONFIDENTIALITY AND THE RIGHT TO PRIVACY

Every patient has the right to have their personal information recognized, respected, and protected. The **Health Insurance Portability and Accountability Act (HIPAA)**, passed in 1996, safeguards the confidentiality of patient information. According to HIPPA, information about the client can be shared with outsiders only if the client grants written authority. Referred to as the "need to know" basis, only those who are directly involved in the client's care should have access to patient information (Taylor et al., 2023). Although HIPAA is a statute, it is simply an expression of a long-held nursing value: shared trust.

In addition, to access client information at your place of employment as an LPN/LVN, you will also do so in a number of agencies as a student in an RN program. In your new role, your adherence to patient privacy is especially important because you will work on documents and treatment plans outside of the facility, in the classroom, and on learning management systems sites (e.g., Blackboard and Canvas). Students must be careful not to take identifiable information from the clinical setting. Once identifying information is traced back to a student or individuals who do not have a "need to know," the agency responsible for the client information may face punishment for any harm caused by the sharing of the client information.

The student nurse is held to the same standard as an RN and has the legal/ethical duty to protect the confidentiality rights of patients during care. How might protected client information be inappropriately shared? A student might innocently misplace or abandon patient assignment sheets, nursing care plans, medication information, and charting references containing the client's name and identifying information. The sharing of client-related information on a social network has become a significant problem as more nurses and students use electronic tools and social media (National Council of State Boards of Nursing, 2018b; Tan et al., 2024). You will want to share any questions or concerns you may have about client privacy issues with your course professors, as they are invaluable resources when it comes to maintaining client confidentiality.

DEFAMATION OF CHARACTER

Defamation of character is closely linked to the principle of confidentiality. Defamation involves the dissemination of false statements that cause harm to an individual's reputation (Potter et al., 2023). Nurses can potentially be held legally responsible for defamation, whether through written (**libel**) or spoken (**slander**) words. Defamation may occur inadvertently. For instance, consider the following example.

EXAMPLE 16.1 The owner of a beauty salon is admitted with a medical diagnosis of pneumonia, but the electronic record discloses that the client actually has multidrug-resistant tuberculosis. If the nurse caring for the client shares with others that the client has active tuberculosis, this unintentional breach of confidentiality can lead to potential legal consequences and a financial impact if the client claims economic losses due to the nursing staff's disclosure about tuberculosis and subsequently files a lawsuit for slander.

As an RN, you must recognize potentially harmful defamation in which other staff are engaged. It is important for the RN to act professionally and responsibly when addressing defamation concerns. Reporting incidents helps maintain a culture of integrity and respect in the workplace while protecting the rights and reputations of individuals involved. Addressing defamation promotes a safe and supportive environment for both staff and patients.

PROFESSIONAL BOUNDARIES

Respecting patient autonomy, promoting open communication, and avoiding any form of exploitation are fundamental principles in maintaining professional boundaries. **Professional boundaries** in nursing refer to the limits and expectations that define the appropriate relationship between healthcare professionals, including nurses, and their patients or clients. These boundaries are essential to maintain the therapeutic nurse–patient relationship and to uphold ethical standards in healthcare practice. Violating professional boundaries can lead to ethical dilemmas, compromised patient care, and potential legal consequences (National Council of State Boards of Nursing, 2018a).

A breach of professional boundaries may occur when a nurse utilizes their position of authority or power to fulfill their own or someone else's needs. Given the intimate nature of nursing, which involves close physical and psychological interaction with potentially vulnerable patients, there is a potential power imbalance. Nurses are responsible for maintaining what is commonly referred to as the "zone of helpfulness." Nurses must find a balance in which the nurse neither becomes too detached nor overly involved with the client, thereby respecting ethical norms and ensuring that the patient's well-being remains the primary focus.

Although some breaches in professional boundaries are intentional and egregious, such as rape or extortion of money, students mostly violate professional boundaries due to their inexperience with nurse–patient relationships (Thomson et al., 2022)—for example, devoting exorbitant time to one client over another or dating a client. Regular self-reflection and adherence to ethical principles are essential for nurses to maintain healthy and professional boundaries in their interactions with patients. When evaluating professional boundaries, the nurse should ask a series of reflective questions (Box 16.10) to ensure ethical and appropriate conduct in the nurse–patient relationship (National Council of State Boards of Nursing, 2018a).

THINKING CRITICALLY

Look up the website for your state, province, or territory's board of nursing. What does the website say about professional boundaries? Does it address defamation or the confidentiality of the nurse–patient relationship? Prepare to use the information you find as a springboard for class discussions.

BOX 16.10

Reflective Questions to Assess Professional Boundaries

1. Am I following the constituents of the nurse practice act?
2. Is my behavior within the ANA *Code of Ethics*?
3. Are my actions in the best interest of this client/family?
4. Would another nurse find my actions acceptable?
5. Am I maintaining patient confidentiality?
6. Is there a balanced level of involvement in the nurse–patient relationship?
7. Do I recognize and manage power differentials appropriately?
8. Am I maintaining professional objectivity?
9. Are there any conflicts of interest or dual relationships?
10. Am I providing unbiased and culturally sensitive care?
11. Is my communication professional and therapeutic?
12. Have I set appropriate professional limits?
13. Do I recognize and address transference and countertransference?
14. Have I sought supervision or consultation when faced with challenging situations?

Source: National Council of State Boards of Nursing. (2018a). *A nurse's guide to professional boundaries* [Brochure]. https://www.ncsbn.org/public-files/ProfessionalBoundaries_Complete.pdf

CONCLUSION

Legal responsibilities apply to everything a nurse performs. Therefore, nurses need to be familiar with relevant legal concepts such as licensure requirements, negligence, malpractice, and other liability issues. Legal accountability is ensured through methods such as document correctness or procedural performance, as well as by professional accountability and responsibility.

When making the transition from LPN/LVN to RN, you will recognize that there are additional legal consequences for the work RNs perform. If a nurse does not practice as defined by legal standards and the client is harmed, the nurse is liable. The most important concern for nurses is the rights of clients, followed by the rights and responsibilities of the nurses' colleagues.

STUDENT *Exercises*

Exercise 16.1

As an RN, you have been hired to be the evening supervisor in a 50-bed, long-term care facility. After an orientation to the role and responsibilities, you are officially the evening charge nurse. There are two units in this agency, one of which is designated for clients with Alzheimer disease. Each unit has one LPN/LVN who acts as the charge person, one certified nursing assistant (CNA) with advanced training to administer oral medications, and three CNAs to provide basic care to the clients.

1. As the RN supervisor, what do you need to know from a legal perspective to do your job? Think in terms of delegating, competencies of other personnel, and your responsibility for the care that clients receive.
2. From a legal perspective, what is your responsibility if an employee practices unsafely?

REFERENCES

American Nurses Association. (2021). *Nursing: Scope and standards of practice* (4th ed.).
Catalano, J. T. (2024). *Nursing now! Today's issues, tomorrow's trends* (9th ed.). F.A. Davis.
DeBrew, J. (2022). "Looks can be deceiving": An innovative way to teach nursing students about substance use disorder. *Creative Nursing, 29*(1), 1–6. doi: 10.1177/107845352202900102
Evans, C., Jabla, J., Gardner, G. A., Rathore, T., & Scruth, E. A. (2022). Speaking up for patient safety: Will nurses report errors now a nurse has been convicted of a criminal act? *Clinical Nurse Specialist: The Journal for Advanced Nursing Practice, 36*(5), 230–232. doi: 10.1097/NUR.0000000000000688
Finkelman, A. (2021). *Professional nursing concepts: Competencies for quality leadership* (5th ed.). Jones & Bartlett Learning.
Graber, C. (2013). *The good nurse: A true story of medicine, madness and murder*. Hachette Book Group.
Guido, G. (2020). *Legal and ethical issues in nursing* (7th ed.). Pearson.
Harrington, L. (2023). The RaDonda Vaught case: A critical conversation on nursing practice and technology. *AACN Advanced Critical Care, 34*(1), 11–15. doi: 10.4037/aacnacc2023873
Huston, C. J. (2023). *Leadership roles and management functions in nursing: Theory and application* (11th ed.). Wolters Kluwer.
Johnson, S. (2022). Legal and ethical issues. In D. L. Huber & M. L. Joseph (Eds.). *Leadership and nursing care management* (7th ed., pp. 112–130). Elsevier.

Maher, V., & Cwiek, M. (2022). Criminal liability for nursing and medical harm. *Hospital topics*, 1–8. Advance online publication. doi: 10.1080/00185868.2022.2101571

Mahlmeister, L. R. (2023). Legal issues in nursing and health care. In B. Cherry & S. R. Jacob (Eds.). *Contemporary nursing: Issues, trends, & management* (9th ed., pp. 124–165). Elsevier.

National Council of State Boards of Nursing. (2018a). *A nurse's guide to professional boundaries [Brochure]*. https://www.ncsbn.org/public-files/ProfessionalBoundaries_Complete.pdf.

National Council of State Boards of Nursing. (2018b). *A nurse's guide to the use of social media*. https://www.ncsbn.org/public-files/NCSBN_SocialMedia.pdf

Potter, P., Perry, A., Stockert, P., & Hall, A. (2023). *Fundamentals of nursing* (11th ed.). Elsevier.

Shearer, E., & Bundorf, M. K. (2023). Changes in emergency department use associated with Medicaid expansion under the Affordable Care Act: A comparison of waiver and traditional expansion states. *Journal of the American College of Emergency Physicians Open*, 4(6). doi: 10.1002/emp2.13060

Tan, M. Y. N., Ni, Z., Liu, A. S. H., & Shorey, S. (2024). The influence of social media on student nurses: A systematic mixed-studies review. *Nurse Education Today*, 132, 106000. doi: 10.1016/j.nedt.2023.106000

Taylor, C., Lynn, P., & Bartlett, J. L. (2023). *Fundamentals of nursing: The art and science of nursing care* (10th ed.). Wolters Kluwer.

The case of nurse RaDonda Vaught - How administering the wrong medication resulted in a criminal conviction. (2022). *Colorado Nurse*, 122(4), 18–20.

The Joint Commission. (2024). *National Patient Safety Goals® Effective January 2024 for the hospital program*. https://www.jointcommission.org/-/media/tjc/documents/standards/national-patient-safety-goals/2024/npsg_chapter_hap_jan2024.pdf

The Joint Commission. (n.d.). *Sentinel event policy and procedures*. https://www.jointcommission.org/resources/sentinel-event/sentinel-event-policy-and-procedures/#:~:text=The%20Sentinel%20Event%20Policy&text=A%20sentinel%20event%20is%20a,intervention%20required%20to%20sustain%20life

Thomson, A. E., Smith, N., & Karpa, J. (2022). Strategies used to teach professional boundaries psychiatric nursing education. *Issues in Mental Health Nursing*, 43(10), 895–902. doi: 10.1080/01612840.2022.2083737

Westrick, S. (2024). *Essentials of nursing law and ethics* (3rd ed.). Jones & Bartlett Learning.

Wilson, R. C. (2023). Workforce engagement through collective action and governance. In P. S. Yoder-Wise & S. Sportsman (Eds.). *Leading and managing in nursing* (8th ed., pp. 268–289). Elsevier.

SUGGESTED READING

Foli, K. J., Zhang, L., & Reddick, B. (2021). Predictors of substance use in registered nurses: The role of psychological trauma. *Western Journal of Nursing Research*, 43(11), 1023–1033. doi: 10.1177/0193945920987123

Gabele, D., Keels, K. M., & Blake, N. (2023). Out of the shadows and into the light: Destigmatization of substance use disorder in nursing. *Nurse Leader*, 21(4), e97–e101. doi: 10.1016/j.mnl.2023.04.003

Lancaster, R. J., Vizgirda, V., Quinlan, S., & Kingston, M. B. (2022). To err is human, just culture, practice, and liability in the face of nursing error. *Nurse Leader*, 20(5), 517–521. doi: 10.1016/j.mnl.2022.06.010

On The WEB

American Association of Legal Nurse Consultants: http://www.aalnc.org

Compassion and Choices: https://www.compassionandchoices.org/

The Joint Commission, Hospital: 2024 National Patient Safety Goals: https://www.jointcommission.org/standards/national-patient-safety-goals/hospital-national-patient-safety-goals/

NCSBN, substance use disorders: https://www.ncsbn.org/sud

NCSBN, professional boundaries: https://www.ncsbn.org/nursing-regulation/practice/professional-boundaries.page

Partners in Care: https://www.picf.org/

Study.com, Ethics & Legal Issues in Nursing | Overview & Examples: https://study.com/academy/lesson/legal-issues-in-nursing-concepts-and-terms.html

Ethical Issues

CHAPTER 17

LEARNING OUTCOMES

By the end of this chapter, the student will be able to:
1. Differentiate ethics, law, and religion.
2. Compare and contrast ethics, bioethics, and nursing ethics.
3. Identify common nursing ethical dilemmas.
4. Distinguish ethical dilemmas from moral distress.
5. Describe three ethical theories.
6. Summarize factors that influence ethical decision-making.
7. Apply the nursing process in analyzing ethical dilemmas.
8. Differentiate between the RN and LPN/LVN roles in decision-making.

KEY TERMS

autonomy	ethics	nursing ethics
beneficence	feminist ethics	paternalism
bioethics	feminist theory	teleology
code of ethics	fidelity	utilitarianism
deontology	justice	values
ethical dilemma	moral distress	veracity
ethical theory	nonmaleficence	

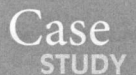**Case STUDY**

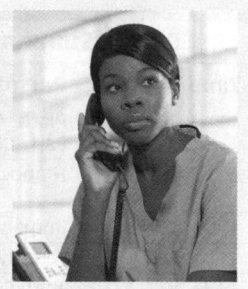

You are the acting charge RN of a busy long-term care facility. Janet Bieber, LPN, calls to notify you that Dr. Brown has made rounds and has ordered a placebo for Mr. Peters. This client was admitted to your unit several weeks ago after an open reduction and internal fixation of the left hip. Janet says she cannot give the placebo because it is against her beliefs and values. You know that Mr. Peters is an older adult who is frail; he has many physiologic reasons for his pain. You also know that various pharmacologic methods have been tried and that nothing so far has been able to stop Mr. Peters' pain.

401

What ethical dilemma is presented in the case study? What principles of nursing ethics are involved? Would moral courage be needed to advocate for Mr. Peters? What arguments could be presented to Dr. Brown against administering the placebo in favor of a different plan for pain management? What kind of plan could the nurse develop to solve this ethical dilemma?

ETHICS AND HISTORY

Ethics are the principles and values that guide individual and group behavior (Guido, 2020). Ethics provide a framework for distinguishing between right and wrong or what is considered acceptable and nonacceptable behavior. Ethical principles, which are based on knowledge rather than emotion or opinion, guide decision-making, especially in situations in which there may be conflicting interests. At times, ethical principles are used to determine the lesser of two evils (Ellis, 2024).

Although ethical principles are often the foundation for legal frameworks, ethical decisions and legal requirements are not mutually exclusive. Laws, which are standards or rules of behavior to protect society, vary from country to country and from society to society (Taylor et al., 2023). Laws refer to general situations and set minimum standards for behavior. Ethical decisions, on the other hand, are flexible and adaptable to specific circumstances. Depending on the situation, individuals may strive for a higher moral standard and act beyond legal requirements. Ethics originated from various sources dating back hundreds of years and have evolved into present-day theories that guide nurses in making ethical decisions.

Ethics developed from philosophy (Table 17.1). Grecian thinkers such as Socrates and Plato took a logical approach to defining what was good or right in human conduct. The Greek physician Hippocrates wrote the Hippocratic Oath, the first written code of ethics for physicians (National Library of Medicine, n.d.). Physicians and philosophers still debate the tenets of the Hippocratic Oath. Theory development continued with the utilitarian work of English philosophers Jeremy Bentham and John Stuart Mill and the deontological work of Immanuel Kant (for more information on these types of philosophies, see the "Teleology" and "Deontology" sections later in this chapter). In addition, Florence Nightingale advocated for core nursing principles such as clean air, decent hygiene, increased nutrition, and hospital cleanliness—ideas not typically recognized at the time by the medical community (Rich, 2023b).

TABLE 17.1 Summary of Nursing Ethics History

Time	Person	Achievement
400–300 BC	Plato, Aristotle, Early Christians	Virtue Ethics
400–300 BC	Hippocrates	Hippocratic Oath, Father of Modern Medicine
1724–1804	Immanuel Kant	Theory of Deontology
1738–1782	Jeremy Bentham	Principle of Utilitarianism
1806–1873	John Stuart Mill	Refined Utilitarianism
1800–1900	Florence Nightingale	Florence Nightingale Pledge
1960s	Feminists	Emotional, intuitive, and relationship aspects of caring

Source: Rich, K. (2023b). Introduction to ethics. In J. B. Butts & K. L. Rich (Eds.), *Nursing ethics: Across the curriculum and into practice* (6th ed., pp. 3–26). Jones & Bartlett Learning.

Originating in the 1960s, the **feminist theory** of ethics critiqued conventional ethical ideas and practices that have historically excluded, disregarded, or oppressed women and other underrepresented groups, and it emphasized the importance of an emotional aspect in decision-making (Taylor et al., 2023). Emotional support, a concept for which Florence Nightingale advocated, is often the tie that binds many nurses to those in their care. (For more information on this topic, see the "Feminist Theory of Ethics" section later in this chapter.)

A **code of ethics** is a document that practitioners in a profession develop and use to guide decision-making. The document is the profession's moral code that serves as a public declaration about the profession's duties. Like laws, ethical codes evolve to keep pace with changes in professions. Nursing's first code of ethics was born from the Florence Nightingale Pledge (Maxwell & Pope, 1910). In contrast to the original pledge, which in one of its principles devalued the status of the nurse to that of the loyal "handmaiden" of the physician, the ethical code has evolved with the nursing profession such that it now includes having the authority to challenge a physician's orders, encouraging collegiality and collaboration in physician–nurse relationships, and supporting patient autonomy (Rich, 2023b).

ETHICAL DILEMMAS AND MORAL DISTRESS

An **ethical dilemma** is a situation in which an individual faces conflicting moral principles, values, or obligations that make it difficult to decide on the most acceptable course of action. Ethical dilemmas often involve weighing the consequences of situations in which a decision could be both positive and negative. An ethical dilemma in nursing can occur when a nurse's personal/professional values and morals conflict with those of a patient, patient's family, provider, another healthcare worker, or the institution where the nurse works, or conflict with a law (Rich, 2023b).

In the case study, acting as a patient advocate, Janet is committed to meeting Mr. Peters' pain control needs and does not believe that Mr. Peters' pain will be controlled with the placebo ordered by Dr. Brown. This presents Janet with an ethical dilemma. There may be other variables that could add to Janet's dilemma. Perhaps other healthcare staff have pressured Dr. Brown into ordering the placebo. Perhaps the family thinks more needs to be done to manage Mr. Peters' pain and is pushing for a solution beyond medication.

Box 17.1 lists common nursing ethical dilemmas.

BOX 17.1

Common Nursing Ethical Dilemmas

How to respond to client's refusal of treatment/medications
Whether to tell the truth
Whether to perform futile care
Participating in research protocols with which the nurse disagrees
Whether to breach confidentiality for what the nurse considers a good reason
Whether to report incompetent or unethical practices by colleagues
Whether to put patients in danger by working overtime when fatigued

Source: Rich, K. (2023a). Ethics in professional nursing practice. In J. B. Butts & K. L. Rich (Eds.), *Nursing ethics: Across the curriculum and into practice* (6th ed., pp. 67–104). Jones & Bartlett Learning.

Moral distress is characterized by recognizing a morally right course of action but feeling constrained or unable to pursue that action due to external or institutional constraints; an individual perceives a conflict between their ethical values and the actions required by their role or organizational policies (Rich, 2023a). An example of moral distress would be if a nurse believes that a particular treatment plan is not in the best interest of the patient, yet they feel compelled to follow established protocols or provider orders. Because nurses have close relationships with their patients, they can experience a range of emotions when making ethical decisions, including generalized anxiety, uncertainty, and outright moral suffering. Moral distress can impact well-being, job satisfaction, and the overall quality of care provided (Guido, 2020).

> ## THINKING CRITICALLY
> Although a code of ethics will never fully answer the multiple dimensions of ethical dilemmas a nurse may encounter, it is important for nurses to examine the ethical codes that are relevant to their practice. Review the classical version of the Hippocratic Oath at https://www.nlm.nih.gov/hmd/topics/greek-medicine/index.html#case1. Write down the ideas you find within the Oath. Compare the Oath to the American Nurses Association (ANA) Code of Ethics for Nurses at https://www.nursingworld.org/practice-policy/nursing-excellence/ethics/code-of-ethics-for-nurses/coe-view-only/ and the International Council of Nurses (ICN) Code of Ethics at https://www.icn.ch/resources/publications-and-reports/icn-code-ethics-nurses. What are the similarities? What are the differences?

ETHICS AND THE LAW

Ethical principles reflect the collective values of a society and are often the foundation of laws. Laws and their relationship to nursing were explored in Chapter 16; examining the connection between laws and ethics is important to understand these two unique concepts. *Laws* are formalized rules that set minimum standards for acceptable conduct (Taylor et al., 2023). As a framework for acceptable behavior, laws may be subject to ethical critique if they are thought to be unfair or fail to address changing moral concerns. In essence, to establish a just and equitable social order, ethics and laws have a symbiotic relationship wherein each influences and is influenced by the other (Rich, 2023b). Ethics may provide a foundation for the creation of laws, and laws can influence ethical considerations. Table 17.2 summarizes the differences between law and ethics.

ETHICS AND RELIGION

Religion is often the starting point for the development of moral thinking and virtues. As with laws, not every religious value or belief provides clear guidelines for ethical decision-making. Throughout history, religious beliefs have been a significant factor in many conflicts and wars. Although strong convictions about religious beliefs can contribute to tensions and lead to violent conflicts, others promote peace, understanding, and coexistence. Nurses must recognize the connection between ethics and religion and how that connection can significantly influence healthcare practices and interactions

TABLE 17.2 Differences Between Laws and Ethics

Laws	Ethics
Clear rules of conduct	Unclear, ambiguity exists
Impartial	Individual
Black and white	Gray areas
Courts decide	Individuals decide
Do not keep pace with society	Change with societal attitude changes
Doing things right	The right things to do
Legal counsel provides legal advice and representation to individuals, organizations, or entities and ensures compliance with applicable laws and regulations	Ethics committees review research and clinical practices to ensure adherence to ethical principles and guidelines
Regulated by authorized organizations	Ethical guidelines do not have a formal enforcement and law officers system

Source: Rich, K. (2023b). Introduction to ethics. In J. B. Butts & K. L. Rich (Eds.), *Nursing ethics: Across the curriculum and into practice* (6th ed., pp. 3–26). Jones & Bartlett Learning.

with patients. Many ethical principles in healthcare—such as autonomy, beneficence, and nonmaleficence (discussed later in this chapter)—often align with religious teachings (Marek & Walulik, 2021).

NURSING ETHICS

Nursing ethics is a set of rules that govern the behavior of nurses in their interactions with patients, their families, other healthcare professionals, policymakers, and society as a whole (Cherry & Jacob, 2023). It is important for nurses to reflect on how their personal values and beliefs relate to the ethical standards of nursing. A nurse's personal philosophy about healthcare forms the foundation for their ethical decision-making and professional conduct. A nurse's behaviors are guided by two sets of ethics: personal and professional. Personal ethics, developed from **values** and behaviors learned at an early age, provide the foundation from which professional ethics are built. Just like ethical codes, personal codes can change and become more defined as an individual grows and is exposed to various circumstances throughout their life (Potter et al., 2023b).

Professional ethics are developed and refined in nursing school, implemented in the clinical environment, and operationalized upon graduation and employment as an LPN/LVN. Nurses are expected to uphold high ethical standards, maintain trustworthiness, and sustain transparency in their professional interactions. Like Janet in the case study, as an LPN or LVN, you already have experience with professional ethics and may have strong beliefs about the use of placebos. Ethical principles help guide decisions regarding the administration of placebos and medications in both research and clinical settings, ensuring that the well-being and rights of participants or patients are prioritized.

Nursing ethics falls within the larger umbrella of **bioethics** (Fig. 17.1). A nurse's ethical decisions are not black and white; each client is unique and no two client care circumstances are the same. Although the *Code of Ethics for Nurses* (ANA, 2015) provides guidelines for behaviors and interventions, nursing ethical challenges are so varied that there is no one solution that works for all situations. To assist in making sound ethical decisions, nurses should apply the *ANA Scope and Standards of Practice* (ANA, 2021a, 2021b) in addition to the *Code of Ethics for Nurses* (ANA, 2015). Although a nurse acquires the

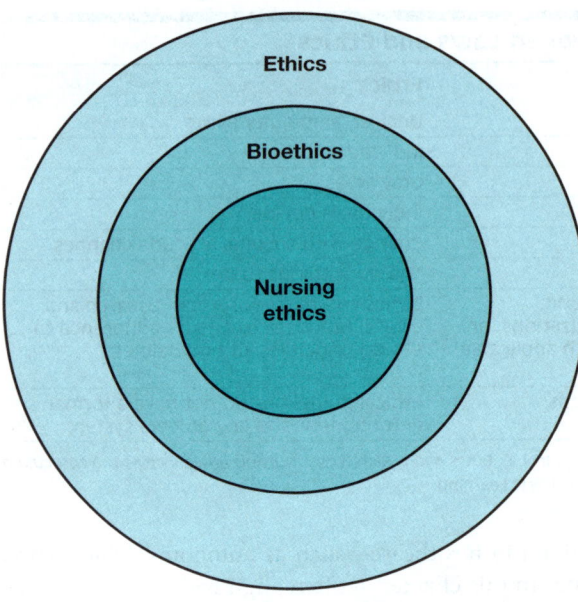

FIGURE 17.1. Model of ethics.

technical abilities necessary to performs skills competently during their education, complete mastery requires integration of science and nursing ethics (Cherry & Jacob, 2023).

Box 17.2 outlines definitions relevant to nursing ethics.

>
> # THINKING CRITICALLY
> The nurse's ethical behaviors and decisions are shaped by their personal history and are often influenced by significant individuals during their early childhood. Reflect on your philosophy about life and health. Who or what was the most influential in your formation of this philosophy? Was religion a factor? How has your philosophy about life and death influenced your professional perspectives?

BOX 17.2

Definitions Related to Ethics

Code of ethics: Standards of conduct and values as defined by a profession; forms the basis for ethical decision-making by a profession

Values: The ideals and beliefs held by an individual or group that are usually influenced by family, society, and religion; have a great impact on behavior

Morals: An individual's standards of right and wrong that are formed in childhood (see Chapter 2); also influenced by family, society, and religion

Bioethics: Ethical questions surrounding life and death; questions and concerns regarding the quality of life as it relates to advanced technology

Ethical dilemma: A situation in which an individual must choose between two alternatives that are not desirable; often involves examining rights and obligations of particular individuals; no clear choice or correct course of action

Source: Guido, G. (2020). *Legal and ethical issues in nursing* (7th ed.). Pearson.

ETHICAL THEORIES IN NURSING
Ethical theories can be a complex philosophical endeavor. This section provides a basic overview of the ethical theories nurses use when making decisions. In general, **ethical theories** are a tool to determine if an action is right or wrong. Because each patient's situation can be complex, it may be necessary to apply more than one ethical theory when making decisions and planning care. In nursing, the most common theories are teleology, deontology, and feminist ethics.

Teleology
Teleology (also called **utilitarianism**, which refers to an end or an outcome) has two principles (Guido, 2020):

- The greatest good for the greatest number
- The end justifies the means

Teleology, which evolved from a humanistic and outcome-oriented approach to a decision-making approach implies that the consequences of actions must be considered—that is, the benefits to many will outweigh the harm to a few. For instance, the allocation of funds might be determined by the number of individuals who benefit from a particular service. Over the years, the United States has experienced several shortages of flu vaccines. The government rationed the vaccine to the young, physically debilitated, and healthcare workers because it determined that vaccinating these individuals would benefit the majority of society.

The advantage of using teleology is that the needs of the majority are prioritized. For instance, in medical research, teleology promotes studies that investigate the causes of widespread diseases or the development of treatments that have a substantial positive impact on a large population. However, teleology also has drawbacks. One concern is the potential to overlook individual rights and liberties in the pursuit of overall goals. The emphasis on achieving positive outcomes might diminish the rights of certain individuals or underrepresented groups for the perceived greater good. The risk of sacrificing individual autonomy in the name of collective benefit raises ethical questions about fairness, justice, and the potential for unintended consequences (Tseng & Wang, 2021).

Deontology
The second most applied theory when making ethical decisions, **deontology** is based on a clear and consistent moral framework, with guidelines of what is inherently right or wrong regardless of the consequences. A central theme in deontological ethics is that individuals should act according to principles. Influenced by the writings of Immanuel Kant, deontological ethics promote a sense of duty and personal responsibility that encourage individuals to act in ways that align with universally applicable moral rules. The rules contribute to a stable moral foundation and foster a society in which individuals prioritize ethical principles, even when faced with challenging situations. Nurses may apply the principles of deontology when prioritizing respect for the individual as their primary consideration (Barrow & Khandhar, 2023).

An advantage of applying a deontological approach is that obligation to duty and moral thinking are foremost, so the decisions made in similar situations will be the same. However, deontology also has drawbacks, such as its potential rigidity in certain situations. Strict adherence to moral rules and duties may lead to moral dilemmas in which following a rule may result in unfavorable consequences, or ignoring a duty may lead to a morally better outcome. It may be difficult to apply the deontological method when the consequence of the decision can be harmful to an individual. For example, the decision to maintain life for any patient regardless of the outcome (futile care) may be difficult when the patient is in constant pain, requiring many invasive and expensive procedures to survive in a vegetative state (Gibson, 2023).

One of the most pressing ethical concerns today is ensuring universal access to healthcare through health insurance. The deontological dilemma regarding access to healthcare for all people who live in the United States revolves around the ethical principle that all individuals have a right to healthcare by virtue of their humanity. Advocates argue that all individuals deserve access to healthcare because it is a fundamental human right and a basic necessity, regardless of socioeconomic status, including employment status or ability to pay. The dilemma arises when considering the practical implications of ensuring universal access to healthcare and balancing individual rights with societal responsibilities. It is possible that providing universal healthcare coverage may impose undue burdens on taxpayers or lead to inefficiencies in the healthcare system (Wester, 2023).

Feminist Theory of Ethics

The feminist theory of ethics offers a perspective on understanding and addressing issues of morality, justice, and power by recognizing the interconnectedness of gender with other social identities such as ethnicity, class, sexuality, and ability. **Feminist ethics** is a framework for moral reasoning and action that emerged from feminist perspectives on ethics and justice. The feminist ethical approach examines how power operates in a society, and it analyzes and critiques conventional ethical ideas and practices that have historically excluded, disregarded, or oppressed women and other underrepresented groups.

One of the core principles of feminist ethics is that patriarchal systems and structures foster gender inequity and oppression and need to be dismantled to promote gender equity by examining how power operates in society. This ethical framework emphasizes the importance of recognizing and valuing diverse perspectives and experiences, particularly those of individuals who have been historically underrepresented or silenced (Gilligan, 1982).

Another key principle of feminist ethics is the ethics of care, which prioritizes relationships, empathy, and interconnectedness in moral decision-making. Feminists believe that virtues such as emotions, compassion, comfort, nurturing, intuition, and empathetic caring have value when making ethical decisions. This approach highlights the importance of fostering caring relationships and attending to the well-being of others, challenging the notion that moral reasoning should be detached or impartial (Morberg Jämterud, 2022).

> **THINKING CRITICALLY**
>
> Review the case study at the beginning of the chapter. Using teleology, deontology, or feminist theory, list the advantages and disadvantages of applying the principles of the chosen ethical theory to the scenario when making a decision. Be specific regarding the impact on the client and the nurse.

FACTORS THAT INFLUENCE DECISION-MAKING IN NURSING

Although selecting an ethical system should simplify the process of decision-making, in practice, a single ethical theory may not be appropriate to a given situation, and there are multiple factors and frameworks that influence decision-making. Circumstances that influence decisions are dynamic and may frequently overlap or be independent of one another.

Legislative and Societal Influences

The development of morals and values is influenced by the expectations of society. Changes in societal thinking affect a person's view of what is right and wrong. Societal thinking and the resulting legislative and judicial decisions have an impact on the ethical decision-making process, as the following examples demonstrate.

EXAMPLE 17.1 The Definition of Death

The issue of declaring death may present a dilemma (Potter et al., 2023a). In 1940, death was defined as the loss of circulation and respiratory function. However, over time as the ability to maintain cardiac and respiratory function increased, medicine and society were compelled to redefine death. In 1968, Harvard University published a report titled "A Definition of Irreversible Coma," in which death was defined as the absence of neurologic function or brain death. By the late 1970s, several states had differing definitions of death. A patient could be declared legally dead in one state while still being considered alive in another. In 1981, the Uniform Determination of Death Act (UDDA), drafted by the Uniform Law Commission (a volunteer organization that provides clarity and consistency in crucial aspects of state statutory law) provided a legal definition of death and the concept of brain death, which includes unresponsiveness and a lack of receptivity, absence of movements or breathing, no reflexes, and a flat electroencephalogram reading (Biel & Durrant, 2020; Omelianchuk et al., 2022). Since the UDDA was introduced, all 50 states have adopted the UDDA; however, specific language may vary from state to state.

Associated ethical issues for nurses may relate to their own beliefs about the dignity of life, the prolonging of a persistent vegetative state, the harvesting of donor organs from an individual who is brain dead, and supporting the family who may be asked to make decisions (Biel & Durrant, 2020). The legality of brain death within each state and the forms donors sign before death have removed some of the uncertainties for nurses regarding ethical considerations.

EXAMPLE 17.2 The Rights of the Individual

The passage of the Equal Rights Amendment in 1972, which guaranteed protection against sexual discrimination for women, and the continuing equal rights movement have increasingly called for an end to bullying and sexual harassment and have had an impact on behavior and societal views of what is acceptable. The importance of the rights of individuals has increased, and the demand to have input in one's healthcare is now seen as a right (Potter et al., 2023a; see also information about the Patient's Bill of Rights in the next section).

EXAMPLE 17.3 Reproductive Rights and the Provider–Client Relationship

With the Supreme Court's June 2022 decision in Dobbs v. Jackson Women's Health Organization, eliminating the federal right to abortion, healthcare providers who believe in a patient's right to choose abortion as part of their reproductive healthcare may face a difficult decision about whether to comply with what they consider to be restrictive laws or to continue to provide what they believe are essential medical services to their clients (Reingold et al., 2022).

Scientific and Technological Advances

Developments in science and technology have also created ethical issues that did not previously exist (Cherry & Jacob, 2023). The dilemmas created by science and technology contribute to the complexity of decision-making in which nurses are involved. The duty to the client is often obscured by the need to promote science and progress.

EXAMPLE 17.4 In Vitro Fertilization

In vitro fertilization (IVF) raises several ethical dilemmas that revolve around various aspects of reproduction, healthcare, and the beginning of human life. IVF often results in the creation of multiple embryos, not all of which are used for implantation, raising questions about the status and rights of these unused embryos. Decisions regarding whether to freeze, donate, discard, or use these embryos for research can be emotionally challenging and ethically complex. In addition, IVF can be expensive, making it inaccessible to many individuals and couples due to financial constraints raising concerns about equity in access to reproductive technologies and whether healthcare resources should be allocated to assist with fertility treatments when other medical needs may be more urgent (Siermann et al., 2022).

EXAMPLE 17.5 Genetic Engineering

Genetic engineering involves altering the genetic makeup of organisms, which can include humans. Genetic engineering offers the potential to enhance human capabilities and traits, such as intelligence, strength, or appearance. However, the pursuit of human enhancement raises concerns about equity, access, and the creation of genetic "haves" and "have-nots." It also raises questions about what traits are desirable to enhance and who gets to make those decisions. Fears related to genetic engineering may influence research and testing, leading to unreliable results (Lorenzo et al., 2022).

Healthcare Reform

Cost control, managed care, shorter hospital stays, and exploration of alternative healthcare provisions have an impact on ethical decision-making. The Affordable Care Act (ACA) of 2010 represented a significant step toward fostering ethical healthcare practices and enhancing access to affordable and comprehensive healthcare services for all individuals in the United States. The ACA led to a Patient's Bill of Rights, which prohibited patients from being denied healthcare coverage and has created access to healthcare for many individuals who did not have access previously (Potter et al., 2023a). The ACA's emphasis on preventive care and wellness programs is a proactive approach to healthcare that aligns with ethical principles that prioritize the promotion of well-being and the prevention of harm. The ACA's provisions not only address systemic inequities within the healthcare system but also uphold ethical principles of justice, beneficence, and autonomy by striving to provide equitable access to quality care for all individuals.

Since its development, the ACA has faced opposition and several calls to alter or eliminate it. One notable criticism of the ACA is its complex regulatory framework, which may lead to administrative burdens and increased bureaucratic inefficiencies within the healthcare system. Critics contend that the ACA's extensive regulations and compliance requirements have imposed significant administrative costs on healthcare providers and insurers, potentially diverting resources from direct patient care and contributing to rising healthcare expenditures (Kishore et al., 2023). Issues related to the ACA's allocation of healthcare funds to those who need them most or to those who have the greatest potential to have a positive outcome are also ethically challenging. The implementation of the ACA underscores ongoing debates regarding the balance between regulatory oversight and healthcare accessibility and affordability.

Professional Values and Client Values

Professional values are beliefs concerning the work that a person does. Some of those values do not differ from personal values, and some may derive from a person's education in a particular profession. Several values guide the decisions that nurses make. These values, which are also called principles of nursing ethics, are beneficence, nonmaleficence, autonomy, justice, fidelity, and veracity (see Box 17.3).

Beneficence

Beneficence is the duty to do good (Rich, 2023b). Beneficence in client care entails both technical proficiency and a humanistic and comprehensive approach. Within healthcare, beneficence guides practitioners to act in the best interests of their clients, striving to maximize positive outcomes and to alleviate suffering. For healthcare professionals, beneficence extends beyond merely avoiding harm and includes actively pursuing opportunities to improve the health and quality of life of those under their care. Beneficence can be demonstrated through handwashing, teaching, and maintaining isolation methods.

There may be a disagreement between the nurse and the client about what is "good." **Paternalism** occurs when a nurse or other member of the healthcare team overrides the client's wishes.

Nonmaleficence

Nonmaleficence is the ethical principle that emphasizes the obligation to avoid causing harm to others (Cherry & Jacob, 2023). Nonmaleficence guides healthcare practitioners in their decision-making processes, encouraging them to assess potential risks and benefits of interventions, to prioritize client safety, and to minimize harm to the greatest

---

BOX 17.3 Principles of Nursing Ethics

Beneficence: Actively do good
Nonmaleficence: Do no harm
Autonomy: The right to make decisions
Justice: Fairness to all people
Fidelity: Faithful to commitments
Veracity: Truth-telling

Source: Boggs, K. U. (2023). *Interpersonal relationships: Professional communication skills for nurses* (9th ed.). Elsevier.

extent possible. It is difficult to discuss nonmaleficence without including beneficence because the choice of treatment for a client may initially cause harm, although the outcome is potentially good. For example, a client with colon cancer undergoes a colostomy, enduring the pain of surgery and the reality of a change in body image; in addition, chemotherapy and radiation therapy are suggested. Although the patient is harmed by these treatments, they serve the ultimate goal, which is for the patient to be cancer free. However, such treatment choices are difficult to make, especially if the treatment is likely to be futile (Gibson, 2023).

Autonomy

Autonomy is a client's right to self-determination or the freedom to make choices and decisions (Guido, 2020). Based on the client's values, preferences, and understanding of relevant information provided by healthcare professionals, autonomy emphasizes a client's ability to make informed decisions about their medical treatment. Healthcare practitioners uphold autonomy by facilitating meaningful client–provider communication, offering comprehensive information about diagnosis and treatment options, and honoring clients' decisions, even if they may differ from the healthcare provider's recommendations.

One egregious violation of autonomy was the 1932 Tuskegee Study of syphilis in the Black male. Study participants were not informed of the advent of a treatment (penicillin) that would have prevented deformity and death (Reverby, 2009). The men's rights to autonomy were violated. Nurses must respect each client's right to informed consent, even if the client's decision is in direct conflict with the nurse's values.

Justice

Justice is the obligation to be fair, equal, and impartial in distributing resources, opportunities, and rights within society. The principle of justice emphasizes the equitable allocation of healthcare resources, ensuring that all individuals have access to necessary medical services regardless of socioeconomic status, ethnicity, gender, or geographic location (Rich, 2023b). Justice addresses systemic disparities and structural barriers that may prevent underrepresented groups from receiving adequate healthcare and strives to promote equal opportunities for health and well-being for all members of society. Justice in healthcare includes advocating for policies and practices that preserve human rights, remove prejudice, and promote social equity, which result in a more fair and equitable healthcare system for individuals and communities.

Fidelity

Fidelity is the principle of faithfulness, loyalty, and honoring commitments in professional relationships (Guido, 2020). In healthcare, fidelity is the obligation of healthcare practitioners to uphold the trust placed in them by clients, colleagues, and the community. This principle emphasizes the importance of maintaining confidentiality, respecting patient privacy, and safeguarding sensitive information shared during care. Health practitioners apply fidelity by fulfilling professional duties and responsibilities with integrity, transparency, and honesty, ensuring that patients receive accurate information and competent care. Expectations of fidelity include keeping the patient informed, teaching the client self-care skills, and maintaining confidentiality.

The NCLEX-RN *Might Ask* 17.1

The nurse is caring for a client with terminal cancer. The patient is seeking the truth about the prognosis of her disease, but her partner wants all healthcare workers involved to avoid talking about this illness. The nurse's duty to tell the truth in this situation is the principle of nursing ethics called:

a. nonmaleficence.
b. beneficence.
c. veracity.
d. justice.

• See Appendix A for correct answer and rationale.

Veracity

Veracity is the duty to be truthful, honest, and transparent in communication and decision-making (Boggs, 2023). Veracity requires that healthcare practitioners provide accurate and complete information to clients, enabling them to make informed decisions about their care. This principle emphasizes the importance of disclosing relevant medical information—including diagnoses, treatment options, risks, and benefits—in a clear and understandable manner.

THINKING CRITICALLY

Review the ANA's Code of Ethics for Nurses at https://www.nursingworld.org/practice-policy/nursing-excellence/ethics/code-of-ethics-for-nurses/. Determine the principle that is addressed by each statement. Examine the Core Values of the National League for Nursing (NLN) in Box 17.4. Compare the Code of Ethics to the NLN's Core Values. Are any values not addressed? Do you believe that any should be added? Discuss this with a group of your classmates and determine if these values and principles are the same or different for LPN/LVNs.

Awareness of the many factors involved in an ethical decision assists the student nurse in examining ethical issues more broadly and with less bias. Letting go of former ways of thinking, not personalizing issues, and working with emotional intelligence are particularly important in making ethical decisions. Transitioning from an LPN/LVN to an RN will add the responsibility and obligation to be a client advocate. The increased responsibility will require the demonstration of a greater understanding of ethical decision-making.

BOX 17.4 Core Values of the National League for Nursing

Caring
Integrity
Diversity and inclusion
Excellence

Source: National League for Nursing. (2024). *Core values.* https://www.nln.org/about/about/core-values

ETHICAL DECISION-MAKING IN NURSING

Applying ethical theories to practice requires critical thinking. To solve problems when providing care to clients, nurses follow the nursing process. The same problem-solving approach with the incorporation of ethical theories can be used to work through ethical dilemmas in the following steps:

1. **Assessment:** Identify the problem and describe it. Determine what values are involved, who are the stakeholders, and who will be affected by the decision. Are there legal ramifications? Obtain as much information as possible to understand the situation. Recognize personal biases that might affect assessments.
2. **Diagnosis:** A statement of the dilemma will assist in seeing the issue as concisely as possible.
3. **Planning:** List *all possible options* for solving the dilemma; do not get involved with determining the consequences at this point. This process is referred to as brainstorming. Identify any time constraints and the nurse's relationship to the situation. Examine all the advantages and disadvantages of each option. Consider the effects on individuals if the teleological, deontological, or feminist perspectives would be used. Consultation with a more experienced nurse, nurse manager, nurse practitioner, or ethics committee may take place at this point. Evaluate similar cases.
4. **Implementation:** Make the decision and follow through on it.
5. **Evaluation:** Evaluate the decision in terms of effects and results. Evaluate how comfortable all stakeholders are with the decision. Have the outcomes been met or not?

The NCLEX-RN *Might Ask* 17.2

An RN is reviewing the expected outcomes in a case involving care of a terminally ill child. The nurse is using which step of the ethical decision-making process?
a. Assessment
b. Diagnosis
c. Planning
d. Evaluation

• See Appendix A for correct answer and rationale.

Using a methodology for solving ethical dilemmas may be challenging at first. The following situation provides some practice for the application of the decision-making process.

EXAMPLE 17.6 Applying the Ethical Decision-Making Process

Early on a Saturday evening, Pat, a 25-year-old RN, was on their way to work a 12-hour shift at the local hospital. As they drove down a road about 2 miles from the hospital, a car came toward them rapidly, weaving from side to side. The road was narrow, and visibility was poor. Eventually, the other car crossed onto her side of the road, hitting

Pat's car on the driver's side and pushing the car into a telephone pole. Pat was killed as a result of the two impacts. Pat had tried to avoid the car, but the other driver was going too fast. The driver of the other vehicle (Chris) was not fatally injured but did sustain multiple orthopedic injuries and a closed head fracture. Chris was taken to the local hospital. Blood levels revealed that they were intoxicated at the time of the accident. Local police also stated that Chris was driving without a driver's license; it had been suspended because on another occasion Chris was driving while under the influence of alcohol.

Both Pat and Chris were brought to the local emergency room. Chris was taken to surgery and then admitted to the intensive care unit. Pat's body was identified by their roommate, also a nurse, who had been working in the maternity unit. The roommate notified Pat's family and helped make initial arrangements for Pat's body to be moved to a funeral home in their hometown. Employees at the hospital were shocked and grief-stricken; even those who had not known Pat were in anguish.

Two weeks later, Chris was moved to a step-down unit in the orthopedic unit. When Casey, RN, arrived for their 11 p.m. to 7 a.m. shift, they were assigned to work in the step-down unit. When Casey realized that they were assigned to Chris, they told the charge nurse that they refused to care for Chris: "I will not take care of the lousy drunk who killed a friend of mine; why did Chris live and Pat die? Chris should be taken out behind the hospital and shot." Casey was unaware that Chris's sister was nearby and heard the entire conversation.

You are the charge nurse. What is the best way to deal with this situation? You had assigned Casey to the care of Chris because of their expertise and because the other most experienced nurse had called in sick.

- Use the steps described for making an ethical decision.
- Write a statement for the ethical dilemma after you have identified the relevant facts for this situation. Do you need other information?
- Determine possible actions for this dilemma. Examine these choices in relation to teleology and deontology. How would a feminist perspective influence actions?
- What are the consequences of each action?
- What decision did you make?
- What effect does this decision have on Chris, Chris's sister, or the other nursing staff?
- In reviewing the ANA's (2015) *Code of Ethics for Nurses*, are there times when nurses may refuse an assignment?

Working to resolve ethical problems is never an easy task. Consider other ethical issues with which an LVP/LVN may be challenged; these may include observing inadequate care of a client, recognizing that a healthcare provider lacks skills or knowledge for the job undertaken, or observing a fellow nurse refusing to care for a client because that client is of a different ethnicity or gender. Nurses develop ethical practice through education, reflection, and ongoing professional development. Ethical principles and codes of conduct established by nursing organizations and regulatory bodies provide guidance. Formal education and training programs help nurses develop the skills necessary to navigate complex ethical dilemmas and to make informed decisions in clinical practice. Reflective practices, such as ethical case discussions and journaling, allow nurses to critically examine their own values, biases, and experiences, fostering self-awareness and moral sensitivity.

CONCLUSION

As a registered nurse embarking on a new professional journey, practicing ethically is paramount to providing high-quality client care and to upholding the integrity of the nursing profession. First and foremost, familiarize yourself with the ethical codes and standards of nursing practice set forth by reputable nursing organizations such as the ANA or the ICN. These guidelines serve as foundational principles to guide your conduct and decision-making in various clinical scenarios.

Foster self-awareness and moral growth by prioritizing ongoing education and professional development in ethical decision-making, seeking out opportunities for further training, attending workshops, and participating in mentorship programs. Embrace reflective practices to regularly assess your values, biases, and ethical dilemmas encountered in your practice. Cultivate strong communication skills, ensuring open and honest dialogue with clients, families, and interdisciplinary team members, and advocate for client autonomy, dignity, and rights. Remember, ethical nursing practice is not a static concept but a dynamic process that requires continuous learning, self-reflection, and compassionate care for the well-being of those entrusted to your care.

STUDENT *Exercises*

Exercise 17.1

Mrs. Smith, age 23, has had frequent episodes of nosebleeds, easy bruising, and one infection after another. She has been caring for her mother and ill father along with an 18-month-old infant. After a bone marrow biopsy, she is informed by the oncologist she has acute lymphocytic leukemia. She has a dazed look about her as the provider describes the next step of treatment, which will be aggressive chemotherapy. The provider leaves with the consent form signed, but when you question her, you realize she didn't hear a word of what transpired.

1. As the RN, would you consider this an informed consent?
2. From an ethical perspective, what are the items in her history that you would like to have more information about?
3. How would you proceed as the client advocate in this case?

Exercise 17.2

You are a nurse starting your shift in a busy hospital unit. As you prepare to care for your assigned clients, you receive the report from the outgoing nurse. The outgoing nurse warns you that one of the clients, Mr. Johnson, is demanding and mean, and the nurse provides examples of past interactions in which Mr. Johnson has been difficult to manage. As you approach Mr. Johnson's room to introduce yourself and to begin your assessment, you can hear him yelling at the nursing assistant who is trying to help him with his morning routine. As you enter, he looks at you with a scowl and begins to complain about the care he's received so far, stating that no one has been attending to his needs promptly enough. Despite your attempts to calm him down and reassure him that you are here to help, Mr. Johnson remains irritable and uncooperative.

1. How would you respond to Mr. Johnson's initial hostility and complaints?
2. What communication techniques could you use to establish trust and rapport with Mr. Johnson?

3. How might you address Mr. Johnson's specific concerns about his care?
4. What steps could you take to ensure that Mr. Johnson's needs are met while also attending to the needs of other patients on the unit?
5. Reflect on the impact of the outgoing nurse's characterization of Mr. Johnson on your perception of him and your approach to caring for him. Consider the ethical implications of labeling patients based on past behavior and the importance of providing patient-centered care regardless of previous interactions.
6. What questions might you ask a client if you wanted to better understand the client's values?

REFERENCES

American Nurses Association. (2015). *Code of ethics for nurses with interpretive statements* (2nd ed.). https://www.nursingworld.org/practice-policy/nursing-excellence/ethics/code-of-ethics-for-nurses/coe-view-only/

American Nurses Association. (2021a). *Nursing: Scope and standards of practice* (4th ed.).

American Nurses Association. (2021b). *Position statement: Nurse's professional responsibility to promote ethical practice environments.* https://www.nursingworld.org/~4ab6e6/globalassets/practiceandpolicy/nursing-excellence/ana-position-statements/nursing-practice/nurses-professional-responsibility-to-promote-ethical-practice-environments-2021-final.pdf

Barrow, J. M., & Khandhar, P. B. (2023, August 8). Deontology. In *StatPearls*. StatPearls Publishing. Retrieved, from https://www.ncbi.nlm.nih.gov/books/NBK459296/

Biel, S., & Durrant, J. (2020). Controversies in brain death declaration: Legal and ethical implications in the ICU. *Current Treatment Options in Neurology, 22*(4), 12. doi:10.1007/s11940-020-0618-6

Boggs, K. U. (2023). *Interpersonal relationships: Professional communication skills for nurses* (9th ed.). Elsevier.

Butts, J. B., & Rich, K. L. (2023). *Nursing ethics: Across the curriculum and into practice* (6th ed.). Jones & Bartlett Learning.

Cherry, B., & Jacob, S. R. (2023). *Contemporary nursing: Issues, trends, and management* (9th ed.). Elsevier.

Gibson, J. (2023). The case against futility. *Nursing, 53*(9), 40–42. doi:10.1097/01.NURSE.0000946792.03627.74

Gilligan, C. (1982). *In a different voice: Psychological theory and women's development.* Harvard University Press.

Guido, G. (2020). *Legal and ethical issues in nursing* (7th ed.). Pearson.

Kishore, S., Johnson, M., & Rosenbaum, S. (2023). Medicaid expansion: The unfinished promise of the Affordable Care Act. *American Journal of Public Health, 113*(5), 482–483. doi:10.2105/AJPH.2023.307258

Lorenzo, D., Esquerda, M., Palau, F., Cambra, F. J., Bioética, & G. I. e. (2022). Ethics and genomic editing using the Crispr-Cas9 Technique: Challenges and conflicts. *Nanoethics, 16*(3), 313–321. doi:10.1007/s11569-022-00425-y

Marek, Z., & Walulik, A. (2021). What morality and religion have in common with health? Pedagogy of religion in the formation of moral competence. *Journal of Religion and Health, 60*(5), 3130–3142. doi:10.1007/s10943-021-01279-6

Maxwell, A. C., & Pope, A. E. (1910). "The Florence Nightingale Pledge". *Practical nursing: A text-book for nurses and a handbook for all who care for the sick* (2nd ed., p. 17). G. P. Putnam's Sons. https://www.google.com/books/edition/_/HK8yAQAAMAAJ?hl=en&gbpv=1

Morberg Jämterud, S. (2022). Acknowledging vulnerability in ethics of palliative care—A feminist ethics approach. *Nursing Ethics, 29*(4), 952–961. doi:10.1177/09697330211072361

National Library of Medicine. (n.d.). *Ancient Greek medicine.* National Institutes of Health. https://www.nlm.nih.gov/hmd/topics/greek-medicine/index.html#case1

Omelianchuk, A., Bernat, J., Caplan, A., Greer, D., Lazaridis, C., Lewis, A., Pope, T., Ross, L. F., & Magnus, D. (2022). Revise the Uniform Determination of Death Act to align the law with practice through neurorespiratory criteria. *Neurology, 98*(13), 532–536. doi:10.1212/WNL.0000000000200024

Potter, P., Perry, A., Stockert, P., & Hall, A. (2023a). Ethics and values. In *Fundamentals of nursing* (11th ed., pp. 327–343). Elsevier.
Potter, P., Perry, A., Stockert, P., & Hall, A. (2023b). Legal implications in nursing practice. In *Fundamentals of nursing* (11th ed., pp. 316–326). Elsevier.
Reingold, R. B., Gostin, L. O., & Goodwin, M. B. (2022). Legal risks and ethical dilemmas for clinicians in the aftermath of Dobbs. *JAMA, 328*(17), 1695–1696. doi:10.1001/jama.2022.18453
Reverby, S. M. (2009). *Examining Tuskegee: The infamous syphilis study and its legacy*. The University of North Carolina Press.
Rich, K. (2023a). Ethics in professional nursing practice. In J. B. Butts & K. L. Rich (Eds.), *Nursing ethics: Across the curriculum and into practice* (6th ed., pp. 67–104). Jones & Bartlett Learning.
Rich, K. (2023b). Introduction to ethics. In J. B. Butts & K. L. Rich (Eds.), *Nursing ethics: Across the curriculum and into practice* (6th ed., pp. 3–26). Jones & Bartlett Learning.
Siermann, M., Claesen, Z., Pasquier, L., Raivio, T., Tšuiko, O., Vermeesch, J. R., & Borry, P. (2022). A systematic review of the views of healthcare professionals on the scope of preimplantation genetic testing. *Journal of Community Genetics, 13*(1), 1–11. doi:10.1007/s12687-021-00573-w
Taylor, C. R., Lynn, P. B., & Bartlett, J. L. (2023). *Fundamentals of nursing: The art and science of nursing care* (10th ed.). Wolters Kluwer.
Tseng, P. E., & Wang, Y. H. (2021). Deontological or utilitarian? An eternal ethical dilemma in Outbreak. *International Journal of Environmental Research and Public Health, 18*(16), 8565. doi:10.3390/ijerph18168565
Wester, G. (2023). Health, health care, and equality of opportunity: The rationale for universal health care. *Cambridge Quarterly of Healthcare Ethics, 32*(1), 26–33. doi:10.1017/S0963180122000469

SUGGESTED READING

Andersson, H., Svensson, A., Frank, C., Rantala, A., Holmberg, M., & Bremer, A. (2022). Ethics education to support ethical competence learning in healthcare: An integrative systematic review. *BMC Medical Ethics, 23*(1), 1–26. doi:10.1186/s12910-022-00766-z
Čartolovni, A., Stolt, M., Scott, P. A., & Suhonen, R. (2021). Moral injury in healthcare professionals: A scoping review and discussion. *Nursing Ethics, 28*(5), 590–602. doi:10.1177/0969733020966776
Ellis, P. (2024). *Understanding ethics for nursing students* (4th ed.). Sage.
Koonce, M., & Hyrkas, K. (2023). Moral distress and spiritual/religious orientation: Moral agency, norms and resilience. *Nursing Ethics, 30*(2), 288–301. doi:10.1177/09697330221122905
Malka, S. (2007). *Daring to care: American nursing and second-wave feminism*. University of Illinois Press.
Mousavi, S. R., Hassanvand, P., Mahmoudi, A., Hosseinigolafshani, S. Z., Rajabi, M., & Rashvand, F. (2023). The relationship between emotional intelligence and the moral performance of nurses. *Journal of Nursing & Midwifery Sciences, 10*(4), 1–10. doi:10.5812/jnms-141609
Pullen, A., & Vachhani, S. J. (2021). Feminist ethics and women leaders: From difference to intercorporeality. *Journal of Business Ethics, 173*(2), 233–243. doi:10.1007/s10551-020-04526-0

On the WEB

American Journal of Bioethics: http://www.bioethics.net

The ICN Code of Ethics for Nurses: https://www.icn.ch/resources/publications-and-reports/icn-code-ethics-nurses

National Library of Medicine—Greek Medicine (includes the Hippocratic Oath): https://www.nlm.nih.gov/hmd/topics/greek-medicine/index.html#case1

Answers to "The NCLEX-RN Might Ask" Questions

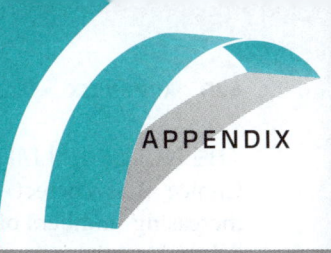

APPENDIX

CHAPTER 2

THE NCLEX-RN MIGHT ASK 2.1
Choice **D** is correct. **Rationale:** Benner's model identifies the stages a nurse progresses through to become an expert in their area of clinical practice. Preceptors should be an expert in their clinical area because they are able to grasp situations and understand needs without reliance on preplanning to guide their actions.

THE NCLEX-RN MIGHT ASK 2.2
Choice **D** is correct, because this is what the nurse would be *incorrect* in stating. **Rationale:** Be careful reading this because the stem (question) is asking for an incorrect statement by the nurse. The professional role is merged with both personal and professional ideas. A, B, and C are acceptable according to Cohen's theory.

CHAPTER 3

THE NCLEX-RN MIGHT ASK 3.1
Choice **B** is correct. **Rationale:** A transformational change refers to a radical difference in how a group is handled as a result of the change. This is a planned change, so C and D are incorrect. There has been no mutual agreement by the stakeholders, so A is incorrect.

THE NCLEX-RN MIGHT ASK 3.2
Choice **B** is correct. **Rationale:** A slight increase in vital signs and blood sugar are characteristic of stimulation of the sympathetic nervous system found in the alarm reaction stage. The changes are not normal and do not indicate those seen in resistance or exhaustion (which can lead to death).

THE NCLEX-RN MIGHT ASK 3.3
Choice **B** is correct. **Rationale:** The client is exhibiting denial by refusing to look at the site and be involved in the dressing changes. If the client had accepted the mastectomy, she would be involved in her care. Bargaining would be indicated by the client saying something like "If only I had stopped smoking." Depression would be indicated by withdrawal behaviors.

CHAPTER 4

THE NCLEX-RN MIGHT ASK 4.1
Choice **A** is correct. **Rationale:** All of these factors impact nursing, but only aging will impact the supply and demand for nurses. An aging population increases the demand for nurses, whereas retiring nurses will impact the supply of nurses.

THE NCLEX-RN MIGHT ASK 4.2
Choice **B** is correct. **Rationale:** Demographic changes of patient populations and increasing numbers of cultural groups in the United States has increased the need for cultural proficiency in nursing practice. The baby boomer population increases the need for nurses but is not culturally significant. Immigration has increased. A decrease in access to healthcare is not based on culture.

CHAPTER 5
THE NCLEX-RN MIGHT ASK 5.1
Choice **B** is correct. **Rationale:** Teaching a client how to irrigate an ostomy involves manipulating and practicing a new skill. Cognitive skills would be more about how and why the stoma functions. Affective learning would explore how the client feels about having the device and how it affects their lifestyle. Communication is not a learning domain.

THE NCLEX-RN MIGHT ASK 5.2
Choice **D** is correct. **Rationale:** Because the LPN is a student studying to be an RN, they are held to the level of an RN.

CHAPTER 7
THE NCLEX-RN MIGHT ASK 7.1
Choices **D, E, F,** and **G** are correct. **Rationale:** The four main categories in the NCLEX-RN test blueprint are (1) safe, effective care environment; (2) health promotion and maintenance; (3) psychosocial integrity; and (4) physiological integrity.

CHAPTER 8
THE NCLEX-RN MIGHT ASK 8.1
Choice **A** is correct. **Rationale:** The nurse practice acts are regulations legislated by state law. They do not include permissive language. Policies and standards are proclaimed from national nursing organizations.

THE NCLEX-RN MIGHT ASK 8.2
Choice **D** is correct. **Rationale:** When the RN is working with others, the RN is collaborating for client care. Independence and autonomy are working and making decisions alone. In the advocacy role, the RN would be working for the client.

THE NCLEX-RN MIGHT ASK 8.3
Choice **D** is correct. **Rationale:** Only minimal safety and competency levels are demonstrated by the RN-level candidate when the NCLEX-RN test is successfully completed. Average, specialty, and excellent practice levels are not demonstrated by passing this examination.

CHAPTER 9
THE NCLEX-RN MIGHT ASK 9.1
Choice **A** is the *incorrect* statement. **Rationale:** Be careful, this question asks you to identify the *wrong* answer. Critical thinking involves recognizing and overcoming feelings as a basis for decisions. It also involves exploring options, problem solving, and not letting age, culture, or personal background influence decisions.

APPENDIX • Answers to "The NCLEX-RN Might Ask" Questions

THE NCLEX-RN MIGHT ASK 9.2
Choice **C** is correct. **Rationale:** C demonstrates that the student needs additional clarification. Critical thinking is based on facts and evidence, not how the student feels about a given situation.

CHAPTER 10
THE NCLEX-RN MIGHT ASK 10.1
Choice **A** is correct. **Rationale:** You are looking for the only *wrong* answer to this question. If the new nurse states that the nursing process is an extension of the medical plan, they need additional help understanding that the nursing process is independent of the medical plan. The other choices are correct and are characteristics of the nursing process.

THE NCLEX-RN MIGHT ASK 10.2
Choice **C** is correct. **Rationale:** Only Choice C meets all three requirements in the NCLEX-RN question: (1) it is a *nursing* (not medical) diagnosis; (2) it is an *actual* (not a risk/potential) diagnosis; and (3) it has *all three* PES components, that is, a **P**roblem statement (stem), **E**tiology (cause), and **S**igns/symptoms (assessment data).

THE NCLEX-RN MIGHT ASK 10.3
Choice **D** is correct. **Rationale:** Airway problems always take top priority. C indicates a "risk for" diagnosis; it can wait. A and B are lower in Maslow hierarchy.

THE NCLEX-RN MIGHT ASK 10.4
Choice **B** is correct. **Rationale:** This outcome stresses the immediate needs of the patient in that the problem involves the airway and needs a short target date. A does not relate to the nursing diagnosis but may be appropriate for a risk for impaired cardiac output nursing diagnosis. C is related to the nursing diagnosis but is not a priority at this time. D is an intervention because it is an assessment.

CHAPTER 11
THE NCLEX-RN MIGHT ASK 11.1
Choices **A & B** are correct. **Rationale:** A is correct – providing general leads is a useful technique for leading an interaction. B is correct – Active listening lets the client know the nurse is interested in what the client has to say. C is incorrect – close-ended questions narrow the depth of information and can close down communication. D is incorrect – A nurse can be professional in appearance but can be cold and uncaring.

THE NCLEX-RN MIGHT ASK 11.2
Choices **C, D, & E** are correct. **Rationale:** C – Therapeutic communication is the foundation for a trusting relationship; D – communication provides information for the nurse to plan care that leads to positive outcomes; and E – allows the client to verbalize thoughts and feelings. B is incorrect as client secrets may not be necessary in a professional association. A is incorrect because one of the goals of communication is to foster client independence.

CHAPTER 12
THE NCLEX-RN MIGHT ASK 12.1
Choices **A** and **E** are correct. **Rationale:** Severe pain and preoccupation with worries about cost/paying for healthcare can block a client's concentration and decrease learning ability. B, C, and D are usually considered to be positive factors for effective learning.

THE NCLEX-RN MIGHT ASK 12.2
Choice **B** is correct. **Rationale:** B is the correct answer and the easiest to do in the home setting. A is not practical, costs money, and may be demeaning to the client. C and D may also make the client feel inferior.

THE NCLEX-RN MIGHT ASK 12.3
Choice **B** is correct. **Rationale:** The cause of the impaired ability to manage medication regime is related to the client's learning need. A, C, and D are correct for the nursing diagnosis but do not clearly state a learning need.

CHAPTER 13
THE NCLEX-RN MIGHT ASK 13.1
Choice **B** is correct. **Rationale:** B is more global and individualized than A; A will give only partial information and may not be uniquely applicable to this client. C ignores the problem and does not help the nurse. D is not client centered.

THE NCLEX-RN MIGHT ASK 13.2
Choice **D** is correct. **Rationale:** The nurse's ability to step outside their own culture to understand another is called cultural relativism. Acculturation is assimilating something outside one's culture. A and C are the opposite of cultural relativism.

THE NCLEX-RN MIGHT ASK 13.3
Choice **B** is correct. **Rationale:** The client speaks only Chinese. There are no data to support the etiologies of the other nursing diagnoses in this scenario.

CHAPTER 14
THE NCLEX-RN MIGHT ASK 14.1
Choice **B** is correct. **Rationale:** The first step in any decision-making process is assessment. A is incorrect because monitoring and assessing outside the normal is not the sole responsibility of the RN. C is incorrect because the nurse needs to trust members of the healthcare team. D is incorrect because the nurse cannot assume a task is completed. They are responsible for the level of care. E is very important for the nurse but not for determining assignments to team members.

THE NCLEX-RN MIGHT ASK 14.2
Choices **A** and **E** are correct. **Rationale:** Both A and E are common time wasters for nurses. B and C are strategies that make the nurse more efficient. D is a legal and ethical responsibility.

THE NCLEX-RN MIGHT ASK 14.3
Choice **B** is correct. **Rationale:** This is a problem with interpretation of the RN's assignment. There are no data to support any of the other answers.

CHAPTER 15
THE NCLEX-RN MIGHT ASK 15.1
Choices **C** and **E** are correct. **Rationale:** When a nurse tries to explain what the client's wishes are, they are acting in the roles of advocate and spokesperson.

THE NCLEX-RN MIGHT ASK 15.2
Choices **B**, **C**, **D**, and **E** are all correct. **Rationale:** The RN must use current knowledge and evidence-based research in designing plans of care for communities. RNs practice with autonomy and are accountable for applying their current knowledge and evidence-based research in planning care for clients and assisting them with preventative methods for self-care. A is incorrect because although traditions are important, the RN must deviate from them when scientific research proves that traditional practices detract from quality client care.

CHAPTER 16
THE NCLEX-RN MIGHT ASK 16.1
Choice **A** is correct. **Rationale:** This is a civil court case initially due to the accidental occurrence of this error. However, if the patient or family loses the case, in some instances, the case could be tried under criminal law. Intent is the determining factor.

THE NCLEX-RN MIGHT ASK 16.2
Choice **A** is correct. **Rationale:** The state nurse practice acts define the scope of nursing practice. Professional organizations develop standards. Hospitals and providers need to adhere to the practice acts and standards.

THE NCLEX-RN MIGHT ASK 16.3
Choices **C**, **D**, and **E** are correct. **Rationale:** To be informed comprehensively, the client needs to be informed about benefits, risks, and alternatives associated with the procedure the provider wants to perform. A client may withdraw consent at any time. A is incorrect because the nurse has an ethical responsibility to the client to ensure that they understand the provider's explanations and must be present to hear them. B is incorrect because not all information gained from a client involves research. A research study would require special permission from the client.

CHAPTER 17
THE NCLEX-RN MIGHT ASK 17.1
Choice **C** is correct. **Rationale:** The nurse must tell the truth. The prognosis is something the client probably knows already but is attempting to confirm. Nonmaleficence is the duty to do no harm, and beneficence is the duty to do good. Justice is fairness to all patients.

THE NCLEX-RN MIGHT ASK 17.2
Choice **D** is correct. **Rationale:** In nursing diagnosis, the expected outcomes are evaluated, not the interventions (planning). A would be correct if the statement included gathering information about the situation. B would be correct if the nurse was clustering data to come up with a statement. C would be correct if the nurse was exploring alternatives and deciding on choices.

Index

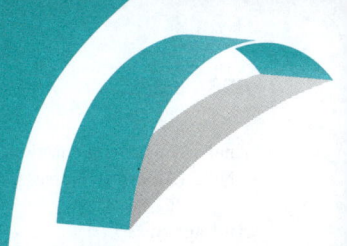

Note: Page numbers followed by *b* indicate boxes; those followed by *f* indicate figures; those followed by *t* indicate tables.

A

AACN (American Association of Colleges of Nursing), 98
Abstract conceptualization, 14
Accommodation
  as conflict resolution, 345
  for disabilities, 141
Accountability, 281*b*, 359–362, 386–389, 387*b*. *See also* HIPAA; Legal accountability
  to colleagues, 362
  to self, 359–361
Acculturation, 323
Acquired roles, 41–42, 42*t*
Acronym, 185–186, 186*b*
Acrostics, 185
Active experimentation, 14
Active learner, 9
Active learning, 139, 144
Active listening, as part of nonverbal communication, 265–266
Addressing age, gender, sexual orientation, cultural differences, 142–143, 143*b*
Administrative law, 382
Administrators and physicians, interactions with, 277
ADN (associate degree nursing) programs, 107–108
  competencies of, 207–208
  LPN/LVN and, education comparison of, 147–149
  roles of, 207–208
  student
    differentiating LPN/LVN practice roles and, 147–149
    generic, 146
ADN student, transition needs of. *See* LPN/LVN
Adult Learner-Centered Teaching, 140*b*
Adult learners, 161–162
  characteristics, 132*b*
Adult learning styles, 14–15
Adult learning theory, 131–134
Advance directives, 393–394
Advanced practice registered nurses (APRNs), 97, 102
Advocacy, 357–359
  health care, nursing relating to, 125
  political, nursing relating to, 125

Affective (values), 299–300
Affective domain, 145
Affective learning, 135
  domain, 208–209
  objectives, 304
African Americans, in nursing, 93
Against medical advice (AMA), 395
Age
  gender, sexual orientation, cultural differences and, addressing of, 142–143, 143*b*
  re-entry process relating to, 6
Agency for Healthcare Research and Quality (AHRQ), 277
Aggressive behaviors, 279, 279*t*, 346
AHNA (American Holistic Nurses Association), 123
Alarm reaction, as stage of general adaptation syndrome, 72, 72*t*
Ambivalence, change relating to, 73–74
American Association of Colleges of Nursing (AACN), 98
American Association of Critical-Care Nurses, 200–201
  regulatory frameworks relating to, 200–201
  social policy statement of, 200–201
American Holistic Nurses Association (AHNA), 123
American Nurses Association. *See* ANA
American Nurses Credentialing Center, 361
American Nurse Today, 95–96
AMT method, of nursing interventions, 255–256, 256*b*
ANA (American Nurses Association), 226, 240
  Code of Ethics for Nurses, 359, 405–406
  Code of Ethics for Nurses with Interpretative Statements, 103, 227–228
  legal accountability relating to, 386, 388–389
  licensure and, 100–102, 101*t*
  Nursing: Scope and Standards of Practice for Nursing, 97, 230
  professional responsibilities relating to, 361
  Scope and Standards of Practice, 254
  social policy statement of, 102–103
  standards of practice and, 104
  stem cell research and, 120
  transitions relating to, 105–109
  website, 125

Index

Analysis/analyzing questions, 180–181
ANCC (American Nurses Credentialing Center), 361
Andragogy, 295
Appearance, as part of nonverbal communication, 267
Application/applying questions, 179–180
APRNs (advanced practice registered nurses), 97, 102
Articulation agreement, 107–108
Ascribed roles, 41, 42*t*
Assault and battery, definitions of, 394*b*
Assertive behaviors, 279*t*
Assertiveness, 19
   in communication, 279, 279*t*
Assessment, 308–310
   of ADN competencies, 208
   adult learners, 161–162
   caring interventions and, of nursing process, 242–247, 244*t*
   of cultural uniqueness, 325*b*
   decision making and, 350
   ethical decision-making, 414
   focused, 244–245, 249
   learning, 162–164
   of learning styles, 161
   legal accountability, 391
   managing conflict relating to, 347–348
   managing time relating to, 331–332
   nursing care process, uniqueness into, 324
   in teaching-learning process, 302, 303*b*
   tests
      for general education, 162–163
      integrated nursing, 163
      for nursing and support curricula, 163
   of time, 333*t*
   tool
      body systems, 244*t*
      evidence-based use of, 243–245
Assistive personnel, 104–105
Associate Degree Nursing. *See* ADN
Attention deficit, 142*b*
Attitudes, 315
   change relating to, 80
Auditory learning, 291
Auditory perceptual problems, 142*b*
Automation in healthcare and health information technology, 121
Autonomous nursing practice, 202–203
Autonomy, 99, 412
   parameters and, for instructor supervision, 148–149
   self-improvement and, desire for, 67
Avoidance, as conflict resolution, 345–346

B

Baby boomers, 111
Baccalaureate of Science in Nursing. *See* BSN
Background assumptions, 216–217
Balance, 44
Barriers
   to communication, about sexuality, 321, 321*b*, 322*b*
   to discussion, of sexual issues, 321*b*, 322*b*
   overcoming fears and, 5–11
Battery. *See* Assault and battery, definitions of
Beliefs, 314, 316
   challenging of, 214
   religious, 324
   values and, 319
Beneficence, 411
Benner, Patricia, 51–52, 51*t*
Bioethics, 119–121, 405–406, 406*b*
Biomedical technology, 125
Biotechnology, 65
Bioterrorism, 119
Blogs, 366*t*
Bloom's Taxonomy of Educational Objectives, 177–182
Body, 226
   posture, as part of nonverbal communication, 266–267
   systems assessment tool, 244*t*
Boundaries, professional, 396–397
Bowen, Murray, 49
BSN (Baccalaureate of Science in Nursing), 108
Bullying, 279–280

C

Career advancement, 108–109
Care provider role, competencies in, 207
Caring behaviors, 273
Caring characteristics and tips, to prevent malpractice claims, 274*t*
CAT (computerized adaptive testing), 174, 174*b*
CCNE (Commission on Collegiate Nursing Education), 106
CEUs (continuing education units), 109
Change
   adapting to, 63–84
   adjusting to, 79–81
   definition of, 64–65
   effects of, 71–79
   improving reception to, 75*b*
   individual and organizational, 65–66, 65*t*
   motivating factors of, 66–67
   paradoxes of, 64, 64*b*
   positive outcomes of, 81–82
   process of, 65
   types, 67–69
Change agent, 68
Charting, focus on, 308*b*
Christian origins, of nursing, 87–88
Chunking, 341
Civil law, 382–383

Civil War, nursing and, 91–92
Clarification, in verbal communication, 269
CLEAR communication, 282b
CLEAR direction, 282
Client
　as cultural being, 318–319
　　customs, beliefs, and values, 319
　　verbal and nonverbal communication, 318–319
　care of. See Managing unique client care
　educational challenge of, 288–289
　learning style, 291–292, 291t
　motivation, 290–291
　need categories of, 175, 175t, 176b
　as sexual being, 321–323
　as social being, 319–321
　as spiritual being, 323–324
　strengths and resources, capitalize on, 293
　teaching documentation of, 307–308
Client expected outcomes, 254
Client's uniqueness
　aspects of, 318–324
　sensitive assessment, 316–317
Clinical example, data analysis for, 249b
Clinical imagination, 223
Clinical judgment, 182–184, 183t, 222–225
　analyze cues, 225
　evaluate outcomes, 225
　generate solutions, 225
　prioritize hypotheses, 225
　recognize cues, 224
　take action, 225
Clinical reasoning, 5, 222–224, 224b
Clinical setting, for teaching strategies, 298b
Cloning, 120
Closed-loop communication, 278
CNEA (Commission for Nursing Education Accreditation), 94–95, 106
CNSA (Canadian Nursing Students Association), 374
　professional responsibilities relating to, 374
Code of ethics, 403, 406b
Code of Ethics for Nurses, 405–406
Code of Ethics for Nurses with Interpretive Statements, 103, 227–228
Cognitive (knowledge), 298–299
Cognitive development, 45
Cognitive domain, 135, 144–145
Cognitive learning achievement levels, 136
Cognitive learning domain, 208–209
Cognitive learning objectives, 304
Cognitive skills, 217t
Cohen, 50, 50t
Collaboration, 276, 346–347
Collaborative nursing practice, 203
Collaborative practice, 116–118, 125–126
Colleague, 362

Collegial communication, 276
Commission for Nursing Education Accreditation. See CNEA
Commitment, 43
Common law, 381–382
Communication conflict, 343
Commission for Nursing Education Accreditation. See CNEA
Communications. See also Nurse, as communicator
　CLEAR, 282b
　collegial, 276
　conflict, 343
　poor, 340
Communication techniques, therapeutic, verbal, 268t
Community, 314–315, 319
Competencies, 275, 315
　in care provider role, 207
　computer, for technologically current nurse, 364–365, 365b
　in member of discipline role, 207
Competition
　as conflict resolution, 346
　for experienced nurses, 114
Comprehension/understanding questions, 179
Compromise, as conflict resolution, 346
Computer competencies, for technologically current nurse, 364–365, 365b
Computer exams, 189–190, 192
Computerized adaptive testing. See CAT
Computer literacy, 121–122
Conceptual models, philosophies and, 134–135
Concrete experimentation, 17
Confidentiality, right to privacy and, 395–396
Conflict. See also Managing time, conflict and nursing environment
　change relating to, 66
　chronic, RTSS relating to, 11t, 12
　communication, 343
　ethical or value, 344
　goal, 343–344
　management strategies, 349b
　personality, 344
　resolution of, 344–347, 344b, 347t
　RTSS relating to, 11t, 12
Constitutional law, 380
Constitution, U.S., 380
Contextual learning, 214
Continuing Education, 52
Continuing education units (CEUs), 109
Continuous quality improvement (CQI), 118
Contract law, 385–386
Coping strategies, change relating to, 80–81
Correct option, 176
Cost awareness, 351
Cost containment, 116, 352
Course syllabus, 21
COVID-19, 280

CQI (continuous quality improvement), 118
Creating questions, 182
Creative problem solving, 214, 226
Creative thinking, 8, 218
Criminal Act, 384
Criminal law, 383–385
Crisis, change relating to, 66
Critical reflection, 219
Critical thinking abilities, 213
Critical thinking, in nursing, 5, 220–221
 abilities/proficiencies, 213
 and accountability, 227–228
 characteristics, 217b
 clinical judgment and, 222–225
 clinical reasoning in, 222–224, 224b
 cognitive skills used in, 217t
 creative thinking and, 218
 definition of, 213–215·
 dispositions, 214
 feeling v., 216–217
 and holistic nursing, 225–227
 intellectual traits or virtues essential for, 216b
 intuition, 222–224
 modes of, 219, 221
 need for, 212–213
 problem solving, 221–222
 teaching and learning exercises, 231b
Critical thinking skills, 213, 221–222, 226, 230–231
Critical Thinking Skills for Dummies, 215
Cryogenics, 120
Cultural blindness, 114t
Cultural competence, 115
Cultural destructiveness, 114t
Cultural diversity, 367
Cultural humility, 115
Cultural incapacity, 114t
Cultural precompetence, 114t
Cultural proficiency, 114–116, 114t
Cultural sensitivity, 266
Culture, 226, 293, 314–315
 competence, 315
 differences, addressing of, 142–143, 143b
 humility, 315
 relativism, 315–316
 resistance factors, 75
 sensitivity, 266
 social, and spiritual nursing diagnoses, 326b
 uniqueness, assessment of, 314–316, 325b
Curricular content, learning domains and, 135–136
Curricular frameworks, 135
Curriculum threads, 21
CUS, 278
Customize teaching, based on client's learning style, 291–292, 291t
Customs, 314, 316
 beliefs, values and, 319
Cyberterrorism, 125

D

Data
 for clinical example, analysis of, 249b
 collection of, 242–243
 documenting, 247
 objective, 245
 organization of, 245–247, 246b
 patterns or clustering, identification, 249
 primary source, 243
 reporting of, 247
 secondary sources, 243
 subjective, 245
 validation of, 245
Decision making, 349–351
 Deontology, 407–408
 ethical, in nursing, 414–415
 ethical issues' influence on, 409–413
 governance and, 373
 informed, 358
 nursing process and, 350, 350t
 process of, 350, 350t
Deductive reasoning, 223
De-escalation of high-stress situations, 280–281
Defamation of character, 396–397
Defendant, 382–383
Delegation, 335–336
 managing time relating to, 335–336
 nursing process and five rights of, 281, 282t
 team member relating to, 281–283
 terms associated with, 281b
Demographic changes, 367
 chronic conditions, 367
 cultural diversity, 367
 older adults, 367
Demonstration exams, 190
Demonstration/return demonstration, 300
Deontology, 407–408
Development. *See also* Personal and adult development; Role development
 change, 67
 family, 47–49, 48t
 stage, 295–296, 295t, 296b
 of study skills, 28–32
Diagnosis, 325, 326b. *See also* Nursing diagnosis; Nursing diagnostic statements
 actual, 250
 as ADN competency, 208
 decision making and, 350
 ethical decision-making, 414
 legal accountability, 391
 managing conflict relating to, 348
 medical v. nursing, 252, 252t
 in nursing process, 248–252
 risk, 251
 statements, 250–251, 250b
 syndrome, 251

teaching-learning process, as steps in, 302–303
validation of, 250
wellness, 251
Diagnostic-related groups. *See* DRGs
Diagnostic statements, formulation of, 250–251, 250*b*
Diploma programs, 107
Directed nursing practice, 202
Disabilities, 141, 142*b*
Disappointment, change relating to, 66
Disaster preparedness, 119
Discussion, 299
Disintegration, 12
Distress, change relating to, 71–73
Diverse learning styles, 13–18
Diversity, 4, 6–8, 114–116
Diversity, Equity, and Inclusion, 52–53
Documentation
   actions, implementation, of nursing process, 259
   of client teaching, 307–308, 308*b*
   efficient, tips for, 338*b*
   legal accountability relating to, 387–388
   streamline, 337
DPA (durable power of attorney), 393
DRGs (diagnostic-related groups), 116–117
Driving forces, 70
Durable power of attorney. *See* DPA
Duvall's theory, 48–49

E

EBP (evidence-based practice), 5, 105, 198, 219, 256*b*, 365–366, 366*b*
Ecological intelligence, 120
Economic pressures, 114
Economic status, 320
Educating Nurses: A Call for Radical Transformation, 222
Educationally mobile, 11
Educational mobility, 108–109
Effectiveness, 336
Effective team, qualities of, 277*b*
Efficient and effective use, of time, 336–337
Efficient documentation, tips for, 338*b*
Emotion, 226
Emotional intelligence, 114–116, 348
Emotional intelligence (EI), 214
Energetic, 226
Engenders trust, 273
Enhanced learning, in older adults, 296*b*
Entrepreneur, 124
Entrepreneurism, nursing, 124–125
Entry-level educational programs, 97
Environment
   modify, 296
   teamwork, 336–337
Environmental well-being, 227

Ethical concerns, legal accountability relating to, 380
Ethical decision making, 414–415
Ethical dilemmas, 403–404, 406*b*
   common, 403*b*
   ethics and law, 404
   ethics and religion, 404–405
   moral distress, 403–404
Ethical issues
   decision making influenced by, 409–413
   history of, 402–403, 402*t*
   learning objectives for, 401
Ethical theories, 407
Ethical value or conflict, 344
Ethics
   definitions related to, 406*b*
   development of, 402
   feminist, 407–408
   history and, 402–403, 402*t*
   laws and, 404, 405*t*
   model of, 406*f*
   nursing, 407
   and religion, 404–405
Ethnicity, re-entry process relating to, 6–8
Ethnocentrism, 315
Eustress, change relating to, 71–73
Evaluation, 208
   of care provider role competencies, 208
   decision making and, 350
   ethical decision-making, 414
   legal accountability, 391
   managing conflict relating to, 349
   in managing unique client care, 327
   of nurse, as teacher, 307
   of nursing process, 259
Evaluation/creating questions, 182
Evidence-based practice. *See* EBP
Evidence-based research, 256, 365–366
Evidential discovery, 122–123
Exams
   common issues, 190–191
   completion, 189–191
   day, 188
   decompressing, 192
   review, 192
   types, 189–190
Exhaustion or recovery, 72*t*, 73
Expected outcomes, 242
   establishment of, 254–255, 254*t*
   learning objectives and, 304–306
Experiences, past, 297
Experiential knowledge, 39, 132
Experiential learning, 16, 162
Experiential wisdom, 122–123
   and evidence-based practice, in nursing, 122–123, 198
Experimentation, concrete, 17
Expert witness, 388–389

External degree programs, 109
Eye contact, as part of nonverbal communication, 266–267

F

Faculty role, principles of, 140*b*
Failure, fear of, 10–11
False assurances, as verbal communication blocks, 270
Family, 319
  constraints of, re-entry relating to, 9–10
  development, 47–49, 48*t*
  interpersonal relationships, 319–320
  structures, changes in, 118–119
  tips for effectively working with, 320*b*
Fear
  of failure, 10–11
  of nursing faculty, technology, today's classroom, 8–9
Feedback mechanism, 154, 264, 283
Feeling, critical thinking v., 216–217
Felony, 383–384
Feminist ethics, 407–408
Feminist theories, 403, 408
Fidelity, 412
Financial and/or family constraints, re-entry relating to, 9–10
Financial obligations, 9
Flexibility, change relating to, 80
Flexible spending account. *See* FSAs
Focused assessment, 244–245, 249
Forced change, 67
Friends, impact of, 319
FSAs (flexible spending account), 118
Functional literacy, 289

G

Gender, 6–8, 142–143, 143*b*, 296
  issues, re-entry process relating to, 6–8
Gender equity, 111
Gender identity, 322–323
General adaptation syndrome, stages of, 72–73, 72*t*
General leads, communication relating to, 268
Generic ADN population, 146
Generic ADN student, 146
Genetic engineering, 125, 410*b*
Gestures, as part of nonverbal communication, 266–267
Global community, 368–369
Global economy, advancement of, 119–121
Globalism, advancement of, 119–121
Goals
  conflict with, 343–344
  self-directed, 143–144
  setting of, 326, 332–334
Good Samaritan laws, 381
Gordon's functional health patterns, 246*b*

Governance, decision making and, 373
Guided and independent practice, 301

H

Health care advocacy and service learning, nursing relating to, 125
Healthcare reform, 116–118, 410–411
Healthcare setting, communications in, 276–283
Health Insurance Portability and Accountability Act. *See* HIPAA
Health literacy, 289
Health maintenance organizations. *See* HMOs
Health Resources and Services Administration (HRSA), 113
Health savings accounts. *See* HSAs
Healthy workplace, 373
Heritage, 314
Highlighter, 187
HIPAA (Health Insurance Portability and Accountability Act), 121–122, 395
Hippocratic Oath, 402
HIV/AIDS, 119
HMOs (health maintenance organizations), 116–117
Holistic and spiritual care, in nursing, 123–124, 318
Holistic nursing, 225–227
Homeland security, 119
Honeymoon stage, 11*t*, 12
Hospice nursing, 124
HSAs (health savings accounts), 118

I

ICN (International council of nurses), 98
ICN Code of Ethics for Nurses, 103
Immigration issues, nurses and, 116
Implementation, 306
  of competencies, in care provider role, 208
  decision making and, 351
  ethical decision-making, 414
  legal accountability, 391
  managing conflict relating to, 348–349
  of nurse, as teacher, 306
  of nursing process: overview and steps for, 258–259
  unique client care, 326
Implicit (unconscious) biases, 52–53
Incident reports, 391–392
Incivility, 279–280
Incremental change, 68
INDEN (International Network for Doctoral Education in Nursing), 105
Independent practice, 301
Independent study, 299
Individual and organizational change, 65–66, 65*t*
Individualized plans, 304, 306*b*
  of care, 256–258
  preoperative plan, 309*b*

Individual loss, change and, 76, 77t
Influential factors, of trends and transitions, in nursing, 109–121
Informal logic, reasoning and, 222
Informed consent, 394–395
Informed decision making, 358
Instructor-student partnership, 164–165
Instructor supervision, autonomy and parameters for, 148–149
Integrated nursing assessment tests, 163
Integration problems, 142b
Intentional torts, 383b
Interaction, with administrators and physicians, 277
Interactive tools, 187–188
International Classification for Nursing Practice (ICNP), 104–105
International council of nurses (ICN), 98
International Network for Doctoral Education in Nursing (INDEN), 105
Interpersonal relationships, 319–320, 320b
Interpersonal role conflict, 57–58
Interprofessional collaborative team, 24
Interprofessional practice, 276
Interruptions, 337–339
Interventions
   assessment and, of nursing process, 235–260
   for culturally competent nurse, 326b
   for managing conflict, 348
   nursing, AMT method of, 255–256, 256b
   teaching, 298–301, 298b, 306
Intrapersonal sense, 321
Intuition, 222–224
   decision-making, 215

J

JAN (Journal of Advanced Nursing), 105
Job analysis studies, 204
Johns Hopkins program, 92–93
Johns Hopkins School of Nursing, 92
Joint Commission Sentinel Event Policy, 392b
Journal of Advanced Nursing. See JAN
Judgmental, being, as verbal communication blocks for nurse, as communicator, 270–271
Judicial and legislative factors, decision making relating to, 409
Justice, 412

K

Kinesthetic learning, 291
Knowledge
   base, current, maintenance of, 363–364
   critical thinking, skills, and abilities required to, 229b
   difficulty levels of questions and, Bloom's Taxonomy relating to, 177–182
   experiential, 132
   new, meaning and relevance of, 132–133
   roles and, mechanisms for identifying differences in, 203–205
   skills, abilities, of LPN/LVN v. RN, 208–209
Knowledge/remembering questions, 178
Korean War, 110

L

Laminectomy, 305b
Language
   impact of, 313, 319
   permissive, 199, 200b
   in regulations, 199, 200b, 209
   restrictive, 199, 200b
   simplify, 293–295
Laws, 380
   classifications of, 382–386
   Good Samaritan, 381
   licensure relating to, 100–102, 101t
   sources of, 380–382, 381b
Leadership, provided through professional organizations, 373–374
Learners
   adult, 161–162
   proactive, 156
   styles of, 15–18
   successful, characteristics, 32, 33t–34t
Learning. See also Teaching-learning process
   achievement levels of, 136
   active, 14–15, 139, 144
   adult. See Adult learning
   affective, 298b
   aides, for children and adolescent, 295t
   auditory, 291, 291t
   cognitive, 298b
   domains of, 135–136, 208–209
   kinesthetic, 291, 291t
   lifelong learning. See Lifelong learning; Lifelong learning world, basic skills and competencies
   LPN/LVN and ADN relating to, 146–147
   in older adults, 296b
   outcomes of, 21
   perceiving and processing tasks, 15, 16
   prior, assessment of, 162–164
   process of, 138
   psychomotor, 298b
   service, nursing relating to, 125
   styles, 15–18, 291–292, 291t
   teaching and, defined, 289
   techniques of, 156
   visual, 291, 291t
Learning achievement levels, 136, 136b
   analysis, 136
   application, 136
   comprehension, 136
   evaluation, 136

Learning achievement levels (*Continued*)
    knowledge, 136
    synthesis, 136
Learning domains, 135–136, 208–209
    affective, 135
    cognitive, 135, 144–145
    psychomotor, 135, 145
Learning management systems (LMS), 365
Learning strategies for success
    active learning, 33, 144
    self-awareness, 141–143
    self-directed goals, 143–144
    techniques to stimulate thinking, 144–145, 208–209
Learning styles, 13–18, 161, 291–292, 291*t*
    diverse, 13–18
Learning Styles Inventory, 141
Lectures, 298
Legal accountability
    accountability, 386–389, 387*b*
    confidentiality and right to privacy, 395–396
    defamation, 396–397
    documentation relating to, 387–388
    ethical concerns relating to, 380
    informed consent, 394–395
    law, classifications of, 382–386
    law, sources of, 380–382, 381*b*
    legally sensitive areas that affect nursing practice, 393–395
    liability, 389, 389*b*
    malpractice, 390, 390*b*
    negligence, 389–390, 389*b*
    professional boundaries, 396–397, 397*b*
    risk management, 391–392, 392*b*
    standards of practice, 388–389
Legal precedent, 381–382
Legislative and societal influences, decision making relating to, 409–410
Liability, 148, 389, 389*b*
Libel, 396
Licensed practical nurse/licensed vocational nurse. *See* LPN/LVN
Licensed vocational nurse. *See* LPN/LVN
Licensure
    examinations for, 204
    for nursing, 100–102, 101*t*
    nursing, history of, 100, 101*t*
    requirements and nurse practice acts, 204–205
Lifelong learning
    basic skills and competencies, 5, 6
    diverse learning styles, 13–18
    in nursing, 5
    professional organizations for, 24
    re-entry process: overcoming barriers and fears, 5–11
    student role, successful strategies for, 19–32

Lifelong learning world, basic skills and competencies for, 5, 6
Living wills, 393
Loss and change, 76–77
    individual, 76, 77*t*
    organizational, 76–77, 77*t*
LPN (licensed practical nurse)
    to professional nursing practice, 238–239
    test success for: challenge of NCLEX-RN questions. *See* NCLEX-RN questions, challenge of: test success for LPN
LPN/LVN (licensed practical nurse/licensed vocational nurse), 4
    and ADN education: a comparison, 147–149
    to ADN student, transition needs unique to, 146–147
    differentiating ADN student and practice roles of, 147–149
    to professional nursing practice, 238–239
    RN knowledge, skills, abilities v., 208–209
    to RN role transition, personal education plan for, 166*b*
    roles and competencies of, 206–207
    straight-through LPN/LVN-to-ADN student, 146
    test plan for, 205–206
    time-out LPN/LVN-to-ADN student, 147

M

Magnet hospital designation, 361
Magnet hospitals, 361
Malpractice, 389–390, 390*b*
Managed care, 116–118
Managing conflict, 343–349
    guidelines for dealing with, 347–349
    resolution of, 344–347, 344*b*, 347*t*
    types and causes of, 343–344
Managing resources, 351–352
    cost awareness, 351
    cost containment, 352
    quality management, 352
Managing time, conflict and resources
    learning objectives of, 329
    making decisions, 349–351
    managing conflict, 343–349
    managing resources, 351–352
    managing time, 331–342
Managing unique client care, 312–328
    client as cultural being, 318–319
    client as sexual being, 321–323
    client as social being, 319–321
    client as spiritual being, 323–324
    client's uniqueness
        aspects of, 318–324
        sensitive assessment, 316–317
    definitions of, 314–316
    learning objectives for, 312
    self-assessment, 315–316

uniqueness
  into nursing care process, 324–327
  understanding of, 313–314
Massive Open Online Courses. *See* MOOCs
Master's degree programs, 108
Measurable outcome criteria, 254, 255*b*
Mechanisms for identifying differences, in knowledge and roles, 203–205
Medical surgical unit, worksheet for, 333*t*
Medical v. nursing diagnosis, 252, 252*t*
Memorization, 185–186
Men and women, in nursing, societal roles, 42
Men, in nursing, 110
Mentoring, of new nurses, 371–372, 372*b*
Mentor–mentee relationship, 158, 158*b*
Mentors, 31–32, 157–159
Metacognition, self-regulation and, 218–220
Metaparadigm, 105
Military origins, of nursing, 88–89
Mind, 226
Mindfulness, 219, 265
The Miniature Guide to Critical Thinking Concepts and Tools, 215
Misdemeanor, 383–384
Mnemonics, 185–186
Model
  communication, 264, 264*f*
  conceptual, philosophies and, 134–135
  critical thinking, in nursing, 219, 221
  role, nurse as, 372
  value nursing and, 360–361
MOOCs (Massive Open Online Courses), 140
Moral development, 46
Moral distress, 403–404
Moral reasoning, 408
Moral resilience, 359–360
Motivating factors, of change, 66–67
Motivation, 290–291
Moving, as stage of planned change, 70–71
Multiculturalism, 114–116
Multicultural nature, 313
Multitasking, 339
Mutual goal setting, 154

N
NANDA (North American Nursing Diagnosis Association), 104–105, 239
NANDA-I (North American Nursing Diagnosis Association International), 104, 239, 248, 250, 302, 325
National Council Licensure Examination for Practical Nurses. *See* NCLEX-PN
National Council Licensure Examination for Registered Nurses. *See* NCLEX-RN
National council licensure examinations, 205–206
National Council of State Boards of Nursing. *See* NCSBN
National Database of Nursing Quality Indicators. *See* NDNQI
National Labor Relations Act, 386
National League for Nursing. *See* NLN
National League for Nursing Accreditation Commission. *See* NLNAC
National Student Nurses Association. *See* NSNA
NCJMM (NCSBN Clinical Judgment Measurement Model), 224
NCLEX-PN (National Council Licensure Examination for Practical Nurses), 204–205
NCLEX-RN (National Council Licensure Examination for Registered Nurses), 59*b*, 96–97, 99*b*, 100, 105–107, 138, 145*b*, 149*b*, 199, 204, 206, 206*b*, 221–222, 228, 240
  style exam, 184–192
  test plan, 174–175
NCLEX-RN questions, challenge of: test success for LPN, 172–194
  blueprint, 175
  development of, 173–175
  main categories of, 175, 175*t*
  taxonomy, Bloom's Taxonomy of Educational Objectives and, comparison of, 177–182, 177*t*
NCSBN (National Council of State Boards of Nursing), 96–97, 135, 138, 202, 204–206, 204*b*, 209, 221, 240
NCSBN Clinical Judgment Measurement Model (NCJMM), 183*t*
NDNQI (National Database of Nursing Quality Indicators), 352
Negative humor, 274
Negligence, 389–390, 389*b*
NeN (Nurse Entrepreneur Network), 125
Netiquette, 8
NI (nursing informatics), 118, 121–122, 324
NIC (Nursing Interventions Classification), 254, 256
Nightingale reform, 89–91
Nightingale system of education, 90–91, 90*b*
NLC (Nurse Licensure Compact), 102
NLN (National League for Nursing), 5, 94–95, 115, 200–201, 205, 207–208, 362
  Hallmarks of Excellence in Nursing Education, 120
NLNAC (National League for Nursing Accreditation Commission), 94–95
NOC (Nursing Outcomes Classification) groups, 254
No-interruption zones, 335
Nonmaleficence, 411–412
Nonstandardized tests, 162
Nonverbal communication, 265–267, 265*b*, 318–319
North American Nursing Diagnosis Association. *See* NANDA

North American Nursing Diagnosis Association International. *See* NANDA-I
Note-taking skills, 29–30
NSNA (National Student Nurses Association), 374
Nurse. *See also* ADN; LPN; LPN/LVN; RN
  as communicator, 261–284
    basic communication revisited, 264–275
    communication, in health care setting, 276–283
    communication, nonverbal, 265–267, 265*b*
    communication, verbal, 264–265, 267–269
    competence in communication, across life span, 275
    de-escalation of high-stress situations, 280–281
    effective communication, 263
    learning objectives for, 261
    process recordings, 271–272, 272*b*
    verbal communication blocks, 270–271, 271*t*
  culturally sensitive, interventions for, 326*b*
  ethical code, 357*b*
  immigrating to United States, 108
  new, mentoring of, 371–372, 372*b*
  as role model, 372
  sexual issues discussion of, 321*b*
  technologically current, computer competencies for, 364–365, 365*b*
  therapeutic caring, 273–274
Nurse, as teacher, 287–311
  case studies for, 287*b*
  client education, challenge of, 288–289
  client teaching, documentation of, 307–308
  teaching and learning defined, 289
  teaching interventions, 298–301
  teaching-learning process
    clinical application, 308–310
    principles of teaching, 289–297, 290*b*, 294*b*
    steps in, 301–307
Nurse Entrepreneur Network. *See* NeN
Nurse Licensure Compact (NLC), 102
Nurse practice act, 97, 102, 198–199
Nursing. *See also* Professional responsibilities
  advancements in, 369–372
  African Americans in, 93
  background assumptions, 216–217
  care planning, interventions of, 352
  Civil War and, 91
  clinical judgment in, 211–234
  clinical reasoning in, 211–234
  coalition of organizations within, 98
  collaborative practice and future, 125–126
  core values, 413*b*
  critical thinking in. *See* Critical thinking, in nursing
  development of, 86–93
  discipline of, 102–105
  educational mobility and career advancement, 108–109
  education for, transitions in, 105–109
  entrepreneurism in, 124–125
  ethical decision-making in, 414–415
  ethics of, 405–413, 406*b*, 406*f*, 411*b*, 413*b*
  evidence-based practice in, 365–366, 366*b*
  experiential wisdom and evidence-based practice in, 122–123, 198
  factors, influence decision-making in, 409–413
  healthcare advocacy and service learning relating to, 125
  holistic and spiritual care in, 123–124
  immigrating to the United States, 108
  immigration issues, 116
  intuitive decision-making, 215
  licensure for, 100–102, 101*t*
  lifelong learning in, 5
  medical diagnosis v., 252, 252*t*
  men in, 7
  modeling and professional values, 360–361, 361*b*
  principles of, 411*b*
  problems of, 250
  professional code of ethics, 103
  professional organizations for, 95, 109, 373–374
  professional qualities relating to, 99–100
  as profession, evolution of, 99–102
  recruitment, 371
  scope and standards of practice, 104
  service learning, advocacy and policy making, 125
  social policy statement, 102–103
  state board of, 198–199
  taxonomies, diagnosis, 104–105
  trends and transitions in, 109–121
  in United States, 91–93
  in the United States, 91–93
Nursing care plan, standard, 257*b*
Nursing care process, for unique client care, 324–327
Nursing Community, 98
Nursing diagnosis, 325
  cultural social, and spiritual, 326*b*
  definition of, 248
  establishing priorities for, 253, 253*b*
  nursing process and, 137–138, 137*t*
  syndrome diagnosis, 251
  taxonomies, 239
  wellness diagnosis, 251
Nursing education, 228–231, 229*b*, 230*t*
  programs, types, 106–108
  transitions in, 105–109
Nursing environment, management of. *See* Managing time, conflict and nursing environment
Nursing ethics, 405–413, 406*b*, 406*f*, 411*b*, 413*b*
Nursing informatics (NI), 118, 121–122, 364
Nursing Informatics: Scope and Standards of Practice, 365

Nursing interventions
  AMT method of, 255–256, 256b
  performing or delegating, 258
  planning, 255–256, 256b
Nursing Interventions Classification. *See* NIC
Nursing Outcomes Classification. *See* NOC
Nursing practice
  acts of, 198–199
  collaboration in, 203
  legally sensitive areas affecting, 393–395
  LPN to professional, 238–239
  standards of, 104, 199–200, 362, 369–370, 388–389
Nursing process
  assessment and caring interventions of, 235–260, 241t
  conflict resolution and, 347t
  decision making and, 350, 350t
  five rights of delegation, 282t
  and nursing diagnosis, 137–138, 137t
  planning in, 252–258
  planning your workday and, 334t
  problem-solving method, 240t
  scientific method, problem-solving process and, comparison of, 240t
  teaching-learning process v., 301t
Nursing process: overview and steps for, 239–240, 240t, 241f
  assessment, 242–247
  diagnosis, 248–252
  evaluation, 259
  implementation, 258–259
  planning, 252–258
Nursing research, 370
Nursing review tests, 163–164
Nursing science, evolution of, 99–102
Nursing's code of ethics, 103
Nursing: Scope and Standards of Practice, 97, 200–201, 230
Nursing's Social Policy Statement, 221–222, 362

O

OADN (Organization for Associate Degree Nursing), 97
Objective data, 245, 245t, 259
Observation
  reflective, 14
  sharing of, 269
Occurrence report, 391–392
OERs (Open Education Resources), 140
Older adults, enhanced learning in, 296b
The Online Journal of Issues in Nursing, 95–96
Open Education Resources. *See* OERs
Open-ended questions, in verbal communication, 268
Order of the Virgins, 88
Order of Widows, 88

Organizational and individual change, 65–66, 65t
Organization for Associate Degree Nursing. *See* OADN
Organizations. *See* HMOs; Professional nursing organizations
  of data, 245–247, 246b
  professional, 200–201, 205, 373–374
Orientation, variations in, 315–316. *See also* Sexual orientation
Origins, of nursing, 86–87
Outcomes
  assessment, 118
  criteria, measurable, 254, 255b
  expected outcomes, 242, 254–255, 304–306
  of learning, 21
  positive, of change, 81–82
Outcomes and competencies for graduates of Practical/Vocational, Diploma, Associate Degree, Baccalaureate, Master's, Practice Doctorate, and Research Doctorate Programs in nursing, 205

P

Palliative care, 124
Pandemic flus, 119
Paper and pencil exams, 189, 191–192
Paradoxes, of change, 64, 64b
Paralanguage, as part of nonverbal communication, 266
Paraphrasing, 176–177
Pareto principle, 332
Partnering, 288
Partnering, with learner, 290
Past experiences, new learning to, 297
Paternalism, 411
Patient advocacy, 357
Patient education, effective Internet use for, 299b
Pedagogy, 295
Peer review, self-regulation and, 362
Pennsylvania State Board of Nursing, 199
PEP (Personal education plan)
  design, 5–6
  for LPN/LVN to RN role transition, 166b
Perfectionism, 342
Periodical subscriptions, 22
Permissive language, in regulations, 199, 200b
Personal achievement, and professional achievement, 133
Personal and adult development
  by Erikson, Erik, 45
  by Gilligan, Carol, 46–47
  by Kohlberg, Lawrence, 46
  by Piaget, Jean, 45–46
Personal disorganization, 340
Personal education plan. *See* PEP
Personal effectiveness, tips for, 337b
Personality conflict, 344

Personal professional library, 22
PES format, for writing actual nursing diagnostic statements, 250, 251*b*
Philosophy, 21, 134–135
Plaintiff, 382–383
Planned change, 68–69
    incremental, 68
    rapid, 68
    stages of, 69–71, 70*b*
    transactional, 68
    transformational, 69
Planning. *See also* Test plans
    as competency, 208
    decision making and, 350
    ethical decision-making, 414
    before exam, 185
    goal setting and, 332–334
    legal accountability, 391
    managing conflict relating to, 348
    nursing care, 257*b*
    in nursing process, 252–258
    personal education plan, 166*b*
    phase, 252
    for post-operative laminectomy, 305*b*
    priorities hierarchy, 334*t*
    problem solving relating to, 208
    for role transition, 152–171
    in teaching-learning process, 304–306
    for unique client care, 326
    workday and nursing process, 334*t*
Policy, 199
Political advocacy, nursing relating to, 125
Poor communication, 340
Positive outcomes, of change, 81–82
Posttraumatic stress disorder (PTSD), 110
Posture of involvement, 265–266
PPOs (preferred provider organizations), 116–117
Practical/vocational programs, *vs.* associate degree nursing education, 134–141
Practice
    concerns, of LPN/LVN and ADN student, 147–148
    evidence-based, 105, 198, 365–366, 366*b*
    guided and independent, 301
    repetition and, 297
    scope of, 198
    standards of, 104, 199–200, 362, 369–370
Preferred provider organizations. *See* PPOs
Priorities, 253, 253*b*, 258, 334–335, 334*t*
Prior learning, assessment of, 162–164
Privileged communication, 273
Proactive learner, 156
Problem-solving method, 240*t*
Procrastination, 28–29, 29*b*, 341, 341*b*
Profession
    advancement, 362–369, 363*b*
    boundaries, 396–397, 397*b*
    growth, 362–369, 363*b*
    organizations, 200–201, 205
    qualities of, 99–100
    role development, 42
    role socialization, 53–55, 54*t*
    stewardship, 372–374
    values and client values, 411–413
Professional achievement, 133
Professional code of ethics, 103
Professional nursing organizations
    AACN, 98
    ANA, 95–96
    ICN, 98
    NCSBN, 96–97
    NLN, 5, 94–95
    OADN, 97
Professional responsibilities
    advocacy, 357–359
    conclusion to, 374
    ethical code for nurses, according to, 357*b*
    modeling and value nursing, 360–361
    nursing practice, standards of, 362, 369–370
    nursing research, 370
    professional advancement, 362–369, 363*b*
    professional stewardship, 372–374
Professional role development, 49–55
Professional values, 360–361
Profession of nursing, evolution of, 99–102
Program philosophy, 21
Protestant reformation, 89
Proxemics, 143
Psychological resistance factors, 75
Psychomotor domain, 135, 145
Psychomotor learning, 298*b*, 300–301
    domain, 208–209
    objectives, 304
PTSD (post-traumatic stress disorder), 110

Q

QA (quality assurance), 118
QM (quality management), 352
Quality assurance (QA), 118
Quality management (QM), 352
Quiet time, 335

R

Rapid change, 68
Reading
    before exam, 186–188
    skills, 29–30
Receiver (decodes), 264–265
Reciprocal teaching, 187
Recovery or exhaustion, 72*t*, 73
Recruitment, nursing, 371
Re-entry process, 154
Referral, client advocacy relating to, 358
Reflective observation, 14

Reflective practitioner, 220
Reflective process: assessing adult learner uniqueness, 161–162
Reflective thinking, self-regulation and, 218–220
Refreezing, as stage of planned change, 71
Regulations, 198–199
　permissive language in, 199, 200b
　restrictive language in, 199, 200b
Regulatory frameworks, practicing within
　ADN roles and competencies, 207–208
　autonomous nursing practice, 202–203
　collaboration in nursing practice, 203
　directed nursing practice, 202
　knowledge and roles, mechanisms for identifying differences in, 203–205
　LPN/LVN, RN knowledge, skills, abilities v., 208–209
　LPN/LVN roles, competencies and, 206–207
　national council licensure examinations, 205–206
　nurse practice acts, 201
　nursing practice, 201–203
　policies, 199
　practical/vocational nursing roles and competencies, 206–207
　regulations, 198–199, 200b
　standards, 199–201
Regulatory law, 382
Reimbursement Programs, 118
Reinforcement, newly learned behaviors, 297
Reintegration, 12
Religion, ethics and, 404–405
Religious beliefs, 324
Religious or spiritual symbols or treatments, 324
Repetition, practice and, 297
Research
　evidence-based, 256
　skills for, 22–23
　stem cell, 120
Resistance
　change relating to, 74–75
　factors of, 75
　as stage of general adaptation syndrome, 72–73, 72t
Resolution, 12–13
　biculturalism, 13
　chronic conflict, 12
　of conflict, 344–347, 344b, 347t
　false acceptance, 12–13
　oscillation, 13
　of role conflict, methods of, 57–59
Resonance, change relating to, 78–79
Resource materials
　course syllabus, 21
　faculty and course web pages, 21–22
　learning outcomes, 21
　periodical subscriptions, web resources and, 22
　personal professional library, 22
　program philosophy and curriculum threads, 21
　student handbook, 20–21
　student learning outcomes, 21
　updating research skills, 22–23
Resources
　client strengths and, 293, 294b
　managing of, 351–352
　Web, 22
Responsibility, healthcare setting, communication in, 276
Restating, in verbal communication, 269
Restraining forces, 70
Restrictive language, in regulations, 199, 200b
Returning to school syndrome. See RTSS
Rewards, lack of, 66–67
Rights, clients, protection of, 359
Right to privacy, confidentiality and, 395–396
Risk diagnosis, 251
Risk management, 391–392, 392b
RN (registered nurse), 95, 124–125
　knowledge, skills, abilities of, LPN/LVN v., 208–209
　roles and competencies of, 206–207
　role transition to LPN/LVN, 166b
　test plan for, 206
Robotics, 125
Role, 39. See also Societal trends and changing role of nursing
　of ADN, 207–208
　care provider, competencies in, 206–207
　change, definition of, 40
　conflict, 57–59, 343
　knowledge and, differences in, 203–205
　modeling, 300
　　nurse as, 372
　overload, 58
　personal, 41
　playing, 300
　practice, of LPN/LVN and ADN student, 147–149
　socialization, professional, 53–55, 54t
　societal, of women and men, in nursing, 42, 110
　strain, 57–59
　stress, 57–59
Role change, 40
Role development, 39–40
　barriers, 44
　definition of, 39
　role choice, 43–44
Roles, types of, 41–42
　acquired, 41–42
　ascribed, 41
Role transition, 40, 55–59, 55t
　definition of, 40, 41b
　endings, 55–56
　neutral zone, 56
　new beginnings, 57–59, 57b
　of RN to LPN/LVN, 166b
RTSS (returning to school syndrome), 11–13, 11t.
　See also Student role, returning to

S

SBAR (situation–background–assessment–recommendation), 277
School
　return to. *See* RTSS
　setting of, 155
Science and technological advances, 410
Scope and Standards of Practice, 254
Scope of practice, 198
Self-actualization, 82, 133
Self-assessment, 315–316, 331
Self-awareness, 141–143, 142*b*
Self-directed goals, 143–144
Self-directed, individualized learning, 133–134
Self-improvement, desire for, 67
Self-regulation, 217*t*, 362
　metacognition and, 218–220
　reflective thinking, 218–220
Sender (encodes), 264–265
Sentinel events, 392, 392*b*
Sequence, series of instructions, 296–297
Service learning, nursing relating to, 125
Sexual being, client as, 321–323
Sexual health, 226
Sexual issues, barriers to nurse's discussion of, 321*b*, 322*b*
Sexual misconduct, 384*b*
Sexual openness, variations in, 321–322
Sexual orientation, 6–8, 142–143, 143*b*, 322–323
Shared healthcare records, 121–122
Silence, as part of nonverbal communication, 266
Simulation, 300
Sixties Revolution, 110–111
Skills
　competencies and, for lifelong learning, 5, 6
　note-taking, 29–30
　research, 22–23
　study, development of, 28–32
Slander, 396
SLOs (student learning outcomes), 21, 118
SNAs (state nurses associations), 95
Social being, client as, 319–321
Socialization, 339
　professional role development relating to, 53–55, 54*t*
Social milieu, 41
Social nursing diagnoses, 326*b*
Social policy statement, 102–103, 200–201
Social resistance factors, 75
Social security, 118
Social strengths and resources, of client, 294*b*
Social well-being, 226
Societal changes, responding to
　demographics, 367
　global community, 368–369
　healthcare reform, 367–368
　technology, advancements in, 369
Societal influences, ethical issues relating to, 409–410
Societal roles of women and men, in nursing, 42, 110
Societal trends and changing role of nursing, 111–121, 112*b*
　advancing technology, bioethics, globalism, 119–121
　aging population, 111
　disaster preparedness, bioterrorism, homeland security, 119
　diversity, multiculturalism, emotional intelligence, 114–116
　family structures, changes in, 118–119
　healthcare reform, 116–118
　HIV/AIDS and pandemic flu, 119
　immigration issues, US nurses and, 116
　nursing shortage, 112–114, 371
　shortened lengths of hospital stays, 111–112
　universal complementary and alternative healing practices, 123
Sociocentric thinking, 217
Spatial perceptual problems, 142*b*
Spirit, 226
Spiritual being, client as, 323–324
Spiritual care, in nursing, 123–124
Spiritual nursing care, 123–124
Spiritual nursing diagnoses, 326*b*
Spiritual strengths and resources, of client, 294*b*
Spiritual symbols, 324
Spontaneous change, 68
Stakeholders, 68
Standardized and nonstandardized tests, 162–164
　assessment tests for general education, 162–163
　integrated nursing assessment tests, 163
　nursing review tests, 163–164
　subject area assessment tests for nursing and support curricula, 163
Standardized teaching plans, 304
Standardized test, 162
Standard nursing care plan, 257*b*
Standards
　of nursing practice, 104, 199–200, 362, 369–370
　of practice, 388–389
　of professional organization, 205
Standards of Professional Practice, 240
State board of nursing, 199, 205–206
Statutory law, 381
Stem cell research, 120
Stereotyping, 314
Stewardship, professional, 372–374
Strategic learner, 156
Stress, change relating to, 71–73
Student learning outcomes. *See* SLOs
Student portfolio, 165
Student role
　assessing preparedness for

Index

balancing personal, career, and, 24–25
returning to. *See also* RTSS
   stage 2: conflict, 11*t*, 12
   stage 1: honeymoon, 11*t*, 12
   stage 3: resolution, 11*t*, 12–13
successful strategies for, 19–32
   becoming a proactive strategic learner, 156
   college success courses and resources, 19
   faculty advisor, working with, 19–20
   learning techniques, 156
   networking and developing mentors, 157–159
   resource materials, 20–22
   study groups, 159–160
   study skills, development of, 28–32
   time management, 24–28, 26*b*
Study
   groups for, 31–32, 159–160, 187
   independent, 299
   skills development for, 28–32
Subculture, 314
Subject area assessment tests, for nursing and support curricula, 163
Subject changing, as part of verbal communication blocks, 271
Subjective data, 245, 245*t*
Success, strategies for. *See* Student role, successful strategies for
Summarization, in verbal communication, 267–268
Sympathy, 273–274
Syndrome diagnosis, 251
Synthesis/evaluating questions, 181

T

Taft–Hartley Act, 96
Taxonomy, 239
Taxonomy of Educational Objectives, 136, 136*b*. *See also* Bloom's Taxonomy of Educational Objectives
Teach back method, 358
Teacher. *See* Nurse, as teacher
Teaching
   individualize, materials for, 292–293
   interventions for, 298–301, 298*b*, 306
   strategic, 228
Teaching-learning process. *See also* Nurse, as teacher
   assessment in, 302, 303*b*
   clinical applications of, 308–310
   nursing process v., 301*t*
Team approach, 117
Team building, 276–278
Team development stages, therapeutic relationship stages and, comparison of, 276*t*
Team members, effective, qualities of, 277*b*
TeamSTEPPS (Team Strategies and Tools to Enhance Performance and Patient Safety) strategies, 277–278

Teamwork, environment, 336–337
Technological advances, 410
Technologically current nurse, computer competencies for, 364–365, 365*b*
Technology
   advancements in, 369
   bioethics, globalism and, advancement of, 119–121
   fear of, 8–9
Telehealth, 122
Teleology, 407
Terrorism, 110
Test distracters, 176
Test item formats, 184, 184*t*
Test language: key components to a test, 176–177
Test options, 176
Test Plan for the NCLEX Examination for Practical Nurses, 205–206, 208–209
Test Plan for the NCLEX Examination for Registered Nurses, 206, 208–209
Test plans
   for licensure examinations, 204
   LPN/LVN, 205–206
   for RN, 206
Tests
   for LPNs, NCLEX-RN questions relating to, 172–194
   preparation for, 31
   standardized and nonstandardized, 162
Test stem, 176
The Joint Commission (TJC), 240
Therapeutic caring nurses, effective, characteristics of
   empathy, 273
   therapeutic humor, 274
   trust, 273
Therapeutic communication, 264, 276
   verbal blocks in, 270–271, 271*t*
Therapeutic humor, 274
Therapeutic relationship stages, team development stages and, comparison of, 276*t*
Time. *See also* Managing time, conflict and nursing environment
   assessment of, 331–332, 333*t*
   class-professor, wise use, 185
   efficient and effective use, 336–337
   management of, 24–28, 26*b*, 160–161, 331
   quiet, 335
   for study, 24–28
Time activity log, 332, 333*t*
Time wasters
   common, 339*b*
   interruptions, 337–339
   perfectionism, 342
   personal disorganization, 340
   poor communication, 340
   procrastination, 341, 341*b*
   socializing, 339

Tort, 382, 383b
Total quality management. *See* TQM
Touch, as part of nonverbal communication, 267
TQM (total quality management), 118
Transactional change, 68
Transactional communication model, 264–265, 264f
Transcultural literacy, 143
Transformational change, 69
Transitions. *See* Role development; Role transition
TRIO program, 9
Trust, 290

U
UAPs (unlicensed assistive personnel), 287–288, 335, 386
Underrepresented groups, 313
Unfreezing, 70
 driving forces, 70
 restraining forces, 70
Unintentional torts, 383b
Unique client care. *See* Managing unique client care
Uniqueness, 314
 and culture, 314–316
Unlicensed assistive personnel. *See* UAPs
Unplanned change, 67–68
 forced, 67
 spontaneous, 68
U.S. Bureau of Labor Statistics, 113
Utilitarianism, 407

V
Validation
 data, 245
 of diagnosis, 250
Value conflict, 344
Value nursing, modeling and, 360–361

Values, 315–316, 405, 406b
 customs, beliefs and, 319
 professional and client, 411–413
Values clarification, 286, 299–300
Valuing prior learning, 23–24
Veracity, 413
Verbal blocks, in therapeutic communication, 270–271, 271t
Verbal communication, 264–265, 267–269, 268t, 318–319
Verbal therapeutic communication techniques, 268t
Violations
 criminal law, 384
 of healthcare regulations, 384b
Virtual learning spaces, 140
Visual, auditory, or kinesthetic delivery) system, 14
Visual delivery system. *See* VAK
Visual learning, 291
Visual–motor problems, 142b
Visual perceptual problems, 142b
Vocational programs *vs.* associate degree nursing education, 134–141

W
War's impact, on nursing, 109–110
Web-based resources, 22
WEB 2.0 resources, 366t
Website, of ANA, 125
Wellness diagnosis, 251
Win/win agreements, 26–28
Women and equal rights, 110–111
Women and men, in nursing, 42, 110
Women's movement, 111
Worksheet, 332–335, 333t, 337
Writing skills, 29–30

Y
Yale School of Nursing, 92